DIETITIANS OF CANADA
Cook
Great Food

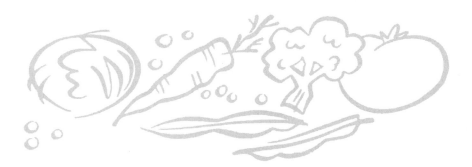

450
DELICIOUS RECIPES

Robert
ROSE

Canadian Cataloguing in Publication Data

Main entry under title:
Cook great food: 450 delicious recipes

Includes index.
ISBN 0-7788-0046-6

1. Cookery. I. Dietitians of Canada.

TX714.C6546 2002   641.5   C2001-903478-4

Disclaimer
The recipes in this book have been carefully tested by our kitchen and our tasters. To the best of our knowledge, they are safe and nutritious for ordinary use and users. For those people with food or other allergies, or who have special food requirements or health issues, please read the suggested contents of each recipe carefully and determine whether or not they may create a problem for you. All recipes are used at the risk of the consumer.

We cannot be responsible for any hazards, loss or damage that may occur as a result of any recipe use.

For those with special needs, allergies, requirements or health problems, in the event of any doubt, please contact your medical adviser prior to the use of any recipe.

Design & Production: PageWave Graphics Inc.
Editor: Judith Finlayson
Photography: Mark T. Shapiro
  Food Stylist: Kate Bush
  Props Stylist: Charlene Erricson
  The publisher and author wish to express their appreciation to the following supplier of props used in food photography in the book: Dishes, cutlery, linens and accessories, HomeFront, 371 Eglinton Avenue West, Toronto; (416) 488-3189; www.homefrontshop.com
Other photography (opposite pages 224, 384 and 385): Fred Bird
Color Scans: Colour Technologies

Cover image: Orange Ginger Pork and Vegetables (see recipe, page 257)

We acknowledge the financial support of the Government of Canada through the Book Publishing Industry Development Program (BPIDP) for our publishing activities.
Canada

Published by: Robert Rose Inc.
120 Eglinton Ave. E., Suite 1000, Toronto, Ontario, Canada M4P 1E2
Tel: (416) 322-6552   Fax: (416) 322-6936

Printed in Canada

1 2 3 4 5 6 7 8 9 10   GP   09 08 07 06 05 04 03 02 01

Contents

Acknowledgements

Cook Great Food is the result of a team effort that reflects the diversity and makeup of our country. From coast to coast, dietitians made valuable contributions to this book in many ways. Dietitians of Canada recognizes the many individuals who have been involved in creating this exciting book.

Thanks go to Helen Haresign, VP Development, Dietitians of Canada for her initiative in getting the project off the ground.

Sincere thanks to the steering efforts of the Advisory Committee, who provided the direction for this book and supported every stage of its development. The committee includes Frances Johnson, British Columbia, Mary Anne Yurkiw, Alberta, Huguette Samson, Manitoba, Lesley Macaskill and Angela Liuzzo, Ontario, Kim Arrey and Anne Gagné, Quebec, and Colleen Goggin, Nova Scotia.

Through the efforts of the Advisory Committee, dietitians across Canada were invited to contribute their expertise to the nutritional content and the chapter introductions. We are very grateful for their outstanding efforts and support in creating this book. They include the following dietitians:

Alexandra Anca, Ontario	Angela Liuzzo, Ontario
Kim Barro, Nova Scotia	Elizabeth Mansfield, Ontario
Silvia Bonome, Quebec	Linda Omichinski, Manitoba
Pierrette Buklis, Ontario	Helen Onderka, Alberta
Janice Daciuk, Ontario	Carla Ross, Alberta
Colleen Goggin, Nova Scotia	Nathalie Roy, New Brunswick
Ramona Josephson, British Columbia	Heather Schnurr, Alberta
Laurence Levy, Ontario	Mary Anne Yurkiw, Alberta

In addition, the sidebar information was reviewed for accuracy and nutrient content by several other dietitians, and we are extremely indebted to them. They include the following:

Barb Anderson, Nova Scotia	Lesley Macaskill, Ontario
Stephanie Buckle, Newfoundland	Shefali Raja, British Columbia
Johanna Fralick, New Brunswick	Debra Reid, Quebec
Joanne Gallagher, Ontario	Maria Sena, Ontario
Kerry Grady-Vincent, Ontario	Ellen Vogel, Alberta
Marian Law-Ledrew, Ontario	Patricia Williams, Nova Scotia
Angela Liuzzo, Ontario	

Thanks to Lynn Roblin and Bev Callaghan, authors of *Great Food Fast* (2000), for the elements of *Great Food Fast* used in this new book. Thanks also to Margaret Howard and Helen Bishop Macdonald, authors of *Eat Well, Live Well* (1990), for their comments used in the introduction. Support from Margaret Carney was invaluable in the early stages of this book.

In addition, the many Canadians, dietitians and chefs who contributed recipes and tips are thanked for their contributions to healthy eating.

Thanks to Judith Finlayson for her editorial guidance.

We also thank our publisher, Robert Rose Inc., in particular Bob Dees and Marian Jarkovich, for their marketing ideas and enthusiasm for the project; Andrew Smith, Joseph Gisini and Kevin Cockburn of PageWave Graphics for their expertise in design and production; and Mark Shapiro for his superb photography. The food was styled with flair by Kate Bush and supported by Charlene Erricson with props that beautifully complement the recipes. Each and every photograph is a beautiful representation of healthy eating.

And last, but not least, thanks to Susan Morgan, who brought all of the above together and coordinated all the pieces.

About Dietitians of Canada

Dietitians of Canada (DC) is the national voice of dietitians, your trusted source of food and nutrition information. DC represents more than 5,000 dietitians working to improve the health of Canadians through food and nutrition.

Dietitians are the ideal source of current, reliable advice. If you need healthy eating information or advice about your diet, contact a registered dietitian. To find a registered dietitian in your community, contact your local department of public health, community health center or hospital. You can also get a list of registered dietitians who work in private practice on the Dietitians of Canada Web site, www.dietitians.ca, or by calling the Consulting Dietitians Network at 1-888-901-7776.

Introduction

In Canada, healthy eating has been an ongoing journey of adventure and discovery for many years. Dietitians are health professionals who help Canadians to enjoy a healthy lifestyle based on nutrition. They play a major role in health care, industry, government and education, influencing the development and promotion of consumer products and managing quality food service operations. They also provide information and advice to help decision makers, including consumers, make informed judgements about food choices and nutrition services.

One of the most successful endeavors undertaken by Dietitians of Canada was the production of three cookbooks that feature healthy eating, by providing an abundance of tasty family-oriented recipes to suit every occasion. The first book of the series, *Eat Well, Live Well,* was published in 1990, and *Healthy Pleasures,* a unique collaboration between dietitians and chefs, followed in 1995. The current cycle was completed in 2000 with the publication of *Great Food Fast,* which focused on meeting the demands of today's time-starved families. *Cook Great Food* combines the best recipes from all three books in one convenient volume.

In *Cook Great Food,* you will find more than 450 mouthwatering recipes to suit every aspect of your lifestyle. More than a cornucopia of delicious recipes, *Cook Great Food* provides a wealth of information on nutrition. Each recipe is accompanied by a nutritional analysis outlining the calories, protein, fat, carbohydrate and dietary fiber in each serving. Useful tips, techniques and menu suggestions prepared by professional dietitians also appear alongside the recipes. On every page of *Cook Great Food,* a dietitian is with you, helping you to make informed choices about food to support a pattern of healthy living.

Everyone knows that good nutrition is a key component of good health. The problem is that people differ in their definitions of good nutrition. In *Cook Great Food,* you'll find some of the answers to the many questions about nutrition and health that dietitians are often asked. The introduction, written by practicing dietitians, provides an overview of current nutritional information, based on the latest research. Since the publication of *Eat Well, Live Well,* by Margaret Howard and Helen Bishop Macdonald, much new research into nutrition has been conducted, but the fundamental message remains the same: consult the advice provided by *Canada's Guidelines for Healthy Eating* and *Canada's Food Guide to Healthy Eating.* Also bear in mind these fundamentals: enjoyment, variety, balance and moderation. To learn more about healthy eating, visit the Web sites we've noted.

Cook Great Food is the perfect cookbook for the everyday cook, the once-in-a-while cook and anyone interested in great-tasting food and healthy eating. It will also serve as a great reference for those interested in learning more about nutrition. Dietitians of Canada hopes that you enjoy this book and that the recipes will help you to "cook great food" every day of the week.

Susan Morgan, RD
Food and Nutrition Consultant

focus on healthy eating

Wondering how to improve your eating habits? Often there are so many things we think we should change that we feel defeated before we start. Dietitians believe that healthy eating is possible for everyone. We recommend that you begin by learning what healthy eating is all about. Then you can identify the changes you want to make and break them down into a series of small steps, which can be taken one at a time.

just the basics

Healthy eating involves three key concepts: variety, balance and moderation. Variety involves enjoying many different foods. It's OK to have favorites, but challenge yourself to expand your culinary horizons. Foods provide different nutrients, so eating a variety of foods will help to ensure that you get all the nutrition you need.

Balance means choosing foods that provide you with the right mix of essential nutrients. Choose foods from the four food groups noted in *Canada's Food Guide to Healthy Eating* (see chart, page 434) most often and eat other foods occasionally to add variety and enjoyment. Balance also means balancing how much you eat with your activity level, as for the most part, the more active you are the greater your food energy requirements (see *Canada's Physical Activity Guide*, page 436).

Moderation means not eating too much of any one food at any one time. Savor one piece, don't devour the whole cake! Practise moderation with foods outside the four food groups, such as those that are higher in fat, salt and calories, but don't deprive yourself. You can enjoy all foods as long as you don't overdo it with any one.

Canada's Food Guide to Healthy Eating has been designed to help you achieve balance, variety and moderation. It emphasizes the importance of eating whole grains, colorful fruits and vegetables, leaner meats and meat alternatives, and lower-fat dairy products more often. Following the recommended servings from each of the four food groups will provide you with all of the nutrients you need on a daily basis.

defining healthy eating

Healthy eating is not about guilt, sacrifice or eating foods you don't like! It is not about avoiding "bad" food and eating only "good" food. Healthy eating is about eating the foods you enjoy. Healthy eating results from the food choices you make over several days, weeks, months and years, not just the choices you make in one day or at one meal.

Healthy eating encompasses more than what we eat. It also involves when we eat, how we eat and with whom we eat. Meals are a time to laugh, share and have fun.

cooking great food

No matter who you are or how old you are, when it comes to nutrition, now is the most important time of your life. Good nutrition helps children to grow, learn and play. Healthy eating helps teens reach their full potential and look good. Paying attention to what you eat as an adult helps you to manage the demands of work and family by contributing to good health and keeping your energy levels high. As you age, healthy eating helps to prevent health problems and enables you to maintain an active, independent life well into your senior years.

how can I get my kids to eat more healthy foods?

Your job as a provider of food for your children is to include balance and variety with the choices you offer. You purchase, prepare and serve the food. It is your child's responsibility to eat the food you provide — in the amounts he or she wants. You can have input into each other's roles. Understanding your roles makes the job easier.

Make food fun and try to understand children's special rhythms. Many adults think kids linger too long over a meal. Is that really so bad? Maybe we could eat slower, too.

The experience and enjoyment of food involves all the senses. A vital part of exploring food is touching, seeing, smelling and, finally, tasting. These activities should be under children's control from the time toddlers are able to grab a fistful of food — even if they are messy!

The best way to ensure healthy eating patterns in our children is to eat well ourselves. So be a good role model. How your kids eat when they can make choices themselves will resemble how you eat. Parents need to look at their own eating habits and make any necessary changes if they want their children to eat well.

make healthy eating economical

Don't get caught up in the myth that healthy eating is too expensive. The following tips can help you to eat well economically.

- Use frozen foods when fresh are not in season. Canned fruits and vegetables are also a good alternative, especially in the winter, when fresh produce is more costly.
- Eat more legumes (such as kidney beans and chickpeas) as a source of protein. They are much less expensive than meat.
- Buy fewer snack foods and other processed foods. They tend to cost more than fresh food.
- Buy in bulk, especially if you are feeding a larger family.
- Check out supermarket flyers and take advantage of the weekly specials.
- Comparison shop. Use shelf labels that tell you the price per unit.

eating well

You are eating well if:

- you eat at least the minimum number of servings recommended by *Canada's Food Guide to Healthy Eating* every day;
- you eat a variety of foods within each group and enjoy regular meals and snacks;
- your clothes fit and you feel good about what you eat.

know what you eat

Look in your cupboards and fridge. Think about your favorite recipe ingredients. Picture your shopping cart. How often do you replace certain foods? What goes out in your garbage? Consider balance, variety and moderation when buying, preparing and eating food. Click the *Eat Well, Live Well* button when you visit the Dietitians of Canada Web site at www.dietitians.ca to analyze your own nutrition profile. While there, take a look at the meal planner, to plan nutritious and tasty meals.

healthy living

One of the cornerstones of healthy living is eating well. Together with other healthy lifestyle habits — such as regular physical activity, minimizing stress, not smoking and using alcohol in moderation — eating well can help to promote longevity and good health. Prevention of chronic diseases such as diabetes, heart disease, some cancers and osteoporosis is a goal of healthy lifestyle habits.

Canada's Guidelines for Healthy Eating and *Canada's Food Guide to Healthy Eating* provide the key principles that can help to reduce your risk of these and other chronic diseases and conditions. These guidelines suggest that you:

- enjoy a variety of foods;
- emphasize cereals, breads, other grain products, vegetables and fruit;
- choose lower-fat dairy products, leaner meats and foods prepared with little or no fat;
- achieve and maintain a healthy body weight by enjoying regular physical activity and healthy eating;
- limit salt, alcohol and caffeine.

build strong bones with calcium

Osteoporosis is a condition in which bones lose calcium, become brittle and break easily. To prevent osteoporosis, men as well as women need to start the process of building strong bones as children and keep it up through life. Maintaining an active lifestyle (see *Physical Activity Guide*, page 436), developing healthy eating patterns and eating plenty of calcium-rich foods will help to prevent this debilitating disease.

Milk and milk products offer the most abundant and easily absorbed sources of calcium. Two to four servings of milk products or their equivalent daily are necessary to meet your calcium requirements. Foods such as canned fish with bones, legumes (beans and lentils) and vegetables such as broccoli and dark leafy greens also provide dietary calcium, but in smaller amounts than milk products. In addition, non-dairy sources of calcium are not as easily absorbed by the body.

Many soy products (such as tofu made with calcium and calcium-fortified soy beverages) are also a source of calcium. Although some are fortified to be equivalent in nutrients to milk, this is not true of all soy products, so read the labels carefully.

milk: not only for children

Milk and milk products are key sources of calcium and protein. Milk is fortified with vitamins A and D. Our bodies need these nutrients to stay healthy and maintain the strong skeleton we built as children. Enjoy two to four servings of milk, cheese, yogurt, and puddings or soups made with milk each day, choosing lower-fat varieties more often.

other bone builders

Vitamin D also plays a crucial role in building bones. A diet too high in salt and protein may impede bone development. Last, but not least, remember that bones are stronger when they are put to the test. Exercise that puts pressure on your bones, like walking or dancing, will help to make them stronger.

a focus on fat

Eating some fat is a good thing because fat:

- cushions and protects the body's vital organs;
- insulates the body against extreme temperatures;
- carries the fat-soluble vitamins A, D, E and K;
- provides essential fats needed to produce hormones and build healthy cells and skin;
- heightens the flavor of food.

But eating too much fat is a problem.

how much fat should I eat?

Most Canadians consume 34% to 37% of their calories from fat. Experts agree that we should reduce our fat intake to no more than 30%. This translates to approximately 60 grams or less for women and 90 grams or less for men per day. Major sources of fat in the Canadian diet include butter, margarine, oils, fat on meats and those found in baked goods.

all fats aren't equal

There are several types of fat. Not all are created equally. Although limiting total fat intake is a goal, additional healthful benefits can be achieved by dramatically reducing the intake of certain fats.

saturated fats

Saturated fats are closely associated with greater health risks, including increased blood cholesterol. They are found mostly in animal products, such as meat, poultry, egg yolks and dairy products, and in fats that are solid at room temperature, such as butter, lard, shortening, hydrogenated or stick margarine, and tropical oils (coconut or palm) found in processed products.

Trans-fatty acids are also thought to raise blood cholesterol. They are formed when liquid oil is processed to make the oil more solid. This process is called hydrogenation. To limit your intake of trans-fatty acids, look for the words "hydrogenated" or "partially hydrogenated" on ingredient lists. Trans fats are found in bakery goods such as cookies, croissants and doughnuts, hydrogenated margarines, fast foods such as french fries, snack foods such as potato chips and crackers, and processed foods such as breakfast waffles and cake mixes.

unsaturated fats

Unsaturated fats provide the essential fats needed for good health. When used in place of saturated fats, they help to reduce the risk of heart disease. There are two types of unsaturated fats.

Monounsaturated fats are found in vegetable oils, such as canola and olive oils, and products made with these oils, as well as in nuts and seeds, avocados, olives and non-hydrogenated margarine.

Polyunsaturated fats include vegetable oils made from corn, sunflowers, safflowers, soybeans, nuts and seeds. This type of fat is also found in soft, non-hydrogenated margarine. Omega-3 fats are a type of polyunsaturated fat found in fatty fish such as salmon, trout, mackerel, Atlantic herring, swordfish and sardines, flaxseeds, walnuts, soybeans and oil made from these foods.

what about cholesterol?

Healthy eating does not necessarily mean limiting your consumption of foods containing cholesterol. It is not the dietary cholesterol found in foods such as eggs, dairy products and shellfish so much as the type and amount of fat in our diet that affects blood cholesterol levels. If your blood cholesterol is elevated, you would be wise to seek the advice of a dietitian.

cut fat and make your fat choices count

- Cut back on the total amount of fat you consume and emphasize monounsaturated and poly-unsaturated fats and oils.
- Choose fish, whole grains, vegetables and fruit more often.
- Choose leaner cuts of meat and lower-fat milk products.
- Limit your intake of fat from oils, spreads, sauces, desserts and greasy snack foods.

increase dietary fiber

Dietary fiber, another important component of healthy eating, helps us to maintain a healthy digestive system and control blood cholesterol, blood sugar and weight. Two types of fiber are important to our health: *insoluble* fiber, which helps promote bowel function, and *soluble* fiber, which plays a role in lowering blood cholesterol levels and controlling blood sugar levels in people with diabetes.

Most Canadians don't consume enough fiber. Adults should consume 25 to 35 grams of dietary fiber per day. For children and teens aged three to 18, daily recommended fiber intake in grams can be calculated as the sum of their age plus 5; so a 10-year-old child, for example, should have 10 + 5, or 15 grams of fiber per day.

weighing in

Weight changes — up or down — are a symptom of imbalance. If your weight has changed rapidly, evaluate whether there has been a significant change in your life that has affected your routines. When routines vary, eating is affected. Weight gain can be your body's way of getting your attention and telling you to restore balance.

achieving a healthy weight

Healthy bodies come in all sizes and shapes. Having realistic expectations about your body and shape and taking a healthy-eating, active-living, feeling-good-about-yourself approach is important. To learn if your weight is within a healthy range, check your body mass index in the Healthy Body Shop at www.dietitians.ca/eatwell.

the value of an active lifestyle

Because inactivity is a risk factor for conditions such as heart disease and diabetes, increasing your activity level is one way to improve your health. Exercise also helps to relieve stress, thereby reducing cravings for sweets and urges to binge. But be aware that if you build muscle, you may actually gain weight while losing inches.

If you are a parent, another benefit to regular activity is the positive message to your family and friends. Regular family outings planned around physical activity can shape behaviors that will last into adulthood.

Visit www.missionnutrition.ca for approaches that will help build healthy habits in youths.

beyond vitamins

Scientists are still discovering how nutrients interact in the body. They are also studying how "non-nutrient" factors in food may benefit health.

Phytochemicals ("plant chemicals") are different from vitamins and minerals, but they, too, seem to play a significant role in our health. These substances occur naturally in all plant foods, including fruits, vegetables, legumes and grains. Unlike for the better-known nutrients, there are no recommendations for how much of these various phytochemicals our bodies need.

Phytochemicals acting as antioxidants help to get rid of cell-damaging free radicals that form in the body and start disease processes. Current research suggests that antioxidants protect your body just as rustproofing protects your car — they come between you and a threat. Antioxidants include vitamin C, beta-carotene (the plant form of vitamin A) and carotenoids such as lycopene and lutein. All these antioxidants are easy to get in the foods you eat. Vitamin E is another antioxidant, which is found primarily in vegetable oils, and margarine, nuts, seeds and wheat germ, and in smaller amounts in leafy green vegetables, sweet potatoes, and whole-grain cereals.

Eating a variety of vegetables and fruits, as well as nuts and seeds, legumes and certain other foods, will help to ensure an adequate supply of these protective factors. When choosing vegetables and fruits, look for color — the brightest ones are often associated with more of these substances. For example, tomatoes, blueberries, carrots, purple grapes, broccoli and red beets are all high in antioxidants.

vitamin and mineral supplements

No supplement can take the place of healthy eating. Generally, healthy Canadians don't need supplements since we have access to a vast array of high-quality food, and more is not necessarily better with regard to most nutrients.

Healthy eating has many advantages over supplements.

- You need more than 50 nutrients daily to stay healthy. Food is full of them.
- No supplement has been made to date that can deliver all your nutrition needs.
- Many foods contain phytochemicals that are believed to provide health benefits beyond basic nutrients.
- Some supplements provide more nutrients than your body can use.
- And food tastes great!

However, vitamin and mineral supplements are sometimes useful. Your dietitian or doctor might recommend a nutritional supplement for:

- serious digestive disorders;
- osteoporosis;
- poor appetite;
- people on strict weight-loss diets;
- breastfed babies;
- pregnant women and women planning a pregnancy;
- vegans (vegetarians who choose not to eat any animal foods).

Supplements are not a substitute for healthy eating. If you think you need a supplement, consult a dietitian.

Principles of Healthy Eating

eat well every time

Everybody has some good eating habits, but we can always improve. After all, the better we nourish our bodies, the better our bodies work for us. For peak performance throughout the day:

- balance your energy intake by eating at regular intervals and never skip meals at mealtime, it's better to eat something rather than nothing;
- build each meal with choices from the four food groups in *Canada's Food Guide to Healthy Eating;*
- choose food you like but also try new dishes sometimes it takes time to acquire a taste.

Enjoy all foods but think about quantity and quality. Build your meals around nutrient-rich foods such as whole grains, vegetables and fruit, milk products and leaner meat and alternatives. Enjoy higher-fat/calorie-dense foods in moderation.

Let *Cook Great Food* inspire you. It is filled with practical information to help you make *great food choices every time you eat*. The recipes have been selected to provide a variety of cooking styles, flavors and textures that will tantalize your taste buds. Most of the recipes have a short preparation time, ingredients that are readily available and easy-to-follow instructions so that all household members can help with meal preparation. Try a familiar favorite or experiment with a new recipe, a new ingredient or a new cooking method.

develop a great plan

You can meet your nutritional needs anytime and every time you eat, even on the go. But *you must be prepared.* To enjoy great food with great taste every day, you need a plan.

A great plan doesn't have to be complicated, but it has to work. Don't let busy schedules keep you from eating well. A great plan considers all the factors that influence your food choices: meeting nutritional needs, taste preferences, access to great recipes, preparation time and food safety.

get organized

The better organized you are, the faster you can prepare great meals. A weekly meal plan that includes everyone's favorite recipes can limit trips to the grocery store, reduce dependence on takeout or commercially prepared foods, and even save on food costs. Post the menu on the refrigerator or memo board and make it flexible. And keep this cookbook handy for everyone to use.

Organize your kitchen so that healthy choices are the most accessible. For example, keep a bowl of fresh fruit on the table and a supply of raw vegetables washed, cut and ready to eat in resealable plastic bags in the fridge.

Try having some meals ready in advance. Prepare extra recipes on the weekend or double a recipe during the week. Freeze the extra, then reheat appropriate servings when required. Remember, a great meal does not have to be a hot meal. A cold meal can be just as nutritionally balanced and delicious. Use commercially prepared ingredients such as frozen vegetables or bottled sauces for shortcuts.

keep a well-stocked pantry

In the cupboard

Beans and lentils: baked beans in tomato sauce, black beans, chickpeas, kidney beans, white (navy) beans, lentils

Breads: whole-grain breads, rolls, pita bread, bagels, biscuit baking mix

Cereals: bran, whole-grain, rolled oats

Condiments and flavorings: mustard, regular and Dijon, vinegar, soy sauce, bouillon cubes, salsa

Fish, canned: tuna, salmon, clams

Flour: white all-purpose, whole-grain

Fruit, canned (packed in juice or light syrup): peaches, pears, mandarin orange segments, applesauce

Fruit, dried: raisins, cranberries, apricots, dates

Grains: wheat bran, cornmeal

Herbs and spices: black pepper, basil, garlic, ginger, oregano, thyme, tarragon, coriander, cumin, curry powder, cayenne pepper or hot pepper flakes

Milk: canned evaporated, powdered skim

Oils: olive oil, vegetable oil such as canola

Pasta: farfalle (bow tie), couscous, fusilli, penne, rotini, spaghetti

Pasta sauces: prepared tomato and vegetable, tomato sauce

Rice: white, brown, quick-cooking

Sweeteners: sugar, honey, syrup, jam

Vegetables, canned: stewed or diced tomatoes, corn kernels, pumpkin, tomato paste

Vegetables, fresh: potatoes, sweet potatoes, onions

Vegetables, pickled: sweet pickles, dill pickles

On the counter

Fruit and vegetables, fresh: bananas, cantaloupe

In the fridge

Cheese: Cheddar, Parmesan, ricotta, mozzarella, cheese slices

Eggs

Fats: butter, soft margarine

Nuts and seeds: almonds, walnuts, peanuts

Fruit, fresh: oranges, apples, grapes, kiwi fruit

Juice: tomato, vegetable, fruit, lemon

Meat and poultry: chicken, turkey, beef, lean ground beef, pork chops (freeze poultry and meat if you can't use it within two days of purchasing)

Milk: skim, 1%, 2%, whole (3.5%) or buttermilk

Vegetables: red and green bell peppers, broccoli, romaine lettuce, celery, spinach, green onions, mushrooms, zucchini

Yogurt: plain and flavored

In the freezer

Breads: pita bread, flour tortillas, flatbread rounds

Frozen fish: sole, perch, halibut, haddock, cooked shrimp

Fruit: strawberries, raspberries, blueberries

Fruit juice concentrate

Vegetables: peas, corn, broccoli, cauliflower, oriental mix

Personalize this list by adding ingredients for your favorite recipes.

With the ingredients in this pantry list, you'll have everything you need to make any recipe marked in the book with a **P**

food safety

Food safety is an important element of healthy eating. Because bacteria cannot be seen or felt, they can easily invade food products. Kitchen surfaces, knives and other utensils carry bacteria that cause food poisoning, which is often dismissed as stomach flu. Here are some helpful rules to keep food safe from harmful bacteria.

cleaning

1) Wash hands in hot, soapy water for at least 20 seconds before handling food. Dry hands thoroughly, as wet hands can transmit bacteria.

2) After preparing food, wash cutting boards, knives, utensils and countertops with hot, soapy water. Dishwasher-safe cutting boards are recommended.

3) Wash meat cutting boards and countertops with hot, soapy water, then disinfect in bleach water (add 2 tbsp/25 mL bleach to 4 quarts/4 liters water).

4) Change dishcloths daily and machine-wash them in the hot cycle. Consider using paper towels for cleaning kitchen surfaces instead.

chilling and storage

1) Keep refrigerators at 40°F (4°C) and freezers at 0°F (–18°C) to prevent bacterial growth.

2) Refrigerate or freeze leftovers in shallow containers (to ensure rapid cooling) within two hours of cooking.

3) Always defrost food in the refrigerator, under cold running water or in a microwave, not on the counter.

4) Marinate food in the refrigerator, not on the counter.

5) Don't overload a refrigerator. Cold air must circulate to keep food safe.

6) Serve food by the expiry date. Remember, once a product is opened, the "best before date" no longer applies.

7) Discard all moldy foods or foods sitting at room temperature for over two hours. *When in doubt, throw it out!*

separating

1) Separate raw meat, poultry, fish and seafood from other foods in your shopping cart and refrigerator. Store in the meat drawer or on the bottom shelf of the refrigerator so that their juices don't drip on other foods.

2) Use one cutting board for raw meat and another for non-meat items and cooked foods.

3) Never place cooked food on a plate that held raw meat, poultry, fish, eggs or seafood.

cooking

1) Cook meat, fish, eggs and poultry thoroughly.

2) Use a clean thermometer and ensure that meat and poultry are cooked all the way through. Meat should be cooked to an internal temperature of at least 145°F (65°C) and poultry to 180°F (80°C). Ground meat should be cooked to at least 160°F (72°C) and not eaten pink. Ground meat is considered a high-risk food because bacteria can spread during the grinding process.

3) Heat leftovers thoroughly to 165°F (74°C). Bring sauces, soups and gravy to a boil if reheating.

> *For additional information on food safety, visit www.canfightbac.org, the Web site of the Canadian Partnership for Food Safety Education.*

learning from labels

Canadian law requires that food labels include an ingredient list and information on how to contact the producer. Many food companies highlight special features of their product by using nutritional claims (such as "low in fat" or "high in fiber"). They may also offer an additional Nutrition Information panel on packages, which outlines the quantity of important nutrients found in a serving of the food, among other information. *To keep updated on nutrition labelling, visit Health Canada's Web site at www.hc-sc.gc.ca/hppb/nutrition/labels/*

nutritional analysis

In every recipe, nutrient values have been provided for protein, fat, carbohydrate, dietary fiber and calories rounded out to the nearest whole number. Almost every recipe includes a message from a dietitian, which often identifies its nutritional strengths or makes suggestions about how to fit the recipe into a meal to maximize its nutritional value. The nutritional guidelines provided in *Canada's Food Guide to Healthy Eating* have been used in the preparation of this information. The computer-assisted nutrient analyses for all recipes were prepared by Info Access (1988) Inc., Don Mills, Ontario. *The nutrient analyses were based on:*

imperial measures and weights (except for foods typically packaged and used in metric);
the smaller number of servings when there was a range;
the first ingredient listed when there was a choice (optional ingredients were not included).

more information

We have provided you with current information on healthy eating. Be inspired to keep searching for updated information. The following are some Web sites that will provide you with an abundance of reliable information.

Dietitians of Canada
www.dietitians.ca
This is an award-winning Web site filled with interactive tools, tips and fact sheets for healthy eating. Check out the Nutrition Profile to get personalized advice about your current food choices. Cruise through the Virtual Kitchen for tips and facts about the food you eat. Take the Nutrition Challenge to test your knowledge on nutrition. The Web site can also help you to find a nutrition professional.

Canadian Health Network
www.canadian-health-network.ca
The Canadian Health Network is a national Internet-based health information service. With content from more than 500 non-profit health organizations, this site provides health information you can trust. Take a look at the collection of healthy eating resources. Dietitians of Canada is an Affiliate Partner of the Canadian Health Network.

Health Canada
www.hc-sc.gc.ca
Health Canada is the department of the Canadian government responsible for helping citizens maintain and improve their health. In this site, you will find links to government publications containing nutrition information, including *Canada's Food Guide to Healthy Eating*, *Canada's Physical Activity Guide*, the *Body Mass Index*, *Nutrition for Healthy Term Infants* and many more resources.

assessing information for accuracy and reliability

As you surf the Web, watch television or read the popular media, you are likely to be inundated with information on nutrition. Not all this information is to be believed. In some cases, it is difficult to distinguish advertising from genuine editorial information. Asking yourself the following five questions can help you to determine the reliability and accuracy of the information you are receiving.

1. Are there any promises made for a quick fix or instant cure?
2. Does the claim sound too good to be true?
3. Do you have to buy special products?
4. Is the recommendation based on personal success stories or testimonials?
5. Does the advice contradict *Canada's Food Guide to Healthy Eating*?

If you answered yes to any of these questions, chances are the information is not trustworthy. Miraculous promises and claims about special products are just too good to be true.

consult a dietitian

If you are seeking advice on healthy eating, you may want to consult a dietitian, a health professional who has unique training to advise you on food, diet and nutrition. You can consult with a dietitian on a variety of topics, ranging from general lifestyle and nutrition counselling to nutrition counselling for special medical needs. Whether you are looking for a consultant to advise you on a wellness program at your workplace or need individual counselling, whether you follow a specific diet or have a desire to improve your eating habits, a dietitian can help you translate scientifically sound nutrition advice into practical strategies that suit your lifestyle.

- Visit Find a Nutrition Professional on the Dietitians of Canada Web site (www.dietitians.ca) to find a dietitian near you.
- Look in the yellow pages under Dietitians.
- Call your local public health department, hospital or community health center.
- Call the Dietitians of Canada Consulting Dietitians Network toll-free at 1-888-901-7776.
- Ask your doctor for a referral to a dietitian.

what is the difference between a dietitian and a nutritionist?

Registered dietitians are your trusted experts for food, nutrition and diet advice. The titles "registered dietitian", "professional dietitian" and "dietitian" are all protected by law. The title nutritionist can be used by people with different levels of training. Some qualified dietitians use the word "nutritionist" or "nutrition consultant" in their job title, so check their credentials to be sure that you are talking to an expert. All registered dietitians must have the credentials RD, R.Dt., P.Dt., RDN or Dt.P., depending on the province.

Nutritious Breakfasts and Breads

The recipes in this section will meet your needs for any breakfast, whether you are on the go or have time for a leisurely repast. We've also included a number of bread and muffin recipes to help you complete your meal, in the morning or at any time of the day.

make breakfast part of your morning routine

As the first meal of the day, breakfast should never be skipped. A nutritious, high-fiber breakfast is an excellent way to kick-start your day. It is unreasonable to expect anyone to study or to work effectively if energy levels are low. Instead of "running on empty," choose to wake up to a healthy start with a well-balanced breakfast that will give you the energy you need.

To create well-balanced breakfasts, consult *Canada's Food Guide to Healthy Eating* (see page 434). Be sure to include at least three of the four food groups so you'll be packing in enough energy, protein, vitamins and minerals to help you meet about 25% of your daily needs.

change your habits

If you are not a breakfast eater, begin gradually. Start off by having a glass of milk or juice, or a piece of fruit. Then add a slice of toast with peanut butter, crackers with cheese or even an egg. After a couple of weeks, you can expect to wake up with an appetite. Still not hungry first thing in the morning? Have your breakfast when you get to work.

make room for bread

Bread is a nutritious addition, not only at breakfast but throughout the day as an accompaniment to meals or a delicious snack. Eating different types of bread will add variety. Healthy eating includes five to 12 servings a day of breads, grains, cereals, pasta and rice.

When buying breads, choose whole grains more often as they provide necessary fiber, and minimize the use of fatty spreads such as margarine, butter and mayonnaise. Try using Fazool, a flavorful spread made from beans, instead. Enjoy higher-fat breads such as croissants and pastries in moderation.

eat breakfast to maintain a healthy weight

Skipping breakfast won't help you to lose weight. In addition to providing you with the nutrients you need to feel energetic and avoid mid-morning fatigue, starting your day with a nutritious breakfast can also make you far less likely to indulge in high-calorie snacks or to overeat at other meals. A balanced breakfast is a priority for anyone working toward achieving and maintaining a healthy weight.

think out of the box

Breakfast doesn't need to be a sit-down affair, nor does it need to include typical "breakfast foods."

caffeine in moderation

All foods can be a part of healthy eating as long as they are consumed in moderation. Recent studies show that a moderate caffeine intake of 400 to 450 mg (about three to four cups of coffee) per day poses no health risk to healthy adults. Just make sure that caffeinated beverages, which include colas as well as tea and coffee, do not take the place of more healthful drinks, such as milk, juice and water.

breakfast dos

- Make breakfast part of your daily routine.
- Include a variety of foods every day; aim to include at least three of the four food groups.
- Vary your menu daily.
- When in a hurry, pack it to go.

quick and e-a-s-y
on-the-go breakfast ideas:

- peanut butter and banana sandwich with a glass of milk
- slice of leftover pizza with a glass of orange juice
- bagel sandwich with a glass of milk
- bran or oatmeal muffin with a fruit smoothie
- bag of mixed dry cereal, dried fruits and nuts with a glass of milk
- toasted English muffin with ham and cheese and a glass of tomato juice

SERVES 1
Makes 1¼ cups
(300 mL)
················
Dairy Farmers of Canada

This shake, like the Banana Berry Wake-Up Shake, is packed with bone-building calcium.

Sunny Orange Shake

¾ cup	lower-fat vanilla yogurt	175 mL
2 tbsp	skim-milk powder	25 mL
½ cup	orange juice	125 mL

1. In a blender, combine yogurt, skim-milk powder and orange juice; blend until smooth.

PER SERVING	
Calories: 262	
Dietary Fiber: Trace	Carbohydrate: 51 g
Fat: 2 g	Protein: 11 g

SERVES 2
Makes about 3¼ cups
(800 mL)
·····················
Ann Merritt

This creamy shake, which can be made the night before, is a great way to use up ripe bananas that have been frozen. When bananas start to get brown, pop them in the freezer and take out as needed.

DIETITIAN'S MESSAGE

Shakes are a great way to increase fruit and milk intake. The skim-milk powder adds thickness to the Sunny Orange Shake and boosts the calcium content to 353 mg per serving. The vanilla yogurt used in these shakes has a slightly higher carbohydrate content than most other yogurts, so people with diabetes may want to choose a lower-carbohydrate brand.

Banana Berry Wake-Up Shake

1	banana	1
1 cup	fresh *or* frozen berries (any combination)	250 mL
1 cup	milk *or* vanilla-flavored soy beverage	250 mL
¾ cup	lower-fat vanilla yogurt (*or* other flavor that complements berries)	175 mL

1. In a blender, liquefy fruit with a small amount of the milk. Add remaining milk and yogurt; blend until smooth. If shake is too thick, add extra milk or soy beverage to achieve desired consistency.

PER SERVING	
Calories: 234	
Dietary Fiber: 3 g	Carbohydrate: 44 g
Fat: 4 g	Protein: 9 g

QUICK SHAKE
Once a week, 12-year-old Amelia Roblin gets up early to treat her dad to a smoothie. She combines ½ cup (125 mL) milk, one 6-oz (175 g) container flavored yogurt and ½ cup (125 mL) fruit in a blender. The flavor combinations are endless. Try peach yogurt and strawberries; lemon yogurt and frozen blueberries and strawberry yogurt and bananas.

Nutritious Breakfasts and Breads

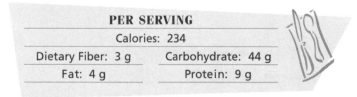

Big-Batch Bran Muffins

Makes 24

P

....

Susanne Stark, Post Cereals

Preheat oven to 375°F (190°C)
Two 12-cup muffin tins, greased or paper-lined

5 cups	all-purpose flour	1.25 L
5½ cups	100% bran cereal	1.375 L
2 cups	packed brown sugar	500 mL
1 cup	chopped dates *or* raisins	250 mL
1 tbsp	baking soda	15 mL
1 tbsp	ground cinnamon	15 mL
4 cups	buttermilk *or* sour milk (see Tip, at right)	1 L
1 cup	vegetable oil	250 mL
4	eggs	4

1. In a large bowl, combine flour, cereal, brown sugar, dates, baking soda and cinnamon.
2. In another large bowl, mix together buttermilk, oil and eggs. Stir into dry ingredients and mix until moistened.
3. Spoon batter into muffin cups, filling to the top. Bake in preheated oven for 25 to 30 minutes or until golden brown. Cool in pans for 5 minutes; remove muffins. Cool on a wire rack. Store in airtight containers; freeze, if desired.

PER MUFFIN	
Calories: 331	
Dietary Fiber: 7 g	Carbohydrate: 57 g
Fat: 11 g	Protein: 7 g

Fresh, nutritious muffins hot out of the oven are a favorite way to start any day.

TIPS

This batter can be prepared and stored for up to 2 weeks in the refrigerator. Pour batter into prepared muffin tins and bake as needed. Or you can bake the whole batch and keep extras in the freezer.

Sour milk can be used instead of buttermilk. To prepare, combine 3 tbsp (45 mL) lemon juice or vinegar with 4 cups (1 L) milk and let stand for 5 minutes.

DIETITIAN'S MESSAGE

Eating bran muffins for breakfast, or as a snack anytime during the day, is a great way to add fiber to your diet. Bran promotes regularity and a healthy digestive system. Pack these muffins with a shake for a quick meal to go.

Serve these delicious muffins with juice or fruit and a quick-cooked egg for a tasty breakfast that is easy to make.

TIPS

These muffins freeze well, so make up an extra batch and store in an airtight container or freezer bag.

Sour milk can be used instead of buttermilk. To prepare, combine 4 tsp (20 mL) lemon juice or vinegar with 2 cups (500 mL) milk and let stand for 5 minutes.

DIETITIAN'S MESSAGE

Eating orange, red and yellow fruits and vegetables, such as squashes, pumpkins, cantaloupe and melon, is an excellent way to boost your intake of vitamin A.

Pumpkin Raisin Muffins

Preheat oven to 375°F (190°C)
Two 12-cup muffin tins, greased or paper-lined

2 cups	whole-wheat flour	500 mL
1½ cups	all-purpose flour	375 mL
1 cup	granulated sugar	250 mL
4 tsp	baking powder	20 mL
1 tsp	baking soda	5 mL
1 tbsp	ground cinnamon	15 mL
1 tsp	ground nutmeg	5 mL
1 tsp	ground ginger	5 mL
¼ tsp	salt	1 mL
1½ cups	raisins	375 mL
1	can (14 oz/398 mL) pumpkin purée (not pie filling)	1
½ cup	vegetable oil	125 mL
2 cups	buttermilk *or* sour milk (see Tip, at left)	500 mL
3	eggs	3

1. In a large bowl, combine whole-wheat flour, all-purpose flour, sugar, baking powder, baking soda, cinnamon, nutmeg, ginger, salt and raisins.

2. In a separate bowl, blend together pumpkin, oil, buttermilk and eggs.

3. Make a large well in center of dry ingredients; pour in wet ingredients all at once. Gently fold together until just combined.

4. Spoon batter into muffin tins. Bake in preheated oven for 18 to 22 minutes or until firm to the touch.

PER MUFFIN	
Calories: 191	
Dietary Fiber: 2 g	Carbohydrate: 33 g
Fat: 6 g	Protein: 4 g

Nutritious Breakfasts and Breads

Fruit and Oatmeal Muffins

Preheat oven to 400°F (200°C)
Two 12-cup muffin tins, greased or paper-lined

2½ cups	all-purpose flour	625 mL
1½ cups	quick-cooking rolled oats	375 mL
1 cup	wheat germ	250 mL
¾ cup	granulated sugar	175 mL
2 tbsp	baking powder	25 mL
½ tsp	salt	2 mL
1 cup	raisins	250 mL
1	medium apple (unpeeled), chopped	1
⅓ cup	shelled sunflower seeds	75 mL
2	eggs	2
1 cup	mashed ripe bananas	250 mL
¾ cup	skim milk	175 mL
2 tbsp	grated orange zest	25 mL
½ cup	orange juice	125 mL
⅓ cup	vegetable oil	75 mL

1. In a large bowl, combine flour, oats, wheat germ, sugar, baking powder and salt; stir in raisins, apple and sunflower seeds.

2. In another bowl, whisk eggs lightly; blend in bananas, milk, orange zest and juice, and oil. Pour into dry ingredients, stirring just until moistened.

3. Spoon about ⅓ cup (75 mL) batter into each greased or paper-lined muffin cup. Bake in preheated oven for about 20 minutes or until firm to the touch. Cool in pans for 5 minutes. Remove from tins and cool on rack. Store in airtight container in freezer.

5pts

PER MUFFIN

Calories: 230

Dietary Fiber: 3 g	Carbohydrate: 39 g
Fat: 7 g	Protein: 6 g

Makes 20
....
Don Costello, Chef
Lisa Diamond, Dietitian

These muffins, which are so moist you won't need to add butter, are chock-full of fruit. They are best eaten warm from the oven. If you must store them, do so in the freezer and thaw as needed.

TIP

Since these muffins freeze well, they are particularly convenient for brown baggers. Pop a frozen muffin into a lunch bag. By the time lunch rolls around, it will be defrosted and ready to eat.

DIETITIAN'S MESSAGE

Serve these muffins along with a Sunny Orange Shake (see recipe, page 20) for a great-tasting breakfast when you are on the go. The wheat germ in these muffins, although high in fat, provides vitamin E, an antioxidant, which promotes health. Wheat germ, once opened, should be stored in the refrigerator because of its high fat content.

Makes 12
....
Laura M. Hawthorn

These tart, tasty muffins can be enjoyed year-round if you freeze fresh cranberries when they are available in the fall. It is unnecessary to thaw cranberries before using in this recipe.

TIP

If fresh or frozen cranberries are unavailable, try soaking ³⁄₄ cup (175 mL) dried cranberries in ½ cup (125 mL) orange juice or water for about 15 minutes, or replace cranberries with blueberries.

DIETITIAN'S MESSAGE

These tangy muffins, along with fresh fruit, cottage cheese and a glass of milk, make a great get-up-and-go start to the day; you get fiber, calcium and many other valuable vitamins and minerals.

Cranberry Oat Muffins

Preheat oven to 400°F (200°C)
One 12-cup muffin tin, greased or paper-lined

³⁄₄ cup	rolled oats	175 mL
1½ cups	all-purpose flour, divided	375 mL
1 cup	granulated sugar	250 mL
2 tsp	baking powder	10 mL
½ tsp	salt	2 mL
½ cup	butter *or* margarine	125 mL
1½ cups	fresh *or* frozen cranberries, chopped	375 mL
2 tsp	grated lemon zest	10 mL
²⁄₃ cup	2% milk	150 mL
1	egg, beaten	1

Topping

2 tsp	ground cinnamon	10 mL
2 tsp	granulated sugar	10 mL

1. In a food processor or blender, process oats until very fine. Combine oats, flour (except for 2 tbsp/25 mL), sugar, baking powder and salt. Cut in butter with a pastry blender or food processor until mixture resembles coarse crumbs.

2. Toss cranberries with reserved flour; stir into flour mixture.

3. Combine lemon zest, milk and egg; mix thoroughly. Add to dry ingredients, stirring just until moistened; do not overmix. Spoon into lightly greased or paper-lined muffin cups, filling three-quarters full.

4. *Topping:* Combine cinnamon and sugar; sprinkle over muffins. Bake in preheated oven for 20 to 24 minutes or until tops of muffins spring back when lightly touched.

PER MUFFIN	
Calories: 227	
Dietary Fiber: 1 g	Carbohydrate: 35 g
Fat: 9 g	Protein: 3 g

Carrot Bran Muffins

Preheat oven to 400°F (200°C)
One 12-cup muffin tin, greased or paper-lined

1¼ cups	whole-wheat flour	300 mL
1¼ cups	high-fiber bran cereal	300 mL
1 tsp	baking powder	5 mL
1 tsp	baking soda	5 mL
1 tsp	ground cinnamon	5 mL
½ tsp	ground nutmeg	2 mL
½ tsp	salt	2 mL
2	eggs	2
1 cup	grated carrots	250 mL
¾ cup	buttermilk	175 mL
⅓ cup	packed brown sugar	75 mL
¼ cup	vegetable oil	50 mL
½ cup	raisins	125 mL

1. In a large bowl, combine flour, cereal, baking powder, baking soda, cinnamon, nutmeg and salt.

2. In a separate bowl, beat eggs thoroughly; blend in carrots, buttermilk, brown sugar and vegetable oil. Add to dry ingredients, stirring just until moistened. Stir in raisins.

3. Spoon batter into greased or paper-lined muffin cups, filling about three-quarters full. Bake in preheated oven for about 20 minutes or until tops of muffins spring back when lightly touched.

3 pts

PER MUFFIN	
Calories: 166	
Dietary Fiber: 5 g	Carbohydrate: 28 g
Fat: 6 g	Protein: 4 g

Makes 12

P

Steve Holodinsky

Two favorites, carrot and bran, are combined in this tasty muffin. A great start to any day!

TIP
When making these muffins, keep wet and dry ingredients separate until you're ready to mix, then mix just enough to blend the 2 components. This produces a coarse crumb that is just fine for these muffins.

DIETITIAN'S MESSAGE
Start your day right by eating one of these muffins for fiber accompanied by a Banana Berry Wake-Up Shake (see recipe, page 20) for calcium and vitamins. The bran in these muffins provides insoluble fiber, which aids in regularity. As you increase your fiber intake, remember to drink more fluids to help the fiber work more effectively.

These tasty muffins replace eggs with egg whites, and sugar with honey and molasses, for an interesting version of a classic bran muffin. Raisins and unsweetened pineapple make these muffins particularly moist and fruity.

TIP

Often older recipes specify that molasses should be non-sulfured. Due to changes in the manufacturing process, all molasses now fits that description. This addresses concerns about the presence of sulfites, which cause allergic reactions in some people.

DIETITIAN'S MESSAGE

Serve these muffins with a glass of orange juice since they contain molasses, a by-product of sugar manufacturing. Molasses provides some iron, and adding orange juice aids in the absorption of this mineral.

Gib's Gourmet Muffins

Preheat oven to 350°F (180°C)
Two 8-cup muffin tins, greased or paper-lined

1½ cups	whole-wheat flour	375 mL
2 cups	natural wheat bran	500 mL
1½ tsp	baking powder	7 mL
¼ tsp	baking soda	1 mL
¼ tsp	ground nutmeg	1 mL
¼ tsp	ground cinnamon	1 mL
1 cup	skim milk	250 mL
2	egg whites, lightly beaten	2
½ cup	safflower oil	125 mL
½ cup	liquid honey	125 mL
½ cup	molasses	125 mL
2 cups	raisins	500 mL
1 cup	crushed unsweetened pineapple, well drained	250 mL

1. In a large bowl, combine flour, bran, baking powder, baking soda, nutmeg and cinnamon.

2. In another bowl, combine milk, egg whites, oil, honey and molasses. Stir in raisins and pineapple. Add to dry ingredients, stirring just until moistened; do not overmix.

3. Spoon into greased or paper-lined muffin cups, filling three-quarters full. Bake in preheated oven for 20 to 25 minutes or until tops of muffins spring back when lightly touched.

PER MUFFIN	
Calories: 243	
Dietary Fiber: 5 g	Carbohydrate: 46 g
Fat: 7 g	Protein: 4 g

Orange Apricot Oatmeal Scones

Makes 12

P

....

Bev Callaghan, Dietitian

These tasty scones are delicious with a relaxing cup of tea.

Preheat oven to 375°F (190°C)
Baking sheet, greased

2 cups	all-purpose flour	500 mL
1½ cups	quick-cooking rolled oats	375 mL
¼ cup	granulated sugar	50 mL
1 tbsp	baking powder	15 mL
2 tsp	grated orange zest	10 mL
½ tsp	baking soda	2 mL
¼ tsp	salt	1 mL
6 tbsp	butter	90 mL
½ cup	chopped apricots	125 mL
1 cup	buttermilk *or* sour milk (see Tip, at right)	250 mL
	Milk	

TIP
Sour milk can be used instead of buttermilk. To prepare, combine 2 tsp (10 mL) lemon juice or vinegar with 1 cup (250 mL) milk and let stand for 5 minutes.

VARIATION
For a change, substitute ½ cup (125 mL) dates, raisins, currants or dried cranberries for the apricots.

1. In a bowl, combine flour, oats, all but 1 tsp (5 mL) of the sugar, baking powder, orange zest, baking soda and salt. Using a fork or pastry blender, cut in butter until mixture resembles coarse crumbs. Stir in apricots. Add buttermilk; stir until mixture is just combined.

2. On a lightly floured surface, knead dough gently 4 or 5 times. Divide into 3 pieces. Shape each piece into a round about 1 inch (2.5 cm) thick. Transfer to baking sheet.

3. Cut each round into quarters. Brush tops with milk; sprinkle with reserved sugar. Bake in preheated oven for 20 to 25 minutes or until lightly browned.

DIETITIAN'S MESSAGE

Try these tasty scones with a shake or a glass of milk and a piece of fruit for a breakfast with a difference. The oats and apricots add fiber to the recipe.

PER SCONE	
Calories: 205	
Dietary Fiber: 2 g	Carbohydrate: 32 g
Fat: 7 g	Protein: 5 g

Keep a supply of these muffins frozen in airtight containers until needed for breakfast, lunch or snacks. Defrost in the microwave for breakfast or pop into a lunch bag directly from the freezer; they'll defrost by the time lunch rolls around.

TIP

Sour milk can be used instead of buttermilk. To prepare, combine 3 tbsp (45 mL) lemon juice or vinegar with 4 cups (1 L) milk and let stand for 5 minutes.

DIETITIAN'S MESSAGE

For a complete meal at breakfast, have a shake (see page 20) with these muffins, or pack them for lunch with a Thermos of Lunch Box Chili (see recipe, page 63) along with a container of milk or yogurt.

Cornmeal Muffins

Preheat oven to 375°F (190°C)
Two 12-cup muffin tins, greased or paper-lined

4 cups	all-purpose flour	1 L
2 cups	cornmeal	500 mL
¾ cup	granulated sugar	175 mL
2 tbsp	baking powder	25 mL
2 tsp	baking soda	10 mL
½ tsp	salt	2 mL
4 cups	buttermilk *or* sour milk (see Tip, at left)	1 L
½ cup	vegetable oil	125 mL
3	eggs	3

1. In a bowl, combine flour, cornmeal, all but 2 tsp (10 mL) of the sugar, baking powder, baking soda and salt.

2. In a separate bowl, whisk together buttermilk, oil and eggs. Add to dry ingredients; stir just until combined.

3. Spoon into muffin cups. Sprinkle with remaining sugar. Bake in preheated oven for 18 to 22 minutes or until firm to the touch.

PER MUFFIN	
Calories: 209	
Dietary Fiber: 1 g	Carbohydrate: 33 g
Fat: 6 g	Protein: 5 g

Granola

Preheat oven to 325°F (160°C)
Large roasting pan

5 cups	large-flake rolled oats	1.25 L
2 cups	barley flakes	500 mL
1½ cups	raw unsalted nuts (almonds, filberts, pecans), chopped	375 mL
1 cup	sesame seeds	250 mL
1 cup	raw unsalted shelled sunflower seeds	250 mL
1 cup	raw unsalted pumpkin seeds	250 mL
1 cup	skim-milk powder	250 mL
1 cup	wheat germ	250 mL
1 cup	unsweetened coconut	250 mL
¾ cup	olive oil *or* canola oil	175 mL
½ cup	molasses	125 mL
½ cup	liquid honey	125 mL
1 tbsp	ground cinnamon	15 mL
2 cups	dried fruit (raisins, apricots, mango, pineapple, banana), chopped	500 mL

1. In a large roasting pan, combine oats, barley flakes, raw nuts, sesame, sunflower and pumpkin seeds, skim-milk powder, wheat germ and coconut.
2. Combine oil, molasses, honey and cinnamon. Stir thoroughly into oat mixture. Bake in preheated oven for about 30 minutes or until golden brown; stir frequently. Cool, stir in fruit. Store, covered, in a cool, dry location.

PER ½ CUP (125 ML) SERVING	
Calories: 241	
Dietary Fiber: 3 g	Carbohydrate: 24 g
Fat: 14 g	Protein: 7 g

STOVE-TOP OATMEAL
Using the ingredients for Creamy Microwave Oatmeal (see recipe, page 30), in a saucepan, combine water, milk, salt, raisins and bran; bring to a boil over medium heat. Add oats and cinnamon, stirring constantly; reduce heat to low and simmer, covered, for 3 to 4 minutes.

Makes 40 Servings

Denise A. Hartley

This is probably one of the best granola recipes you will ever make! Enjoy as a cereal, with yogurt, over fruit or as a snack.

TIPS
You can vary the taste and texture of this granola by trying different grains and adding dried fruits such as apples, pears and dates.

Although sunflower and pumpkin seeds provide fiber, they are also high in fat. This means they become rancid quickly. Be sure to buy them from a store with high turnover, use them quickly, and store in the refrigerator.

DIETITIAN'S MESSAGE

This granola makes a great energy-packed breakfast or healthy snack. Like most granola, it is high in calories and fat, so serve it with skim or a lower-fat milk or yogurt. Add fresh fruit salad for great-tasting breakfast.

Creamy Microwave Oatmeal

SERVES 1

Bev Callaghan, Dietitian

This recipe is easily multiplied to serve 2, 3 or 4 people.

DIETITIAN'S MESSAGE

Here's an easy way to boost your calcium intake: when preparing hot cereal, substitute milk for half of the water called for in the package directions.

This breakfast provides both soluble fiber from oatmeal and insoluble fiber from wheat bran. Including both types of fiber in your diet is beneficial to long-term health.

½ cup	water	125 mL
½ cup	milk *or* soy beverage	125 mL
⅛ tsp	salt	0.5 mL
2 tbsp	raisins	25 mL
1 tsp	wheat bran	5 mL
½ cup	quick-cooking rolled oats	125 mL
¼ tsp	ground cinnamon	1 mL

1. In a 4-cup (1 L) microwave-safe bowl, combine water, milk, salt, raisins and bran. Microwave on High for 2 minutes. Stir in oats and cinnamon; microwave on High for 3 to 4 minutes, stirring at 1-minute intervals, or until oatmeal has thickened. Cover and let stand for 1 minute. Serve with brown sugar or maple syrup, and milk.

PER SERVING	
Calories: 282	
Dietary Fiber: 6 g	Carbohydrate: 51 g
Fat: 5 g	Protein: 11 g

Not Your Same Old Oats

SERVES 7

Michael G. Baylis

This breakfast cereal combines the goodness of oats and oat bran with high-fiber grains like cracked wheat.

TIP

To vary this recipe, try altering the proportion and types of grains.

DIETITIAN'S MESSAGE

This fiber-packed cereal is a new twist on traditional oatmeal. Serve with milk and fresh fruit, and breakfast will set you up for the day.

1 cup	large-flake rolled oats	250 mL
⅔ cup	5-grain cereal	150 mL
½ cup	oat bran	125 mL
⅓ cup	medium bulgur (cracked wheat)	75 mL

1. In a large bowl, combine oats, cereal, oat bran and bulgur. Store in airtight container.

PER SERVING	
Calories: 143	
Dietary Fiber: 4 g	Carbohydrate: 27 g
Fat: 2 g	Protein: 6 g

FOR 1 SERVING OF NOT YOUR SAME OLD OATS
Place ⅓ cup (75 mL) of the oat mixture in a deep bowl. Add ¾ cup (175 mL) water and a pinch of salt. Microwave on High for 2 minutes; stir. Microwave for 1 to 2 minutes longer or cook in small saucepan on top of stove for about 5 minutes.

Muesli Mix

4 cups	quick-cooking rolled oats	1 L
½ cup	flax seeds	125 mL
½ cup	wheat germ	125 mL
½ cup	oat bran	125 mL
½ cup	wheat bran	125 mL
1 cup	dried cranberries	250 mL

1. Mix together all ingredients and pour into an airtight container. Store in a cool, dry place.

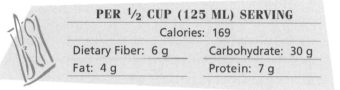

PER ½ CUP (125 ML) SERVING

Calories: 169

| Dietary Fiber: 6 g | Carbohydrate: 30 g |
| Fat: 4 g | Protein: 7 g |

Makes 14 Servings

Stefa Katamay, Dietitian

TIPS

This muesli is also great for camping, backpacking and canoe trips.

Store flax seeds and wheat germ in the refrigerator because of their high fat content.

DIETITIAN'S MESSAGE

To add even more fiber and nutrients to this high-fiber cereal, try serving it with peaches and blueberries, topped with yogurt.

Breakfast Muesli to Go

1 cup	large-flake *or* 3-minute oats (not instant)	250 mL
1 cup	lower-fat plain yogurt	250 mL
½ cup	2% milk	125 mL
2 tbsp	liquid honey *or* maple syrup	25 mL
1 cup	assorted berries (fresh *or* frozen)	250 mL
1	large banana, sliced	1

1. In a plastic container, combine oats, yogurt, milk and honey; gently fold in berries. Add banana before serving or add to sealable container before taking muesli on the go.

PER SERVING

Calories: 423

| Dietary Fiber: 8 g | Carbohydrate: 79 g |
| Fat: 7 g | Protein: 16 g |

SERVES 2 **P**

Renée Crompton, Dietitian

Rushing out in the morning? Divide into 2 sealable containers and leave room to add some banana.

TIP

For variety, try serving this muesli with different types of yogurt and fresh fruit in season. If using vanilla or fruit-flavored yogurt, you can omit the honey or reduce the amount you use.

DIETITIAN'S MESSAGE

This complete breakfast works well for people on the go as it is best if made the night before.

SERVES 6
•••••••••••••••••••••••••••
**Blair Woodruff and
Kurt Zwingli, Chefs
Cathy Thibault, Dietitian**

*A great low-fat breakfast
choice that is ready to eat
in the morning if prepared
the night before. It can be
made ahead and it stores
well, refrigerated, for 2 to
3 days. Garnish with fresh
seasonal fruit if desired.*

DIETITIAN'S MESSAGE

Because it's easily
prepared, eaten and
digested, this muesli is
particularly popular
with athletes who
are on the go.

Bircher Muesli

²/₃ cup	quick-cooking rolled oats	150 mL
2 cups	2% milk	500 mL
¼ cup	granulated sugar	50 mL
¼ tsp	ground cinnamon	1 mL
1½ cups	lower-fat plain yogurt	375 mL
1½ tsp	lemon juice	7 mL
2	medium apples (unpeeled)	2
2	medium bananas	2

1. In a bowl, stir oats into milk; let stand for 15 minutes.
   Stir in sugar and cinnamon.

2. Combine yogurt and lemon juice. Dice apples; stir into
   yogurt mixture. Stir into softened oats. Refrigerate.

3. At serving time, slice bananas and stir into mixture.

PER SERVING	
Calories: 208	
Dietary Fiber: 2 g	Carbohydrate: 39 g
Fat: 3 g	Protein: 8 g

SERVES 6
••••••••••••••••••••••
P

Lise Parisien

*Here's a lower-fat, higher-
fiber version of an
old favorite.*

TIP
Both the whites and the
yolks of eggs provide
such valuable nutrients as
vitamin A, magnesium,
iron and riboflavin, in
addition to protein.

DIETITIAN'S MESSAGE

Sprinkle with fresh berries
and serve with plain yogurt
sweetened with maple
syrup. This will add calcium
and vitamin C to this
breakfast favorite.

French Toast

4	egg whites	4
2 tbsp	skim milk	25 mL
½ tsp	vanilla	2 mL
Pinch	ground nutmeg *or* cinnamon	Pinch
6	slices whole-wheat bread	6

1. Beat together egg whites, milk, vanilla and nutmeg until
   frothy. Pour into large flat dish; dip both sides of bread
   slices into mixture.

2. In a large nonstick or lightly buttered skillet, cook bread
   over medium heat until brown on 1 side. Flip and cook
   other side. Serve immediately.

PER SERVING	
Calories: 80	
Dietary Fiber: 2 g	Carbohydrate: 14 g
Fat: 1 g	Protein: 5 g

Banana Berry Wake-Up Shake ➤
(page 20) and Pumpkin Raisin
Muffins (page 22)

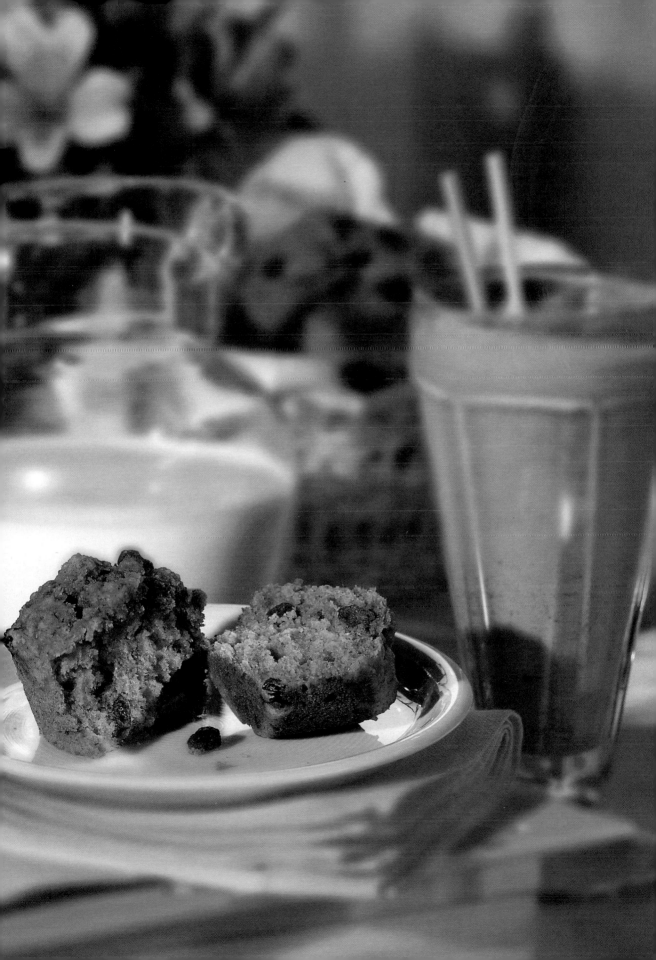

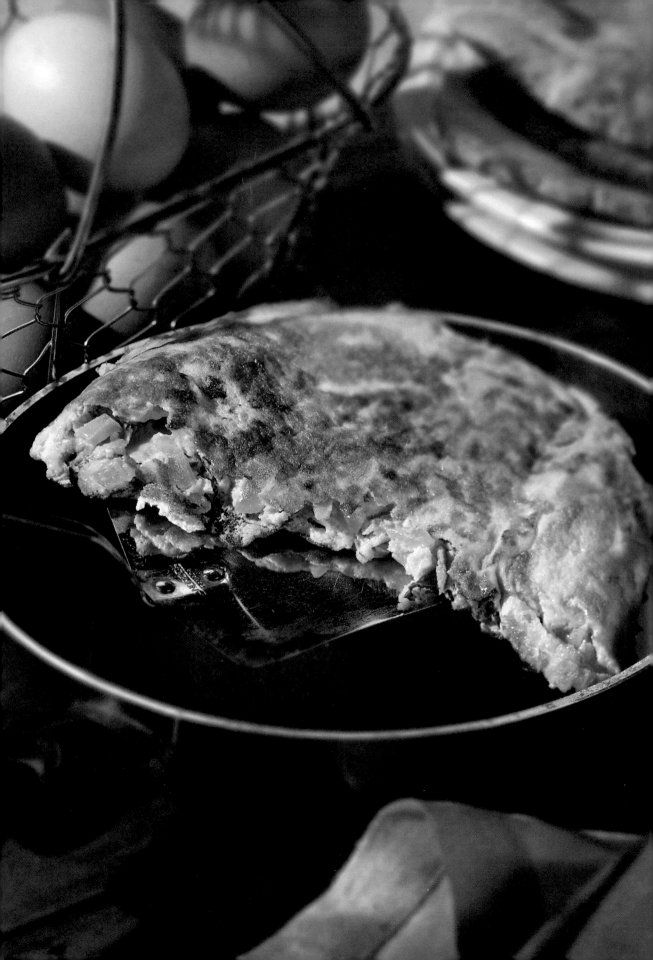

Finnish Apple Pancake

Preheat oven to 425°F (220°C)
8-inch (2 L) square baking pan, greased

2 cups	thinly sliced cored peeled apples	500 mL
1 tbsp	butter, melted	15 mL
3	eggs	3
½ cup	milk	125 mL
⅓ cup	all-purpose flour	75 mL
¼ tsp	baking powder	1 mL
⅛ tsp	salt	0.5 mL
Topping		
½ tsp	ground cinnamon	2 mL
1 tbsp	granulated sugar	15 mL

1. Place apples and butter in baking pan; toss to coat. Bake in preheated oven for 5 minutes.

2. Meanwhile, in a small bowl, whisk together eggs, milk, flour, baking powder and salt until smooth. Set aside.

3. *Topping:* In another small bowl, combine cinnamon and sugar. Set aside.

4. Pour egg mixture over cooked apples; sprinkle evenly with topping. Bake for 15 to 20 minutes or until pancake is puffed and golden brown. Serve immediately.

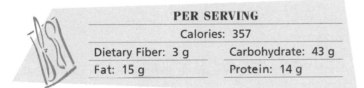

PER SERVING	
Calories: 357	
Dietary Fiber: 3 g	Carbohydrate: 43 g
Fat: 15 g	Protein: 14 g

QUICK SCRAMBLED EGGS FOR ONE
Using a microwave is a great way to teach children how to prepare their own meals.

In a microwave-safe bowl, whisk 2 eggs with 2 tbsp (25 mL) milk and salt and pepper to taste. Cover with plastic wrap, leaving a small steam vent. Microwave on Medium-High for 1 minute 30 seconds to 1 minute 45 seconds, stirring several times during cooking. Cover and let stand for 30 to 60 seconds before serving. Eggs will look slightly moist at first but will finish cooking while covered.

SERVES 2 **P**

Kimberly Green, Dietitian

This is an easy recipe for a special breakfast. And it's a real hit as part of a brunch menu. Serve immediately with maple syrup or your favorite fruit preserves.

TIP
For variety, use peaches or pears to bake this delicious breakfast dish.

DIETITIAN'S MESSAGE

This is a complete breakfast. Accompanying it with a glass of milk and a serving of fruit or juice will add calcium and vitamin C. Be aware that fruit punches and flavored drinks don't deliver the same nutrients as fresh fruit juice or juice from concentrate.

◄ Swiss Chard Frittata in a Pita (page 56)   *Nutritious Breakfasts and Breads*

Fiber-Full Bran Pancakes

¾ cup	whole-wheat flour	175 mL
½ cup	bran cereal flakes, crushed	125 mL
¼ cup	wheat germ	50 mL
1½ tsp	baking powder	7 mL
⅛ tsp	salt	0.5 mL
1 cup	milk	250 mL
1	egg	1
1	egg white	1
1 tbsp	vegetable oil	15 mL

1. In a medium bowl, combine flour, bran flakes, wheat germ, baking powder and salt. Set aside.

2. In a small bowl, blend together milk, egg, egg white and oil; stir into bran mixture until combined. Heat nonstick griddle or frying pan over medium heat. For each pancake, pour about ¼ cup (50 mL) batter onto griddle. Cook, turning once, for about 1 to 2 minutes per side or until golden.

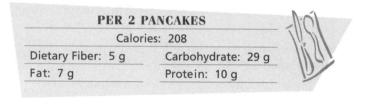

PER 2 PANCAKES	
Calories: 208	
Dietary Fiber: 5 g	Carbohydrate: 29 g
Fat: 7 g	Protein: 10 g

• •

QUICK-COOKED EGG

Break an egg into a small microwave-safe bowl or ramekin; pierce yolk with a fork. Cover with plastic wrap, leaving opening for venting. Microwave on Medium-High for 45 to 60 seconds or until desired consistency is reached. Let stand for 1 to 2 minutes before removing the plastic wrap.

• •

Whole-Wheat Pancakes with Strawberry Purée

Makes 8
....
Caroline Beaurivage

1⅓ cups	whole-wheat flour	325 mL
3 tbsp	brown sugar	45 mL
1 tbsp	baking powder	15 mL
1 tsp	ground cinnamon	5 mL
¼ tsp	salt	1 mL
1¼ cups	2% milk	300 mL
1	egg, beaten	1
3 tbsp	vegetable oil	45 mL
½ tsp	vanilla	2 mL
	Vegetable oil (optional)	

Strawberry Purée

2 cups	fresh strawberries *or* 1 pkg (10 oz/300 g) frozen unsweetened strawberries, thawed	500 mL
	Granulated sugar (optional)	

1. In a bowl, mix together flour, sugar, baking powder, cinnamon and salt.

2. In a separate bowl, beat together milk, egg, oil and vanilla. Add liquid ingredients to dry, mixing until almost smooth (disregard small lumps).

3. Heat skillet or griddle over medium heat; brush with oil (optional for nonstick pans). For each pancake, pour ¼ cup (50 mL) batter into skillet. When underside is brown and bubbles break on top (after 1½ to 2 minutes), flip over and cook for 30 to 60 seconds or until second side is golden brown. Serve hot.

4. *Strawberry Purée:* Wash fresh strawberries; remove hulls. In saucepan, cook fresh or thawed strawberries gently over low heat until softened; cool. In a food processor or blender, purée until smooth. Taste and add sugar, if desired. Serve warm over pancakes. Makes approximately 1 cup (250 mL).

These light-textured whole-wheat pancakes are certain to become a treasured recipe. Serve with sliced fresh fruit or Strawberry Purée for a good start to your day.

TIP
These pancakes can be frozen by layering them between sheets of waxed paper. Freeze in packages of 2 or 4 to suit your needs.

VARIATION
Replace strawberries with fresh or frozen unsweetened raspberries or blueberries or fresh peaches.

DIETITIAN'S MESSAGE
Whole-wheat pancakes are a great way to add fiber to your diet. By adding your favorite fruit as a topping, you will add even more fiber as well as many valuable vitamins and minerals.

PER PANCAKE WITH PURÉE	
Calories: 170	
Dietary Fiber: 3 g	Carbohydrate: 24 g
Fat: 7 g	Protein: 5 g

For variety, try adding a handful of fresh blueberries, frozen cranberries or chocolate chips to the batter when baking this family favorite.

TIP

As this loaf freezes well, why not make an extra one and freeze it for later use? You can also slice and freeze individual servings and have them ready to include in lunch bags.

DIETITIAN'S MESSAGE

To increase the fiber content of this recipe, substitute up to ½ cup (125 mL) whole-wheat flour for the same quantity of all-purpose flour. If your bananas are extremely ripe, you can reduce the sugar to ½ cup (125 mL).

Banana Bread

Preheat oven to 350°F (180°C)
9- by 5-inch (2 L) loaf pan, greased

1¼ cups	all-purpose flour	300 mL
1 tsp	baking soda	5 mL
½ tsp	baking powder	2 mL
¾ cup	granulated sugar	175 mL
1	egg	1
1	egg white	1
¼ cup	lower-fat plain yogurt	50 mL
¼ cup	vegetable oil	50 mL
1 tsp	vanilla	5 mL
1 cup	mashed ripe bananas (about 2 to 3 medium)	250 mL

1. In a bowl, sift together flour, baking soda and baking powder. Set aside.

2. In a large mixing bowl, blend sugar, egg, egg white, yogurt, oil and vanilla. Blend in bananas. Add dry ingredients; mix until just combined. Pour batter into prepared pan. Bake in preheated oven for 1 hour or until a tester inserted in center of loaf comes out clean.

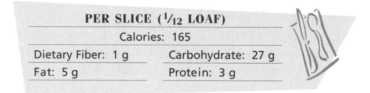

PER SLICE (¹/₁₂ LOAF)	
Calories: 165	
Dietary Fiber: 1 g	Carbohydrate: 27 g
Fat: 5 g	Protein: 3 g

BANANA MUFFINS
To make a muffin version of this recipe, spoon batter into 12 greased or paper-lined muffin cups. Bake at 350°F (180°C) for 18 to 22 minutes or until firm to the touch.

Oatmeal Bannock

Preheat oven to 425°F (220°C)
Baking sheet, ungreased
2-inch (5 cm) round cutter

1 cup	whole-wheat flour	250 mL
½ cup	quick-cooking rolled oats	125 mL
1 tbsp	baking powder	15 mL
1 tsp	granulated sugar	5 mL
½ tsp	salt	2 mL
⅓ cup	each margarine and 1% milk	75 mL

1. In a bowl, combine dry ingredients. Cut in margarine until crumbly. Make well in middle; add milk and mix just until blended.
2. On a floured board, pat dough to ¾-inch (2 cm) thickness. Cut into 9 rounds. Bake in preheated oven for 12 to 15 minutes or until golden.

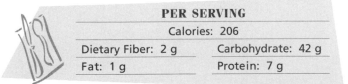

PER BISCUIT	
Calories: 129	
Dietary Fiber: 2 g	Carbohydrate: 14 g
Fat: 7 g	Protein: 3 g

Makes 9 **P**
....
Peter Graham, Chef
Sharlene Clarke,
Dietitian

Bannock bread, originally from Scotland, became a staple in the diet of native North Americans because it is so quick and easy to make. In Scotland, it is usually made from barley. Bannock can be eaten with hot soup, stew, fresh vegetables, wild game and even seasonal fruit. It should be served warm.

Oven Bannock

Preheat oven to 400°F (200°C)
Baking sheet, greased

2½ cups	all-purpose flour	625 mL
2½ tsp	baking powder	12 mL
½ tsp	salt	2 mL
1 cup	skim milk, at room temperature	250 mL

1. In a medium bowl, combine flour, baking powder and salt. Stir in milk until evenly blended. Knead 10 to 12 times.
2. On a floured board, pat into circle 1½ inches (4 cm) thick. Bake in preheated oven for 20 to 25 minutes or until golden.

PER SERVING	
Calories: 206	
Dietary Fiber: 2 g	Carbohydrate: 42 g
Fat: 1 g	Protein: 7 g

SERVES 6
....
Jo-Anne Chalmers, Chef
Christina Scheuer,
Dietitian

VARIATION
Whole-Wheat Bannock:
Use 1½ cups (375 mL) all-purpose flour and 1 cup (250 mL) whole-wheat flour.

DIETITIAN'S MESSAGE

Bannock is traditionally fried; these healthier alternatives are baked. Using whole-wheat flour and oatmeal adds fiber.

*Think bread making is
too time-consuming? Try
this easy-to-make bread.
It's hearty and ideal for
serving with lunch, dinner
or as a snack.*

TIP

If out of buttermilk,
substitute 2 cups (500 mL)
2% milk mixed with
2 tbsp (25 mL) lemon
juice or vinegar.

DIETITIAN'S MESSAGE

You'll be surprised by
how easy it is to make
bread with this recipe,
which doesn't use yeast.
Icelandic in origin, this
bread makes a great
accompaniment for many
of the soups and salads
found in this book.

Three-Grain Bread

Preheat oven to 350°F (180°C)
Two 9- by 5-inch (2 L) loaf pans, greased

½ cup	butter *or* margarine, softened	125 mL
½ cup	packed brown sugar	125 mL
2	large eggs	2
2 cups	whole-wheat flour	500 mL
2 cups	all-purpose flour	500 mL
1 cup	dark rye flour	250 mL
1 cup	quick-cooking rolled oats	250 mL
2 tsp	baking soda	10 mL
1 tsp	salt	5 mL
2½ cups	buttermilk	625 mL

1. In a large bowl, cream butter and brown sugar until light;
   beat in eggs. Combine whole-wheat, all-purpose and dark
   rye flours, oats, baking soda and salt. Add to creamed
   mixture alternately with buttermilk, making 3 additions
   of dry ingredients and 2 of buttermilk. Divide between
   2 greased 9- by 5-inch (2 L) loaf pans.

2. Bake in preheated oven for 55 to 60 minutes or until wooden
   skewer inserted in center comes out clean. Cool in pans for
   10 minutes, then remove from pans and cool on rack. Store
   in airtight container.

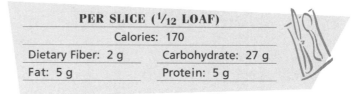

PER SLICE (¹/₁₂ LOAF)	
Calories: 170	
Dietary Fiber: 2 g	Carbohydrate: 27 g
Fat: 5 g	Protein: 5 g

Herb Grain Bread

Preheat oven to 375°F (190°C)
Baking sheet, greased

1 tsp	granulated sugar	5 mL
½ cup	warm water	125 mL
1	pkg (¼ oz/8 g) active dry yeast	1
¾ cup	water	175 mL
½ cup	2% milk	125 mL
⅓ cup	packed brown sugar	75 mL
¼ cup	olive oil	50 mL
¼ cup	7-grain cereal	50 mL
¼ cup	oat bran *or* wheat bran	50 mL
¼ cup	crushed whole-wheat cereal biscuit	50 mL
1 tsp	each salt and dried sage	5 mL
½ tsp	crushed dried thyme	2 mL
½ tsp	celery seed	2 mL
1 cup	whole-wheat flour	250 mL
4 to 5 cups	all-purpose flour	1 to 1.25 L
1	egg	1

1. In a large bowl, dissolve sugar in warm water. Sprinkle in yeast and let stand for 10 minutes or until foamy; stir well.

2. Heat water and milk until lukewarm; add to yeast mixture along with sugar, oil, cereals, cereal biscuit and seasonings. Add whole-wheat flour and 2 cups (500 mL) of the all-purpose flour; blend well. Beat in egg. Add enough of the remaining flour to make soft dough.

3. On a floured board, knead until smooth and elastic, about 5 minutes. Place in greased bowl, turning until coated. Cover and let rise in warm place until doubled in size, 30 to 45 minutes.

4. Punch down dough and divide into 2 rounds. Place on baking sheet. Cover and let rise in warm place until doubled in size, about 30 minutes.

5. Bake in preheated oven for 35 to 40 minutes or until golden brown and loaves sound hollow when tapped on bottom. Remove from baking sheet; let cool on rack.

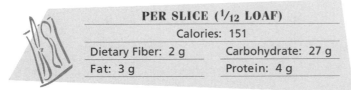

PER SLICE (¹/₁₂ LOAF)	
Calories: 151	
Dietary Fiber: 2 g	Carbohydrate: 27 g
Fat: 3 g	Protein: 4 g

Makes 2 Loaves
....
Janice Mitchell, Chef
Jane Henderson,
Dietitian

This round loaf is made with 3 kinds of cereal and 2 kinds of flour to produce a deliciously different bread.

VARIATIONS
For a finishing touch, brush with milk and sprinkle with sesame seeds before baking. For Italian flavoring, use 1 tsp (5 mL) each dried basil and oregano instead of the seasonings indicated.

TIPS
Yeast causes dough to rise. When it is mixed with flour, water and sugar, it releases carbon dioxide into the mixture, causing it to expand. You can use 1 tbsp (15 mL) active dry yeast instead of the package noted in the recipe.

The first step in making bread is to "proof" the yeast. If it foams, the yeast is still alive. If not, the yeast is dead and you'll need to use a fresh package.

DIETITIAN'S MESSAGE
The variety of grains add fiber to this flavorful bread, which is a delicious accompaniment to soup or salad.

Makes 10 Servings
••••••••••••••••••••••••
Margaret Howard,
Dietitian

This is a bread that Marg's family particularly enjoys. For many years, she has served it as an accompaniment to brunch or a salad supper.

TIP

If you're out of sesame seeds, sprinkle this loaf with chopped walnuts before baking.

DIETITIAN'S MESSAGE

Containing cheese, milk and sesame seeds, this delicious bread is a great way to add calcium to your diet. Serve with a hearty soup for an easy lunch or light supper.

Healthy
Cheese 'n' Herb Bread

Preheat oven to 400°F (200°C)
8-inch (1.2 L) round pan, nonstick or lightly greased

2 cups	all-purpose flour	500 mL
1 cup	whole-wheat flour	250 mL
½ cup	rolled oats	125 mL
1 tbsp	granulated sugar	15 mL
2 tsp	baking powder	10 mL
½ tsp	baking soda	2 mL
1 tsp	dried basil	5 mL
½ tsp	dried oregano	2 mL
½ tsp	salt	2 mL
¼ cup	cold butter *or* margarine	50 mL
1 cup	shredded Swiss cheese	250 mL
1	egg	1
1 cup	buttermilk	250 mL
2 tbsp	sesame seeds	25 mL

1. In a medium bowl, combine flours, oats, sugar, baking powder, baking soda, herbs and salt. Using a pantry blender, cut in butter until mixture resembles fine crumbs. Stir in cheese.

2. Beat together egg and buttermilk; add to butter mixture, stirring with fork to make a soft moist dough. Place dough in a nonstick or lightly greased 8-inch (1.2 L) round pan. Sprinkle with sesame seeds. Bake in preheated oven for 25 to 30 minutes or until tester inserted in center comes out clean. Cut into 10 wedges to serve.

PER SERVING	
Calories: 259	
Dietary Fiber: 2 g	Carbohydrate: 33 g
Fat: 10 g	Protein: 10 g

Apricot Bran Bread

Makes 1 Loaf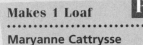
....
Maryanne Cattrysse

Preheat oven to 350°F (180°C)
8- by 4-inch (1.5 L) loaf pan, nonstick or lightly greased

2 cups	bran cereal flakes	500 mL
½ cup	all-purpose flour	125 mL
½ cup	whole-wheat flour	125 mL
½ cup	packed brown sugar	125 mL
2 tsp	baking powder	10 mL
½ tsp	salt	2 mL
½ tsp	ground nutmeg	2 mL
¾ cup	chopped dried apricots	175 mL
1 tsp	grated orange zest	5 mL
1	egg, lightly beaten	1
½ cup	skim milk	125 mL
½ cup	orange juice	125 mL
¼ cup	vegetable oil	50 mL

This tasty and nutritious quick bread freezes well. Keep some in the freezer for unexpected guests.

TIP
Freeze this and other quick breads in individually wrapped single slices. Pop them into lunch bags. They will be defrosted by the time lunch comes around.

DIETITIAN'S MESSAGE
Make your snack count! Since quick breads freeze well, keep frozen slices of this healthful bread on hand. Pack into brown bag lunches or serve with a glass of milk as a delicious after-school snack.

1. Crush cereal to make ¾ cup (175 mL) crumbs. In a large bowl, combine cereal, flours, sugar, baking powder, salt, nutmeg, apricots and orange zest.

2. In a second bowl, beat together egg, milk, orange juice and oil; stir into dry ingredients until well combined. Pour into nonstick or lightly greased 8- by 4-inch (1.5 L) loaf pan. Bake in preheated oven for about 55 minutes or until tester inserted in center comes out clean. Cool for 10 minutes before removing from pan. Cool completely on wire rack.

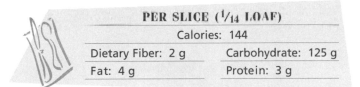

PER SLICE (¹⁄₁₄ LOAF)	
Calories: 144	
Dietary Fiber: 2 g	Carbohydrate: 125 g
Fat: 4 g	Protein: 3 g

This bread was made by our pioneer ancestors and is still a favorite. It's great served with a hearty soup for supper, or as a healthy after-school snack with cheese or peanut butter.

TIP

To sour milk, combine 1 tbsp (15 mL) lemon juice or vinegar with 1½ cups (375 mL) milk and let stand for 5 minutes.

Steamed Brown Bread

Dutch oven or stockpot
Three 19-oz (540 mL) fruit, vegetable or coffee cans, greased

1 cup	all-purpose flour	250 mL
1 cup	whole-wheat flour	250 mL
1 cup	cornmeal	250 mL
½ cup	granulated sugar	125 mL
1½ tsp	salt	7 mL
1 tsp	baking soda	5 mL
1½ cups	sour milk (see Tip, at left)	375 mL
½ cup	molasses	125 mL
2 tbsp	olive oil	25 mL

1. In a large bowl, combine flours, cornmeal, sugar, salt and baking soda.

2. In another bowl, combine sour milk, molasses and olive oil. Add to dry ingredients, stirring just until moistened; do not overmix. Pour into 3 well-greased coffee cans; fill each about three-quarters full. Cover cans with foil; secure with elastic bands.

3. In a large Dutch oven or stockpot, bring about 4 cups (1 L) water to boil. Place cans in water; cover and steam over low heat for 1½ to 2 hours. Remove cans from water and remove foil; cool for 1 hour or until tester inserted in center comes out clean.

4. With a can opener, remove the bottom of each can and push the steamed bread through the open end. Leftovers can be frozen.

PER SLICE (¹/₁₀ LOAF)	
Calories: 82	
Dietary Fiber: 1 g	Carbohydrate: 16 g
Fat: 1 g	Protein: 2 g

Fruit Malt Bread

Makes 1 Loaf
••••••••••••••••••••••••
Margaret Carson, Chef
Pam Lynch, Dietitian

Preheat oven to 400°F (200°C)
8- by 4-inch (1.5 L) loaf pan, greased

1 tsp	granulated sugar	5 mL
1¼ cups	warm water, divided	300 mL
1	pkg (¼ oz/8 g) active dry yeast	1
1½ cups	all-purpose flour	375 mL
1 tbsp	brown sugar	15 mL
1 tsp	salt	5 mL
½ tsp	each ground cinnamon, nutmeg and ginger	2 mL
¼ tsp	ground cloves	1 mL
1 tbsp	vegetable oil	15 mL
1 tbsp	barley malt extract *or* molasses	15 mL
1½ cups	chopped dried fruit (raisins, currants, apricots and pitted prunes)	375 mL
1½ to 2 cups	whole-wheat flour	375 to 500 mL
	Milk	

1. In a bowl, dissolve sugar in ¼ cup (50 mL) of the water. Sprinkle in yeast and let stand until foamy; stir.

2. Combine all-purpose flour, sugar, salt and spices. In a large bowl, combine yeast mixture, remaining 1 cup (250 mL) water, vegetable oil and barley malt extract; gradually beat in flour mixture until smooth. Stir in dried fruit. Add enough of the whole-wheat flour to make moderately stiff dough.

3. On a floured board, knead until smooth and elastic. Place in greased bowl, turning to grease all over. Cover and set in warm place until doubled in size, about 1½ to 2 hours.

4. Punch down dough and shape into 2 balls. Place side by side in prepared pan. Cover and let rise until doubled in size, 1 to 1½ hours.

5. Bake in preheated oven for 30 to 35 minutes or until loaf sounds hollow when tapped on bottom. Brush with milk; remove from pan and cool on rack.

With a flavor reminiscent of hot cross buns, this aromatic bread is perfect for breakfast, a snack or dessert.

TIPS

Place dough in a bowl sprayed with vegetable oil spray and turn to grease all over.

When baking bread, use a baking stone to promote even heating. Heat the stone in the oven for about 45 minutes before adding the dough.

If the top of this loaf becomes too brown while baking, cover loosely with foil.

Barley malt extract provides enzymes that feed the yeast in this dough, helping it to rise.

You can use 1 tbsp (15 mL) active dry yeast instead of the package noted in the recipe.

DIETITIAN'S MESSAGE

This is a rich fruit-filled bread that is particularly delicious for breakfast. Served with cheese and fruit, it makes a great start to the day.

PER SLICE (¹/₁₀ LOAF)	
Calories: 228	
Dietary Fiber: 5 g	Carbohydrate: 49 g
Fat: 2 g	Protein: 6 g

Zucchini Nut Loaf

Preheat oven to 350°F (180°C)
8- by 4-inch (1.5 L) loaf pan, greased

1½ cups	all-purpose flour	375 mL
1 tsp	ground cinnamon	5 mL
½ tsp	baking soda	2 mL
½ tsp	each salt and ground nutmeg	2 mL
¼ tsp	baking powder	1 mL
1	egg	1
¾ cup	granulated sugar	175 mL
⅓ cup	vegetable oil	75 mL
2 tbsp	2% milk	25 mL
1 cup	shredded zucchini (unpeeled)	250 mL
½ cup	chopped walnuts *or* pecans	125 mL
½ tsp	grated lemon zest (optional)	2 mL

1. In a large bowl, combine flour, cinnamon, baking soda, salt, nutmeg and baking powder.

2. In a medium bowl, beat egg; whisk in sugar, oil and milk. Stir in zucchini, nuts, and lemon zest, if desired; stir zucchini mixture into dry ingredients.

3. Pour batter into greased 8- by 4-inch (1.5 L) loaf pan. Bake in preheated oven for 50 minutes or until tester inserted in center comes out clean. Cool for 10 minutes in pan. Turn out onto rack to cool completely.

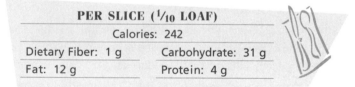

PER SLICE (¹⁄₁₀ LOAF)	
Calories: 242	
Dietary Fiber: 1 g	Carbohydrate: 31 g
Fat: 12 g	Protein: 4 g

Mixed Herb Baguette

Preheat oven to 350°F (180°C)
Baking sheet, greased and dusted with cornmeal

2 tsp	granulated sugar	10 mL
1⅓ cups	warm water	325 mL
1	pkg (¼ oz/8 g) active dry yeast (*or* 1 tbsp/15 mL)	1
2½ to 3 cups	all-purpose flour	625 to 750 mL
¼ cup	mixed chopped fresh herbs	50 mL
2 tsp	butter, melted	10 mL
1 tsp	salt	5 mL
1	egg	1
2 tbsp	milk	25 mL

1. In a large bowl, dissolve sugar in warm water. Sprinkle in yeast and let stand for 10 minutes or until foamy; stir well. Stir in 2 cups (500 mL) of the flour, herbs, butter and salt. Add enough of the remaining flour to make soft dough.

2. Turn out onto floured board; knead for a few minutes or until smooth and elastic. Place in greased bowl, turning to grease all over. Cover and let rise in warm place until doubled in size, 45 to 60 minutes.

3. Punch down dough and cut in half; roll each into long, thin cigar-shaped stick (about 15 inches/38 cm long). Place on cornmeal-dusted greased baking sheet; score tops 3 times on the diagonal. Cover and let rise in warm place until doubled in size, 30 to 45 minutes.

4. Bake in preheated oven for 30 minutes. Combine egg and milk; brush over loaves. Bake for 10 to 15 minutes longer or until loaves sound hollow when tapped on bottom. Cool on racks.

PER SLICE (¹/₂₀ LOAF)

Calories: 37	
Dietary Fiber: Trace	Carbohydrate: 7 g
Fat: Trace	Protein: 1 g

Makes 2 Loaves
....
Peter Ochitwa, Chef
Susie Langley, Dietitian

Baguettes, immortalized in France, are long, thin loaves of crusty bread that are baked on a cookie sheet. The addition of herbs distinguishes this from the traditional version.

TIPS

Instead of fresh herbs, you can substitute a mixture of 1 tsp (5 mL) each dried oregano, thyme, rosemary, sage and tarragon.

People often purchase baking stones to use when making pizza because they promote even heating, but they improve results when baking bread, too. Heat the stone in the oven for about 45 minutes before adding the dough.

DIETITIAN'S MESSAGE

This tasty bread has endless uses. Serve with sliced cheese, a healthful spread such as Fazool (see recipe, page 75) or as the base for a Tuna Salad Melt (see recipe, page 58).

Cottage cheese adds extra nutrients to this uniquely flavored casserole bread. The dill flavor makes it a particularly good choice to serve with fish.

TIP

If your active dry yeast isn't in a package, use 1 tbsp (15 mL) of loose yeast.

DIETITIAN'S MESSAGE

For a calcium-rich lunch, use this savory bread as a base for a grilled cheese sandwich. For one high in protein, serve it with Zucchini Frittata (see recipe, page 57) or a Farmer's Omelette (see recipe, page 55).

Dilly Bread

Preheat oven to 350°F (180°C)
8-inch (1.2 L) round casserole, lightly greased

1 tsp	granulated sugar	5 mL
¼ cup	warm water	50 mL
1	pkg (¼ oz/8 g) active dry yeast	1
1 cup	lower-fat cottage cheese	250 mL
1 tbsp	grated onion	15 mL
2 tbsp	granulated sugar	25 mL
1 tbsp	dill seed	15 mL
1 tsp	salt	5 mL
¼ tsp	baking soda	1 mL
1 tbsp	butter *or* margarine, melted	15 mL
1	egg, beaten	1
2¾ cups	all-purpose flour	675 mL

1. In a bowl, dissolve 1 tsp (5 mL) sugar in warm water. Sprinkle yeast over top and let stand for about 10 minutes or until foamy.

2. In a large bowl, combine yeast mixture, cottage cheese, onion, 2 tbsp (25 mL) sugar, dill seed, salt, baking soda, butter and egg. Gradually stir in flour until smooth (this will be a stiff dough). Turn out onto lightly floured surface and knead until smooth and elastic.

3. Place dough in lightly greased 8-inch (1.2 L) round casserole, turning to grease all over. Cover bowl loosely and let stand in warm place until doubled in size, about 1½ hours. Bake in preheated oven for about 45 minutes. (Do not underbake; a crisp crust is desirable.)

PER SLICE (¹⁄₁₂ LOAF)	
Calories: 148	
Dietary Fiber: 1 g	Carbohydrate: 25 g
Fat: 2 g	Protein: 6 g

Speedy Yam 'n' Egg Rolls

Makes 16
•••••••••••••••••••••••
Linda Terra

Preheat oven to 375°F (190°C)
Baking sheet, nonstick or lightly greased

3 cups	all-purpose flour, divided	750 mL
1½ cups	whole-wheat flour	375 mL
½ cup	oat bran	125 mL
¼ cup	skim-milk powder	50 mL
2 tbsp	grated orange zest	25 mL
½ tsp	salt	2 mL
¾ cup	currants, washed and dried	175 mL
1	pkg (¼ oz/8 g) quick-rise instant yeast	1
¾ cup	mashed cooked yams (cooking liquid reserved)	175 mL
¼ cup	butter *or* margarine, melted	50 mL
¼ cup	liquid honey	50 mL
1 cup	yam cooking liquid	250 mL
2	eggs, lightly beaten	2
	Melted butter	

1. In a large bowl, mix together 2 cups (500 mL) of the all-purpose flour, whole-wheat flour, oat bran, skim-milk powder, orange zest, salt, currants and yeast.

2. In a small saucepan over low heat, heat yams, butter, honey and yam cooking liquid until hot to the touch. Stir mixture and eggs into dry ingredients.

3. Stir in enough of the remaining flour to make a soft dough. Turn out onto lightly floured surface and knead until smooth and elastic. Cover and let rest for 10 minutes.

4. With a sharp knife, cut dough into 16 equal pieces; shape each into smooth ball, tucking ends under. Place seam side down on baking sheet, about 2 inches (5 cm) apart. Cover and let rise until doubled in size, about 1 hour.

5. Bake in preheated oven for about 15 minutes or until golden brown. For shiny tops, brush baked buns with melted butter while still hot.

PER ROLL	
Calories: 220	
Dietary Fiber: 3 g	Carbohydrate: 40 g
Fat: 4 g	Protein: 6 g

These soft and golden fruit buns are tasty and nutritious. Serve warm for breakfast or at tea time.

TIPS

If you use canned yams for this recipe, reserve the liquid. If you cook and mash yams, use the cooking liquid.

Yams are often thought of as sweet potatoes and the two are used interchangeably in North America, although they are actually quite different. Yams are a white starch root and are rather bland in taste. Like sweet potatoes, they can be boiled, baked or fried and are often used in soups and stews. Either can be used in this recipe.

DIETITIAN'S MESSAGE

These rolls are a welcome change from the usual breakfast and brunch fare. The oat bran and yams contribute complex carbohydrates and fiber. To increase the protein and calcium, serve these rolls with fresh fruit and cheese slices.

This nutrition-packed bread can help you to "eat right anytime." It is very easy to make and tastes great served with milk, juice or coffee.

TIP

Wheat germ, the embryo of the wheat berry, is very high in fiber. Use it to replace some of the bread crumbs in recipes such as meat loaf, or when breading meats such as turkey cutlets. Because it contains oils that go rancid quickly, it should be stored in the refrigerator.

DIETITIAN'S MESSAGE

This slightly sweet bread, which is loaded with fiber, can be used as a lower-fat alternative to muffins. Serve with fresh fruit and cheese to get your day off to a good start, or enjoy it with a sharp cheese such as Stilton or old Cheddar for a great-tasting snack.

Super Health Bread

Preheat oven to 350°F (180°C)
9- by 5-inch (2 L) loaf pan, lightly greased

½ cup	boiling water	125 mL
1 cup	raisins	250 mL
1	egg, beaten	1
1 cup	lightly packed brown sugar	250 mL
1 cup	buttermilk	250 mL
1 cup	whole-wheat flour	250 mL
1 cup	rolled oats	250 mL
1 cup	high-fiber bran cereal	250 mL
¼ cup	wheat germ	50 mL
1½ tsp	baking soda	7 mL
½ tsp	salt	2 mL

1. Pour boiling water over raisins; cool. Stir in egg, sugar and buttermilk.

2. In a medium bowl, combine flour, oats, cereal, wheat germ, baking soda and salt. Stir in egg mixture until thoroughly combined. Pour into nonstick or lightly greased 9- by 5-inch (2 L) loaf pan. Bake in preheated oven for about 45 minutes or until tester inserted in center comes out clean. Cool before removing from pan.

PER SLICE (¹/₁₆ LOAF)	
Calories: 151	
Dietary Fiber: 4 g	Carbohydrate: 34 g
Fat: 1 g	Protein: 4 g

Whole-Wheat Pizza Dough

Makes 2 Crusts
....
Melanie Galvin

Preheat oven to 425°F (220°C)
Baking sheets or pizza pans, lightly greased

1¼ cups	all-purpose flour	300 mL
1¼ cups	whole-wheat flour	300 mL
1	pkg (¼ oz/8 g) quick-rise instant yeast	1
1 tsp	granulated sugar	5 mL
½ tsp	salt	2 mL
½ tsp	dried basil	2 mL
½ tsp	dried oregano	2 mL
¼ tsp	garlic powder	1 mL
½ cup	water	125 mL
¼ cup	2% milk	50 mL
3 tbsp	olive oil	45 mL

1. In a bowl, combine flours, yeast, sugar, salt, basil, oregano and garlic powder.

2. In a small saucepan over low heat, heat water, milk and olive oil until hot to the touch (125°F/50°C). Stir into dry ingredients. Knead on floured surface until smooth and elastic. Cover and let rest for 10 minutes.

3. Cut dough in half; roll each half into 12-inch (30 cm) round. Place on nonstick or lightly greased baking sheets or pizza pans. Flute edges to form shells to hold fillings. Cover; let rise in warm place for about 30 minutes.

4. Add desired toppings; bake in preheated oven on bottom rack for about 15 minutes.

PER SLICE (¹⁄₆ SHELL)	
Calories: 122	
Dietary Fiber: 2 g	Carbohydrate: 20 g
Fat: 4 g	Protein: 3 g

Whole-wheat flour and herbs provide a tasty pizza crust to use with your favorite toppings or for Chicken Pizza (page 282). The garlic and herbs may be omitted if a plainer crust is required.

TIP
Making pizza is a great way to get kids involved in the kitchen. Have them help make the dough and use their favorite toppings to make pizza faces.

DIETITIAN'S MESSAGE
This pizza dough is a snap to make and the whole-wheat flour adds fiber to your diet.

Light Meals and Healthy Snacks

The recipes in this chapter are great for light meals and those days when you need a quick bite before dashing out again. If you are trying to instill healthy eating patterns in your children, this chapter is full of ideas. Many of the recipes can be made ahead so that they will be ready for after-school snacks. We've also included some that kids can make for themselves. Use these recipes in conjunction with the dips and spreads in Chapter 3 to ensure that you are eating well even while snacking or on the run.

make grazing count

For many people, eating three square meals a day has given way to a patchwork quilt of light meals and snacks. This "grazing" approach to eating makes it even more important to understand the principles of healthy eating. On the run, it is all too easy to make food choices that are less nutritious.

Eating a small quantity of nutritious food more frequently throughout the day will help to boost your energy levels and keep you productive. Skipping meals or going for long periods without food can lead to poor nutrition. Such habits may also encourage impulse eating or overeating later in the day, which can lead to weight gain.

If you have a "grazing" lifestyle, the meals you eat should still meet your daily requirements of essential nutrients and include the right mix of foods. Make sure your snacks and light meals are comprised of vegetables, fruit, whole grains, milk, cheese or yogurt, meat and alternatives. Combine high-carbohydrate snacks (such as bagels, breads, cereal, fruit and vegetables) with protein-rich foods (such as milk, cheese, yogurt, meat, fish, poultry, eggs, peanut butter, nuts, seeds, beans and lentils) to keep you feeling satisfied longer.

snacking at home or *on the run*

Good snack foods to keep around the house include fruit, vegetables, juice, pita bread, bagels, crackers, bread sticks, yogurt, milk, cheese, muffins, dry cereals, bean dips, hummus, peanut butter, nuts and seeds.

If you are on the run, keep dry cereals, fig bars, whole-grain crackers, cereal bars, dried fruit, nuts or seeds, and individual containers of juice wherever they will be handy.

Often snack foods include low-nutrient, high-calorie choices such as chips, candy and chocolate. While you don't need to eliminate these foods from your diet, you shouldn't let them take over, either.

streamlining nutrition on the go

If, like most people, you are feeling frenzied and looking for ideas on how to get organized as well as what to pack for lunch or make for healthy snacks, here are a few suggestions to get you started.

- Plan lunches on the weekends, as part of your weekly meal planning.
- Make extra servings of dinner dishes such as pasta, soups and stews, which can be heated up quickly in the microwave. Pack leftovers in lunches with a mixture of fresh foods such as muffins and fruit. Also try canned beans, pizza, tortillas or burritos, Lunch Box Chili or Lunch Box Peachy Sweet Potato and Couscous.
- Make sandwiches, salads and dips the night before and chill them in the refrigerator overnight.
- Clean and store fresh fruit and raw vegetables, so they are ready to grab and go. If necessary, cut them up and put them in individual containers.
- If you don't have time to make a meal, fill a cooler bag with fresh fruit, juice, whole-grain bread or crackers, yogurt or cheese.

keep hot foods hot and cold foods cold

If you are packing a lunch, you will need to follow some basic food safety rules. Make an investment in an insulated lunch bag, some small freezer packs and a good Thermos to expand your lunchtime options. Perishable items, such as dairy products, meat and eggs, and sandwich mixes with salad dressing or mayonnaise, need to be kept cold. Transport soups and stews cold and heat them in a microwave when you are ready to eat, or pack them hot in a Thermos.

know thyself

Some people find that eating a series of snacks and smaller meals throughout the day keeps them from feeling hungry and helps them to control their weight. Others find that following this pattern means that they are eating constantly and consuming a larger quantity of food over the course of the day. There's no right or wrong way. Get to know yourself, and do what works best for you.

SERVES 2
••••••••••••••••••••••
Canadian Egg
Marketing Agency

This is an easy meal for older children or teens to prepare for themselves and the family. The ingredients can easily be doubled to serve 4.

TIPS

If you don't have time to make the salsa, use a commercially prepared salsa instead. Use about ½ cup (125 mL) salsa per omelette.

The extra 1 cup (250 mL) Salsa Fresca in this recipe can be used in Hurry-Up Fill-Me-Up Burritos (see recipe, page 63) or as a dip for baked tortilla chips.

VARIATION

Dress up your omelette with chopped ham and green onions, shredded cheese or diced leftover cooked potatoes.

DIETITIAN'S MESSAGE

The Salsa Fresca is rich in vitamins and antioxidants, which work to help the body get rid of cell-damaging free radicals. Serve these omelettes with a Mixed Herb Baguette (see recipe, page 45) or whole-wheat toast. Finish with frozen yogurt and berries for a complete meal.

Individual Salsa Fresca Omelettes

Salsa Fresca

1 cup	diced seeded tomatoes	250 mL
1 cup	diced cucumber	250 mL
⅓ cup	chopped red onions	75 mL
¼ cup	chopped fresh cilantro *or* parsley	50 mL
2 tbsp	lime juice	25 mL
	Salt and black pepper to taste	

Omelettes

4	eggs	4
1 tbsp	water	15 mL
	Salt and black pepper to taste	
1 tsp	butter *or* vegetable oil	5 mL

1. *Salsa Fresca:* In a bowl, combine tomatoes, cucumber, red onions, cilantro, lime juice, salt and pepper. Let stand for 10 minutes. Drain well.

2. *Omelettes:* In a bowl, beat together eggs, water, salt and pepper. In a small (8-inch/20 cm) nonstick skillet over medium-high heat, melt ½ tsp (2 mL) of the butter. Making 1 omelette at a time, pour half of the egg mixture into pan. As eggs begin to set at edges, use a spatula to gently push cooked portions to the center, tilting pan to allow uncooked egg to flow into empty spaces.

3. When eggs are almost set on the surface but still look moist, fill half the omelette with some of the Salsa Fresca. Slip spatula under unfilled side, fold over filling and slide omelette onto plate. Top with additional Salsa Fresca. Repeat with remaining butter, egg mixture and Salsa Fresca.

PER OMELETTE	
Calories: 185	
Dietary Fiber: 1 g	Carbohydrate: 6 g
Fat: 12 g	Protein: 13 g

Overnight Broccoli and Cheese Strata

Preheat oven to 350°F (180°C)
9-inch (2.5 L) casserole, greased

2 cups	chopped fresh broccoli *or* asparagus	500 mL
4 cups	cubed whole-wheat bread (preferably stale)	1 L
2 cups	shredded Swiss *or* Cheddar cheese	500 mL
4	eggs	4
2 cups	milk	500 mL
½ to 1 tsp	dry mustard	2 to 5 mL
	Cayenne pepper to taste (optional)	

1. In a pot of boiling water, cook broccoli just until tender-crisp; drain and pat dry. Set aside.
2. Place bread cubes in casserole dish. Add cheese and broccoli; gently toss together.
3. In a bowl, beat together eggs, milk, mustard and, if using, cayenne; pour evenly over bread mixture. Cover and refrigerate for 2 hours or overnight.
4. Bake in preheated oven for 50 to 60 minutes or until golden brown and just set in center. Let stand for 3 to 4 minutes before serving.

PER SERVING	
Calories: 435	
Dietary Fiber: 4 g	Carbohydrate: 26 g
Fat: 24 g	Protein: 30 g

SERVES 4 **P**
....
Canadian Egg Marketing Agency

This is a wonderful meal to make ahead for a special breakfast or brunch.

TIPS
This recipe is a great way to use up stale bread, which actually works better than fresh in this recipe; it absorbs more of the egg and milk mixture, which makes the strata taste creamier.

Frozen broccoli can easily be used in place of fresh broccoli. Place frozen broccoli in a microwave-safe bowl, cover and microwave on High for 2 minutes. Drain, pat dry and proceed with recipe.

DIETITIAN'S MESSAGE
All food groups are featured in this delicious dish. To boot, the quantities of milk and cheese make it an excellent source of calcium. It is also an excellent source of B vitamins, and vitamins A and C as well as folic acid. When serving this dish, make the remainder of the day's meals lighter, as it is higher in fat.

Brunch Rice Bake

Preheat oven to 350°F (180°C)
6-cup (1.5 L) baking dish, greased

2 cups	lower-fat plain yogurt	500 mL
½ cup	chopped green bell pepper	125 mL
½ cup	diced cooked chicken	125 mL
½ cup	diced cooked ham	125 mL
3 tbsp	ketchup	45 mL
½ tsp	crushed dried oregano	2 mL
¼ tsp	black pepper	1 mL
2 cups	cooked rice	500 mL
1 cup	lower-fat ricotta cheese	250 mL
1 cup	bread crumbs	250 mL
½ cup	grated Parmesan cheese	125 mL
1 tbsp	butter *or* margarine, melted	15 mL

1. In a bowl, combine yogurt, green pepper, chicken, ham, ketchup, oregano and pepper; stir in rice. Spoon half of the mixture into greased 6-cup (1.5 L) baking dish. Spoon ricotta cheese evenly over top. Top with remaining rice mixture.

2. Combine bread crumbs, cheese and butter; sprinkle over casserole. Bake in preheated oven for 25 to 30 minutes or until bubbling and golden brown.

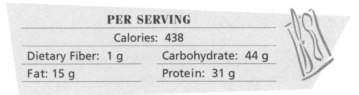

PER SERVING	
Calories: 438	
Dietary Fiber: 1 g	Carbohydrate: 44 g
Fat: 15 g	Protein: 31 g

Farmer's Omelette

Preheat broiler
9-inch (23 cm) ovenproof skillet

1 tbsp	vegetable oil	15 mL
1	medium onion, chopped	1
1	clove garlic, minced	1
½ cup	each chopped red and green bell pepper	125 mL
1	medium potato, peeled, cooked and diced	1
1	medium tomato, seeded and chopped	1
6	eggs	6
⅓ cup	skim milk	75 mL
½ tsp	crushed dried oregano	2 mL
½ tsp	salt	2 mL
¼ tsp	white pepper	1 mL
Pinch	crushed red pepper flakes	Pinch
1 cup	shredded part-skim mozzarella cheese	250 mL

1. In a 9-inch (23 cm) ovenproof skillet, heat oil over medium-high heat; sauté onion, garlic and red and green peppers for 3 to 5 minutes or until softened. Stir in potato and tomato.

2. Whisk together eggs, milk, oregano, salt, pepper and red pepper flakes; pour into skillet and cook until bottom is set. Lift with spatula to allow uncooked portion to flow underneath; cook until almost set. Sprinkle with cheese. Broil until cheese melts, 2 to 3 minutes. To serve, cut into 4 wedges.

PER SERVING

Calories: 285

Dietary Fiber: 2 g	Carbohydrate: 16 g
Fat: 16 g	Protein: 19 g

SERVES 4

Tyrone Miller, Chef
Karen Jackson, Dietitian

P

Fresh herbs and vegetables enhance the flavor and eye appeal of this omelette, which is partially cooked, then sprinkled with cheese and browned under the broiler.

TIP
To tell if an egg is fresh, place it (in its shell) in a bowl of tap water. If the egg is fresh, it will lie flat on the bottom. If not, it will rise to the surface and bob.

DIETITIAN'S MESSAGE

Although eggs contain cholesterol, they are part of a healthy diet. By omitting eggs from your meal planning, you are missing out on an important source of nutrients such as protein, iron, zinc and B vitamins.

This dish makes a delicious quick meal or snack. If you don't have any pita bread on hand, serve it with whole-grain toast.

TIP

Chopped fresh spinach can easily be substituted for the Swiss chard. Experiment with other greens, too, such as collard greens, kale, mustard greens, dandelion greens and rapini; they are all great substitutes for the chard in this recipe.

DIETITIAN'S MESSAGE

While this dish is already a good source of fiber, you can increase the fiber by using whole-wheat pita bread instead of white pita bread.

Swiss Chard Frittata in a Pita

4	eggs	4
1 tbsp	water	15 mL
1 tsp	olive oil	5 mL
¼ cup	chopped onion	50 mL
½ tsp	minced garlic	2 mL
2 cups	packed chopped Swiss chard	500 mL
2 tbsp	chopped fresh basil (*or* ½ tsp/2 mL dried)	25 mL
¼ cup	grated Parmesan cheese	50 mL
2	small (6-inch/15 cm) pita breads	2

1. In a small bowl, whisk together eggs and water. Set aside.

2. In a small (8-inch/20 cm) nonstick skillet, heat oil over medium-high heat. Add onion and garlic; cook for 1 to 2 minutes. Stir in chard and basil (it will cook down; if necessary, add it in 2 batches); cook for 3 to 4 minutes or until chard is wilted. Remove from pan; set aside.

3. Wipe skillet and place over medium heat. Add half of the chard mixture and half of the egg mixture. Cook for 3 to 5 minutes or until browned on the bottom but still not completely set on top; sprinkle with half of the cheese. Flip frittata over; cook for 1 to 2 minutes or until browned and completely set. Remove from pan and cut in half. Repeat with remaining ingredients to make second frittata.

4. Cut pitas in half; place frittata halves inside each half.

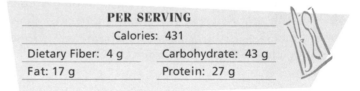

PER SERVING	
Calories: 431	
Dietary Fiber: 4 g	Carbohydrate: 43 g
Fat: 17 g	Protein: 27 g

Zucchini Frittata

SERVES 6
....
Ruth Borthwick

P

Preheat broiler
Ovenproof skillet

2 cups	sliced zucchini	500 mL
1	small onion, minced	1
1 tbsp	butter *or* margarine	15 mL
1½ tsp	olive oil	7 mL
6	eggs, beaten	6
1 tbsp	chopped fresh parsley	15 mL
1 tsp	ground fennel (see Tip, at right)	5 mL
½ tsp	ground dried rosemary	2 mL
½ tsp	salt	2 mL
¼ tsp	freshly ground black pepper	1 mL
2 tbsp	shredded Cheddar cheese	25 mL

1. In a large ovenproof skillet over medium-high heat, cook zucchini and onion in butter and olive oil for about 5 minutes or until tender.

2. In another bowl, combine eggs, parsley, fennel, rosemary, salt and pepper; pour over vegetables. Cook over medium heat, without stirring, until bottom of mixture has set but top is still soft. Sprinkle cheese on top. Place under preheated broiler for about 3 minutes or until cheese is melted and top is brown.

PER SERVING	
Calories: 126	
Dietary Fiber: 1 g	Carbohydrate: 3 g
Fat: 9 g	Protein: 7 g

Zucchini is a sweet summer squash, North American in origin, that has been warmly embraced in Italian cooking. Make this Italian-style omelette when zucchini is in season or vary the recipe using other vegetables — mushrooms, red or green bell peppers and broccoli would also work well.

TIPS

If the handle of your skillet is not ovenproof, wrap it in aluminum foil for protection.

If you don't have ground fennel in your cupboard, use a generous teaspoon (5 mL) of fennel seeds in this recipe. Toast them over medium heat in a dry pan until they release their aroma, then crush finely before adding to the eggs. The flavor will be even better than if you had used the ground spice.

DIETITIAN'S MESSAGE

This meatless light meal is best served with lower-fat accompaniments. A side salad or Italian Broiled Tomatoes (see recipe, page 349), crusty bread and a fruit dessert will complete the meal.

P

Bev Callaghan, Dietitian

Older children and teens can make these tasty treats easily in a toaster oven. The tuna mixture also makes a great filling for sandwiches, wraps and pita bread, as well as a great topping for salad greens or spinach. If desired, substitute salmon for the tuna.

VARIATIONS

Hot Tuna Salad Wrap: Fill flour tortillas with tuna mixture and shredded cheese. Fold up and microwave on High for 30 to 45 seconds or until cheese is melted.

Cold Tuna Salad Wrap: Add any shredded or grated vegetable, such as purple cabbage, carrots, zucchini, arugula, mustard greens, kale or spinach, to the tuna mixture. Roll in a tortilla and serve.

DIETITIAN'S MESSAGE

One way to cut back on fat in tuna or egg salad is to use yogurt or yogurt cheese (see recipe, page 154) as a substitute for some of the mayonnaise.

Tuna Salad Melt

Preheat broiler
Large baking sheet

2	cans (6 oz/170 g) water-packed tuna, drained	2
¼ cup	finely chopped celery	50 mL
¼ cup	finely chopped sweet pickle *or* sweet relish	50 mL
¼ cup	finely chopped red *or* green bell pepper (optional)	50 mL
¼ cup	light mayonnaise	50 mL
2 tbsp	lower-fat plain yogurt	25 mL
1 tbsp	lemon juice *or* pickle juice	15 mL
1	French stick (baguette)	1
½ cup	shredded Cheddar cheese	125 mL

1. In a bowl, stir together tuna, celery, pickle, red pepper, if using, mayonnaise, yogurt and lemon juice. Blend well.

2. Slice French stick in half lengthwise. Cut each half into 4 equal portions, making 8 pieces; place on baking sheet. Toast under preheated broiler for 1 to 2 minutes or until golden.

3. Remove from broiler; spread tuna mixture evenly over each piece. Sprinkle with cheese. Broil for 2 to 3 minutes or until cheese is melted and golden.

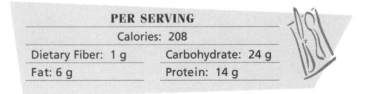

PER SERVING	
Calories: 208	
Dietary Fiber: 1 g	Carbohydrate: 24 g
Fat: 6 g	Protein: 14 g

Salmon Oasis

Preheat broiler
Baking sheet, ungreased

4	whole-wheat English muffins	4
1	can (7½ oz/213 g) salmon, drained	1
¼ cup	light mayonnaise	50 mL
2 tbsp	finely chopped green onion	25 mL
2 tsp	lemon juice	10 mL
½ tsp	curry powder	2 mL
¼ tsp	black pepper	1 mL
8	green bell pepper strips	8
¾ cup	shredded part-skim mozzarella cheese	175 mL
	Paprika to taste	

1. Split muffins in half and toast.
2. Combine salmon, mayonnaise, onion, lemon juice, curry powder and pepper. Spread on muffin halves; top with green pepper and cheese. Sprinkle with paprika. Place on ungreased baking sheet. Broil for about 3 minutes or just until cheese melts.

PER ½ MUFFIN	
Calories: 154	
Dietary Fiber: 2 g	Carbohydrate: 13 g
Fat: 6 g	Protein: 11 g

SERVES 4 **P**
•••••••••••••••••••
Ellen Craig

This tasty combination of English muffins and salmon with a hint of zest makes a satisfying and delicious lunch.

TIP
For a change, try making this with Dilly Bread (see recipe, page 46) instead of the English muffins.

DIETITIAN'S MESSAGE
Team this with Root Vegetable Soup (see recipe, page 114), a glass of skim milk and some fruit for a lunch that will go a long way toward meeting the daily requirement of many vitamins and minerals.

**Murray Henderson, Chef
Carole Doucet Love,
Dietitian**

*Here's a terrific lunch
pizza that uses whole-
wheat pita bread for
the base and emphasizes
vegetables in the topping.*

TIP
Freeze any leftover Lentil
Spaghetti Sauce (see
recipe, page 181) to
have on hand to make a
version of this tasty pizza
with added fiber.

DIETITIAN'S MESSAGE
Soft crumbled goat
cheese, which is called
for in the recipe, is
unripened. It is lower in
sodium than the ripe or
solid versions.

Gathers Lighter Pizza

Preheat oven to 350°F (180°C)
Large baking sheet

½ cup	tomato sauce	125 mL
½ tsp	each crushed dried basil and oregano	2 mL
Pinch	garlic powder	Pinch
4	8-inch (20 cm) whole-wheat pita breads	4
½ cup	soft crumbled goat cheese	125 mL
½ cup	shredded part-skim mozzarella cheese	125 mL
8	medium mushrooms, thinly sliced	8
½ cup	each diced red and green bell pepper	125 mL
4	thin slices onion, separated into rings	4

1. Whisk tomato sauce with basil, oregano and garlic powder. Place pitas on large baking sheet; spread sauce evenly over each.

2. Combine goat and mozzarella cheeses; sprinkle half of the mixture over sauce. Divide mushrooms, red and green peppers and onion rings among pitas; top with remaining cheese. Bake in preheated oven for 5 to 6 minutes or until cheese melts.

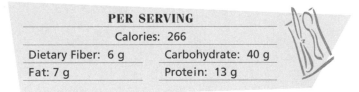

PER SERVING	
Calories: 266	
Dietary Fiber: 6 g	Carbohydrate: 40 g
Fat: 7 g	Protein: 13 g

Cottage Cheese–Filled Crêpes

Makes 8
....
Teresa Feduszczak

Preheat oven to 300°F (150°C)
8-inch (20 cm) nonstick pan

½ cup	all-purpose flour	125 mL
1 tbsp	granulated sugar	15 mL
½ tsp	salt	2 mL
2	eggs	2
⅔ cup	2% milk	150 mL
Filling		
1 cup	creamed lower-fat cottage cheese, drained, *or* pressed cottage cheese	250 mL
1	egg, lightly beaten	1
2 tbsp	granulated sugar	25 mL
¼ tsp	vanilla	1 mL
½ tsp	grated lemon zest	2 mL
1 tbsp	butter *or* margarine	15 mL

1. In a bowl, combine flour, sugar and salt. Beat eggs until light and fluffy. Add milk; mix well. Add dry ingredients to egg mixture; beat with rotary or hand mixer until smooth. Let mixture rest for 30 to 60 minutes.

2. Heat a nonstick 8-inch (20 cm) crêpe or omelette pan. Pour about ¼ cup (50 mL) batter into pan. When bottom looks done, loosen and flip. (This is a test crêpe.) When pan is ready, pour ¼ cup (50 mL) batter into pan; swirl until bottom is coated. Cook until crêpe is brown, then flip out of pan, cooking only 1 side. Repeat with remaining batter.

3. *Filling:* In a medium bowl, combine cottage cheese, egg, sugar, vanilla and lemon zest. Spread filling evenly over uncooked side of each crêpe. Roll up crêpes; place seam side down in nonstick or lightly greased ovenproof baking dish. Dot each crêpe with butter. Cover and bake in preheated oven for about 20 minutes.

These crêpes are similar to cheese blintzes. Serve for brunch or lunch with fresh fruit and yogurt, or as a dessert. Substitute dry-curd or pressed cottage cheese for a drier filling.

TIP
For a delicious change, serve these crêpes topped with a dollop of Raspberry Coulis (see recipe, page 401).

DIETITIAN'S MESSAGE
These crêpes are rich in protein and lower in fat and calories than the traditional version. For extra fiber, vitamins and minerals, serve with Mandarin Orange Salad with Almonds (see recipe, page 143). Finish the meal with Fruit Squares (see recipe, page 431).

PER CRÊPE	
Calories: 121	
Dietary Fiber: Trace	Carbohydrate: 13 g
Fat: 4 g	Protein: 7 g

Bev Callaghan, Dietitian
Lynn Roblin, Dietitian

Tired of the same old sandwiches? This tasty meal to go makes a delicious change of pace for the lunch box crowd.

TIP

The idea here is to pack up the ingredients you need for this meal the night before and, if you have access to a microwave, cook the meal at work or at school.

VARIATION

For a change, substitute curry powder for the ginger and cinnamon. Add some leftover cooked pork strips, if desired.

DIETITIAN'S MESSAGE

This colorful light meal is a great way to add vitamin A and antioxidants, and to ensure that your meals on the go are nutritious and contribute to healthy eating. Add some yogurt or a carton of milk for a third food group.

Lunch Box Peachy Sweet Potato and Couscous

3-cup (750 mL) microwave-safe plastic container

1	small sweet potato (about 6 oz/175 g)	1
¼ cup	couscous (uncooked)	50 mL
2 tbsp	raisins	25 mL
1 tsp	chicken *or* vegetable bouillon powder	5 mL
¼ tsp	ground ginger	1 mL
⅛ tsp	ground cinnamon (optional)	0.5 mL
1	can (5 oz/142 g) diced peaches, with juice	1
¼ cup	water	50 mL

1. Microwave sweet potato on High for 2 to 2½ minutes or until just cooked. Let cool; peel and dice into 1-inch (2.5 cm) pieces. Place in microwave-safe plastic container.

2. Add couscous, raisins, chicken bouillon, ginger and, if using, cinnamon. Refrigerate for up to 1 day.

3. When you are ready to cook, stir in peaches and water. Microwave, loosely covered, on High for 3 minutes. Stir, cover and let stand for 2 to 3 minutes. Fluff with a fork.

PER SERVING	
Calories: 440	
Dietary Fiber: 8 g	Carbohydrate: 101 g
Fat: 1 g	Protein: 10 g

Lunch Box Chili

3-cup (750 mL) microwave-safe plastic container

1 cup	cooked rice	250 mL
3/4 cup	canned kidney beans, drained and rinsed	175 mL
1/2 cup	frozen corn kernels	125 mL
1	medium tomato, chopped	1
1/4 cup	diced green bell pepper	50 mL
2 tbsp	finely chopped onion	25 mL
1/4 tsp	chili powder	1 mL

1. In a microwave-safe container, stir ingredients until combined.
2. Microwave on High, loosely covered, for 2 to 3 minutes or until hot. Stir before serving.

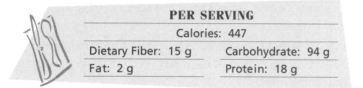

PER SERVING	
Calories: 447	
Dietary Fiber: 15 g	Carbohydrate: 94 g
Fat: 2 g	Protein: 18 g

SERVES 1

Bev Callaghan, Dietitian
Lynn Roblin, Dietitian

Here's a quick, portable lunch that is guaranteed to perk up your taste buds!

TIP
Pack up the ingredients you need for this chili the night before and, if you have access to a microwave, cook the meal at work or school. Be sure to pack this dish in an insulated lunch bag with a small ice pack.

DIETITIAN'S MESSAGE
This great-tasting lunch is perfect when you are on the go. It is low in fat and packed with fiber (an incredible 15 g!) and essential nutrients.

Hurry-Up Fill-Me-Up Burritos

1 cup	cooked rice	250 mL
1	can (14 oz/398 mL) kidney beans, drained and rinsed	1
1 cup	corn kernels, canned *or* frozen	250 mL
3/4 cup	prepared salsa	175 mL
10	large (10-inch/25 cm) flour tortillas, warmed	10
1 1/4 cups	shredded Cheddar cheese	300 mL

1. In a nonstick pan over medium heat, cook rice, beans, corn and salsa, stirring, until hot. Divide evenly among tortillas. Sprinkle with cheese and roll up.

PER BURRITO	
Calories: 318	
Dietary Fiber: 5 g	Carbohydrate: 47 g
Fat: 9 g	Protein: 12 g

Makes 10

Susan Blanchard

These fast and easy burritos make popular after-school snacks. Add sour cream, shredded lettuce and extra salsa, if desired.

VARIATION
Substitute black beans or white kidney beans for the red kidney beans.

DIETITIAN'S MESSAGE
Beans and legumes contain protein and fiber as well as iron, zinc, calcium and vitamin B6. Combining grains with legumes is a great way to get necessary protein.

Stuff this chicken mixture into mini pita breads for a tasty appetizer. It also makes a great sandwich filling for pumpernickel bread.

TIP

If you don't have any cooked chicken on hand, pick up a cooked chicken at the grocery store. One cooked deli chicken yields about 3 cups (750 mL) cubed cooked chicken. You can also substitute cooked turkey for the chicken — a great way to use up Christmas or Thanksgiving leftovers.

DIETITIAN'S MESSAGE

Replace one-third of the mayonnaise in this recipe with lower-fat yogurt or sour cream for a different taste. Complete the meal by serving Chilled Melon Soup with Mango (see recipe, page 96) and finish with yogurt to feature all food groups.

Curried Chicken Salad Wraps

3 cups	cubed cooked chicken	750 mL
1 cup	chopped celery	250 mL
1 cup	halved seedless red or green grapes	250 mL
½ cup	toasted slivered almonds (see technique, page 350)	125 mL
1 tbsp	lemon juice	15 mL
¾ tsp	curry powder	4 mL
⅔ cup	light mayonnaise	150 mL
	Salt and black pepper to taste	
10	lettuce leaves	10
10	large (10-inch/25 cm) flour tortillas	10

1. In a large bowl, stir together chicken, celery, grapes, almonds, lemon juice, curry powder, mayonnaise, salt and pepper.

2. Place 1 lettuce leaf on each tortilla. Divide chicken mixture evenly along center of each lettuce leaf. Fold up bottom and roll up tortilla.

PER WRAP	
Calories: 366	
Dietary Fiber: 3 g	Carbohydrate: 38 g
Fat: 15 g	Protein: 19 g

Light Meals and Healthy Snacks

Lunch Box Chili (page 63) ➤
Overleaf: Whole-Wheat
Pancakes with Strawberry
Purée (page 35)

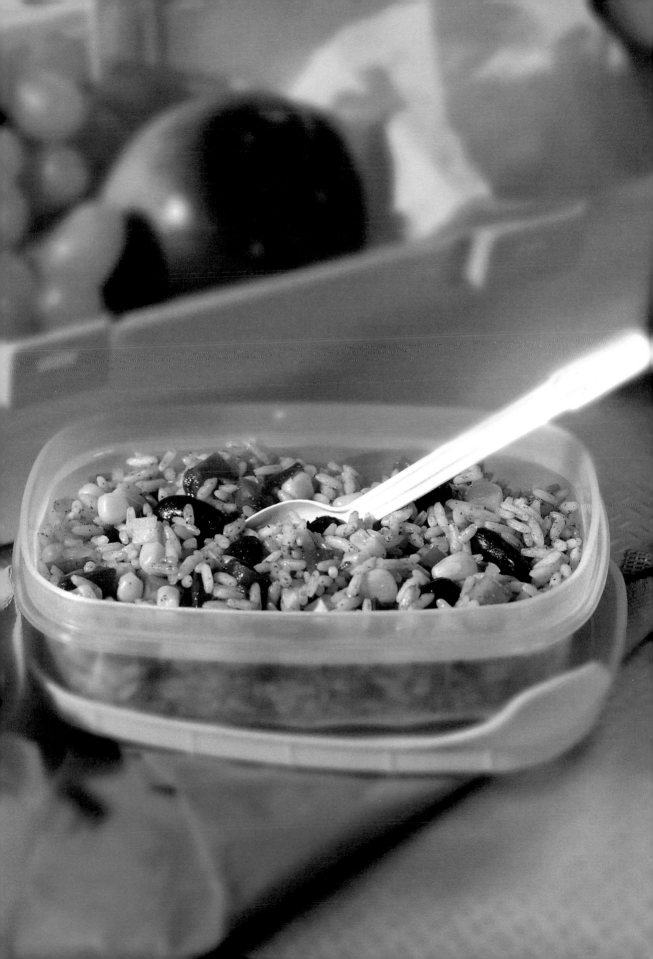

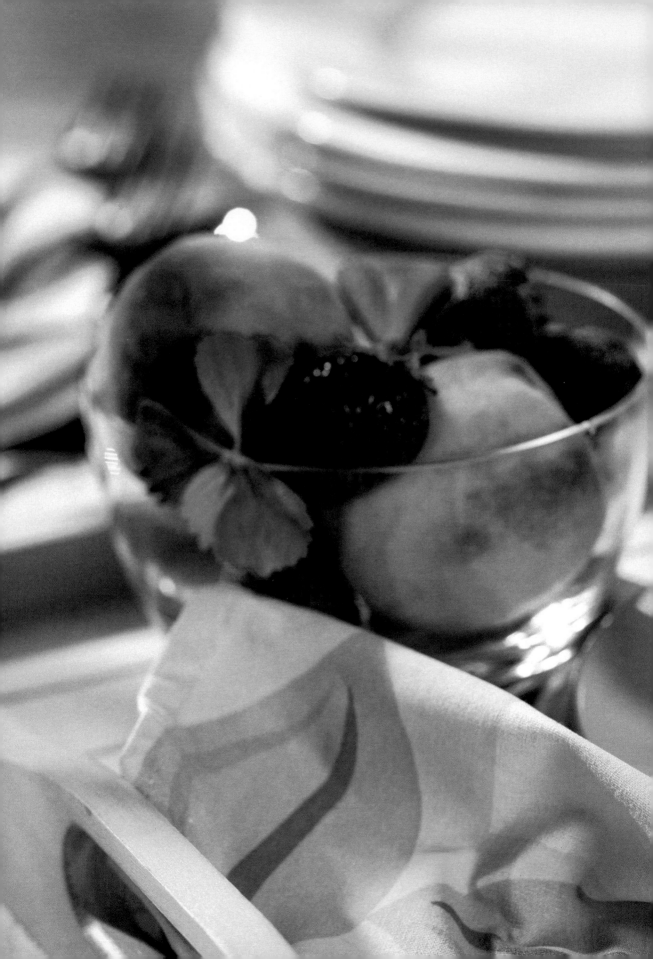

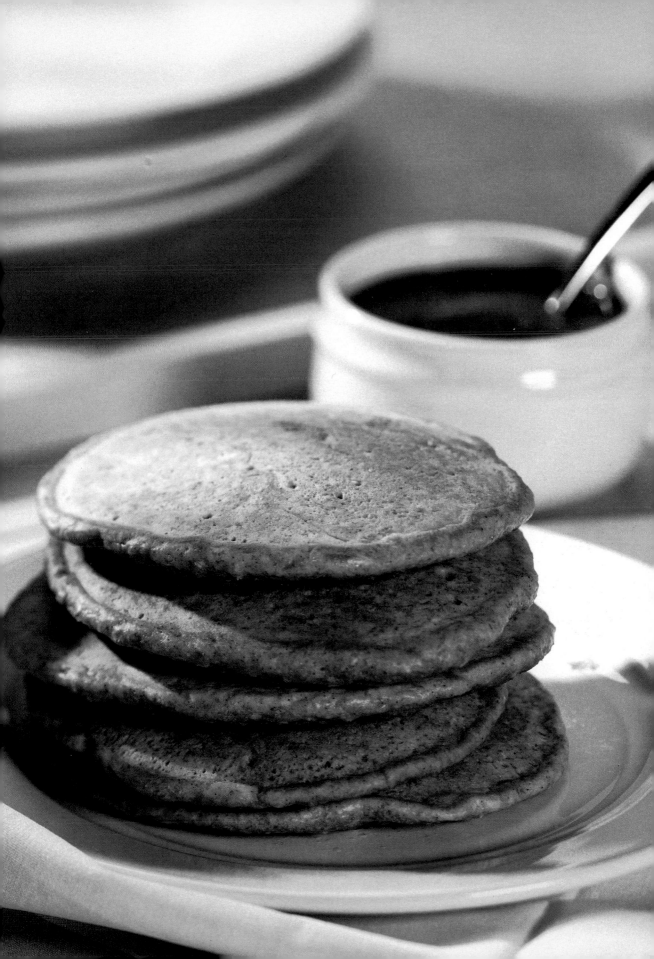

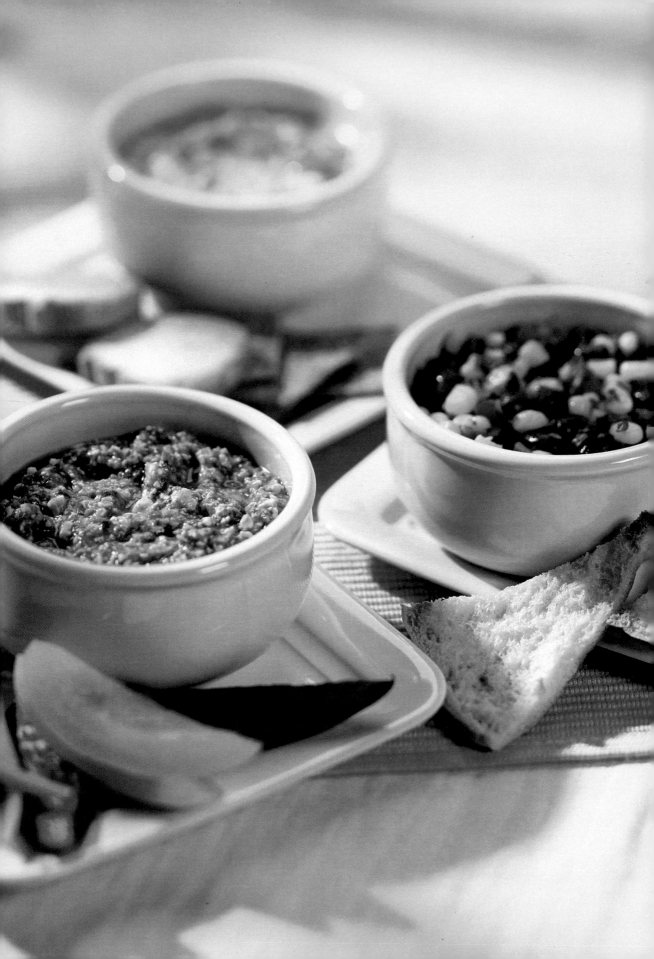

Favorite Chicken Fajitas

Makes 10
....
Cindy Felix

1 lb	boneless skinless chicken breasts, cut into strips	500 g
2 tbsp	balsamic vinegar	25 mL
1 tbsp	soy sauce	15 mL
1 tbsp	Russian-style salad dressing	15 mL
½ tsp	garlic powder	2 mL
½ tsp	crushed red chili peppers (optional)	2 mL
1 tbsp	vegetable oil	15 mL
1 cup	sliced green bell pepper, cut into 2-inch (5 cm) strips	250 mL
1 cup	sliced red bell pepper, cut into 2-inch (5 cm) strips	250 mL
1 cup	zucchini, cut into 2-inch (5 cm) strips	250 mL
1 cup	sliced mushrooms	250 mL
½ cup	sliced onion	125 mL
10	large (10-inch/25 cm) flour tortillas	10

These fajitas are the perfect solution if you are always looking for new ways to work vegetables into your family's diet.

TIP

Serve these with a variety of toppings, including shredded lettuce, diced tomatoes, chopped green onions, grated cheese and sour cream, and let family members assemble their own fajitas.

DIETITIAN'S MESSAGE

Using tortillas as wraps is an easy way to introduce vegetables and grains into your diet. Experiment with grains such as quinoa and couscous, and lower-fat spreads such as Hummus with Tahini (see recipe, page 72) and Fazool (see recipe, page 75).

1. In a medium bowl, stir together chicken, vinegar, soy sauce, salad dressing, garlic powder and, if using, red chili peppers; blend well. Set aside.

2. In a large nonstick skillet, heat oil over medium-high heat. Add green pepper, red pepper, zucchini, mushrooms and onion; cook for 4 to 5 minutes. Add chicken mixture; cook for 5 to 6 minutes or until chicken is no longer pink in the center.

3. Warm tortillas in oven. Divide mixture evenly among tortillas. Add toppings (see Tip, at right) as desired. Roll up tortillas. Serve hot.

PER FAJITA	
Calories: 270	
Dietary Fiber: 2 g	Carbohydrate: 35 g
Fat: 7 g	Protein: 16 g

◄ Lemon Pesto Dip (page 76)
Black Bean Salsa (page 80)
Quick Roasted Red
Pepper Dip (page 81)

Light Meals and Healthy Snacks

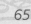

This casserole is a delicious variation on Italian polenta.

TIP

If your cornmeal is "stone-ground," it will have a higher oil content than cornmeal that is processed by more modern methods. So be sure to store it in an airtight bag in the refrigerator (for up to 3 months) or in the freezer (for as long as 6 months).

DIETITIAN'S MESSAGE

Because sweet onions such as Spanish and Vidalia contain fewer sulfur compounds, they cause your eyes to water less when preparing. Use them for salads and in recipes with a delicate flavor such as this casserole. Serve this economical dish with Stir-Fried Vegetables with Tofu (see recipe, page 341). The combined protein from the cornmeal and tofu will be high quality. Serve with yogurt and fresh berries for a complete meal.

Cornmeal Casserole

Preheat oven to 350°F (180°C)
4-cup (1 L) baking dish, lightly greased

1	small onion, chopped	1
1	stalk celery, chopped	1
1 tbsp	butter *or* margarine	15 mL
½ cup	yellow cornmeal	125 mL
½ tsp	salt	2 mL
½ tsp	granulated sugar	2 mL
Pinch	freshly ground black pepper	Pinch
2 cups	2% milk	500 mL
1	egg, well beaten	1

1. In a skillet over medium heat, cook onion and celery in butter until golden. Stir in cornmeal and mix until coated. Add salt, sugar and pepper.

2. Scald milk; stir into cornmeal mixture. Cook over low heat until thickened; let cool. Stir in beaten egg and mix well. Spoon mixture into a lightly greased 4-cup (1 L) baking dish. Bake, uncovered, in preheated oven for 35 to 40 minutes or until top is browned and casserole is set.

PER SERVING	
Calories: 170	
Dietary Fiber: 1 g	Carbohydrate: 20 g
Fat: 7 g	Protein: 7 g

Light Meals and Healthy Snacks

No-Bake Trail Mix

SERVES 12
Makes 6 cups (1.5 L)

Marilynn Small, Dietitian,
Post Cereals

4 cups	Shreddies-type cereal	1 L
1 tsp	ground cinnamon	5 mL
1½ cups	chopped mixed dried fruit	375 mL
½ cup	whole almonds, toasted	125 mL
1 cup	shredded coconut (optional)	250 mL

1. In a large bowl, combine cereal and cinnamon; mix in remaining ingredients.

PER ½ CUP (125 ML) SERVING	
Calories: 153	
Dietary Fiber: 3 g	Carbohydrate: 28 g
Fat: 4 g	Protein: 3 g

Here's a quick and easy snack to make up and take along for a high-carbohydrate energy boost.

TIP
Prepare this snack as needed and store in an airtight container. Mixture will be less crisp after 1 or 2 days.

DIETITIAN'S MESSAGE
Snacking is part of our lifestyle. Too often we take the easy route, indulging in high-fat snacks, then skimping on meals. Choose snacks wisely. No-Bake Trail Mix is a keeper.

1. *Cinnamon Crisps:* Brush tortillas with water; sprinkle with sugar and cinnamon. Cut into wedges. Place on nonstick baking sheet and bake in preheated oven for 5 minutes or until golden and crisp.

2. *Strawberry Apple Salsa:* In a medium bowl, mash strawberries; add apple, honey and, if using, orange zest. Stir to blend well. Serve with Cinnamon Crisps.

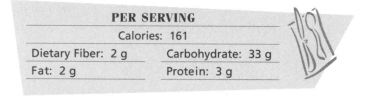

PER SERVING	
Calories: 161	
Dietary Fiber: 2 g	Carbohydrate: 33 g
Fat: 2 g	Protein: 3 g

CRANBERRY CRUNCHERS

The next time you're craving something sweet and crunchy, try one of these crunchers from Susanne Stark of Post Cereals. They're made in under 10 minutes.

In a large microwave-safe bowl, microwave ¼ cup (50 mL) butter on Low for 40 seconds or until melted. Add 1 pkg (8 oz/250 g) marshmallows, tossing to coat well. Microwave on High for 1 to 1½ minutes or until smooth when stirred. Stir in ½ tsp (2 mL) almond extract. Add 6 cups (1.5 L) cranberry almond crunch–type cereal, stirring until coated. Press into a buttered 13- by 9-inch (3 L) baking dish. Let cool. Cut into squares. Makes 24 squares.

Light Meals and Healthy Snacks

Applesauce Snack Cakes

Makes 16   **P**
....
Elaine Durst

Preheat oven to 400°F (200°C)
Two 8-cup muffin tins, greased or paper-lined

½ cup	butter *or* margarine	125 mL
1½ cups	granulated sugar	375 mL
2	eggs	2
1 tsp	vanilla	5 mL
2 cups	all-purpose flour	500 mL
1 tbsp	baking powder	15 mL
1 tsp	baking soda	5 mL
1½ tsp	ground cinnamon	7 mL
1 tsp	ground allspice	5 mL
½ tsp	ground cloves	2 mL
2 cups	unsweetened applesauce	500 mL

1. In a large bowl, cream butter and sugar. Beat in eggs and vanilla until light and fluffy.

2. Sift together flour, baking powder, baking soda and spices. Add to creamed mixture alternately with applesauce, mixing well after each addition.

3. Spoon into prepared muffin cups, filling each about two-thirds full. Bake in preheated oven for about 20 minutes or until firm to the touch.

PER CUPCAKE	
Calories: 200	
Dietary Fiber: 1 g	Carbohydrate: 34 g
Fat: 6 g	Protein: 2 g

These muffin-like cakes are a treat for kids' lunch boxes or for breakfast.

TIP
Make your own applesauce when apples are plentiful and freeze in 2-cup (500 mL) portions.

DIETITIAN'S MESSAGE
For extra fiber, slide a wedge of unpeeled apple into the top of each snack cake before baking.

Appetizers and Dips

If you are ready to serve your family and friends healthy appetizers and dips that taste great, you will find lots of good ideas in this chapter. Hot or cold, from rustic to elegant, whether you are feeding a few people or an entire crowd, you can find a great-tasting recipe that meets your needs. Many of the dips and spreads also do double duty as snacks, so use them to curb hunger after school or work or as part of a nutritious brown bag lunch, as well as in their more traditional role.

Appetizers are the spice of meal planning! Appetizers are an easy way to introduce variety into your diet because they allow you to integrate many different tastes, styles, textures and colors into your meals. They can also add exotic culinary and ethnic influences to your meal planning.

make an **impression**

Most appetizers look as if they require lots of time and effort. In fact, most of the recipes in this chapter are easy to make, and can be whipped up fairly quickly. Moreover, many can be prepared in advance. When ready to serve, transfer from the refrigerator or freezer to a serving dish or pop them into the microwave or oven for a few minutes, if necessary.

Use your creativity to present appetizers with flair. Scoop out large fruits or vegetables to use as serving bowls, or garnish your favorite serving dishes with sprigs of fresh herbs or a swirl of citrus peel to add color and fragrance.

make healthy choices

While appetizers are frequently bite-size, they can still pack a high-fat, high-calorie punch. All too often, appetizers come wrapped in bacon or layers of pastry, are deep-fried, or contain mayonnaise, sour cream or cheese in substantial quantities.

When serving appetizers, keep *Canada's Food Guide to Healthy Eating* in mind and choose appetizers that incorporate vegetables, fruit, grain products, lower-fat dairy products, lean meats, fish and legumes.

Plan for moderation and balance. Make portions small (as appetizers should be!) and limit amounts to about three pieces per person. If the main meal that follows will be heavy, serve lighter, less filling appetizers. Remember, all foods can be enjoyed in moderation, so enjoying higher-fat appetizer choices now and again can be part of healthy eating, too.

great pantry items

Here are a few ingredients to keep on hand so you can make appetizers and dips in a flash:

- Melba toast, mini rice cakes, crisp breads
- frozen tortillas and pita breads
- canned chickpeas, kidney beans, black beans
- jars of flavorful condiments such as salsa, chutney, hot pepper jelly, pesto
- lower-fat yogurt, mayo, sour cream, cream cheese, mozzarella and other cheeses
- smoked salmon, frozen shrimp, tuna
- jars of capers, artichoke hearts, roasted red peppers, tomato paste/sauce
- a variety of dried spices, herbs and garlic

serving appetizers and dips

MORE OFTEN

- Baked, broiled, grilled or steamed choices
- Vegetables or fruits (such as asparagus, melon and dates) wrapped in prosciutto or Black Forest ham
- Veggies and fruits served with dips made with yogurt or lower-fat or fat-free mayonnaise, dressings, sour cream or cream cheese
- Mini pizza wedges made with whole-wheat pita bread and topped with fresh or roasted veggies, part-skim mozzarella or feta cheese and lemon pesto
- Salsa with baked flour tortilla chips; hummus with baked pita chips

LESS OFTEN

- Deep-fried choices such as potato chips, breaded vegetables, egg rolls, wontons, chicken wings
- Bacon-wrapped scallops or liver pieces, pepperoni and other fatty processed meats
- Full-fat mayonnaise, cream cheese and sour cream dips and spreads
- Mini pizzas made with loads of higher-fat processed meats and cheeses
- Nachos with meat, cheese and sour cream; potato chips and chip dip

Brenda Steinmetz

*This version of the Middle
Eastern dip uses yogurt
to replace much of the
traditional olive oil. Serve
hummus as a dip with
vegetable crudités or
pita bread.*

TIP
Tahini, a sesame seed
paste, is widely available
in health food stores. If
you cannot find tahini,
substitute toasted sesame
seeds and process
with chickpeas.

DIETITIAN'S MESSAGE
Chickpeas, also known
as garbanzo beans,
are a great source of
plant protein.

Hummus with Tahini

1	can (19 oz/540 mL) chickpeas, drained	1
2	green onions	2
2 to 4	large cloves garlic	2 to 4
¼ cup	each lemon juice and tahini (see Tip)	50 mL
½ tsp	each ground cumin and salt	2 mL
	Freshly ground black pepper to taste	
½ cup	lower-fat plain yogurt	125 mL
	Chopped onion, tomato, parsley	

1. In a food processor or blender, purée chickpeas, green
onions, garlic, lemon juice, tahini and seasonings until
smooth. Mix in yogurt. Garnish with onion, tomato and
parsley. Chill or serve at room temperature.

PER SERVING (1 TBSP/15 ML)	
Calories: 55	
Dietary Fiber: 2 g	Carbohydrate: 8 g
Fat: 1 g	Protein: 3 g

Rainer Schindler, Chef
Monica Stanton,
Dietitian

*Hummus takes on an
Italian twist with the
addition of Parmesan and
red pimiento.*

TIP
To toast sesame seeds,
spread them on a baking
sheet and place in a
350°F (180°C) oven for
5 to 6 minutes. Watch
closely, as they burn
easily. Serve hummus
with vegetable crudités
or whole-wheat pita to
increase fiber intake and
add vitamins.

Italian-Style Hummus

1	clove garlic	1
½	small onion	½
1	can (19 oz/540 mL) chickpeas, drained and rinsed	1
¼ cup	bottled pimientos, drained	50 mL
3 tbsp	grated Parmesan cheese	45 mL
1 tsp	lightly toasted sesame seeds	5 mL
1 tsp	lemon juice	5 mL
½ tsp	salt	2 mL

1. In a food processor, mince garlic and onion. Add
remaining ingredients and process until blended. Chill.

PER ⅓ CUP (75 ML)	
Calories: 105	
Dietary Fiber: 2 g	Carbohydrate: 16 g
Fat: 2 g	Protein: 6 g

Mediterranean Eggplant Spread

Preheat oven to 375°F (190°C)
Baking sheet, greased

2	medium eggplants	2
2 cups	lower-fat plain yogurt	500 mL
2 tbsp	lemon juice	25 mL
1	clove garlic, minced	1
1 tbsp	red wine vinegar	15 mL
1 tbsp	olive oil	15 mL
½ tsp	crumbled dried oregano	2 mL
½ tsp	salt	2 mL
2	medium tomatoes, seeded and diced	2
½ cup	diced celery	125 mL

1. Cut eggplants in half lengthwise. Place on greased baking sheet, cut side down; cut 2 or 3 slits in skin. Cover with foil; bake in preheated oven for 35 to 45 minutes or until tender. Cool. Remove stalk, peel and seeds; finely chop eggplants.

2. In a bowl, combine eggplants, yogurt, lemon juice, garlic, vinegar, oil, oregano, salt, tomatoes and celery, mixing well. Cover and chill for at least 30 minutes.

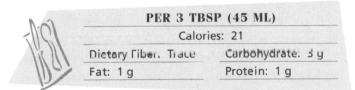

PER 3 TBSP (45 ML)	
Calories: 21	
Dietary Fiber: Trace	Carbohydrate: 3 g
Fat: 1 g	Protein: 1 g

PITA HUMMUS SANDWICH
Stuff hummus into split pitas. If desired, garnish with a choice of raw vegetables such as sliced radish, grated carrot, sliced cucumber, shredded lettuce, red cabbage, alfalfa sprouts and roasted red peppers (see instructions for how to roast peppers, page 127).

Makes 5 cups (1.25 L)

Louis Rodriguez, Chef
Joan Rew, Dietitian

Make this creamy spread when eggplants and tomatoes are in season for maximum flavor and minimum cost. Serve with Melba toast and bread sticks.

TIP
Choose eggplants that feel firm and have a shiny, wrinkle-free skin. The stem should look moist, as if recently cut.

DIETITIAN'S MESSAGE
Experiment using this spread instead of butter or margarine in traditional recipes, or try substituting ¾ cup (175 mL) of the spread for the pickle, yogurt and mayonnaise in Tuna Salad Melt (see recipe, page 58).

Eggplant and Olive Antipasto

Preheat oven to 400°F (200°C)
Baking sheet, greased

1	medium eggplant (*or* 2 Japanese-type eggplants), diced	1
2	medium onions, chopped	2
4	stalks celery, sliced	4
2	small zucchini, sliced	2
3	cloves garlic, sliced	3
1	can (14 oz/398 mL) chickpeas, drained and rinsed	1
1	can (14 oz/398 mL) tomatoes, drained and sliced	1
½ cup	green *or* black pitted olives, halved	125 mL
4	sun-dried tomatoes, softened and sliced (see Tip, at left)	4
3 tbsp	capers, drained	45 mL
2 tbsp	balsamic vinegar	25 mL
2 tbsp	olive oil	25 mL
1 tbsp	granulated sugar	15 mL
¼ tsp	black pepper	1 mL

1. Bake eggplant on greased baking sheet in preheated oven for 10 minutes, turning once. Spoon into bowl.

2. In a steamer, steam onions for 5 minutes. Add celery; steam for 3 minutes. Add zucchini and garlic; remove from heat and let stand, covered, for 2 minutes. Add to eggplant.

3. Add remaining ingredients; toss well. Cover and refrigerate until chilled.

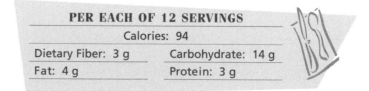

PER EACH OF 12 SERVINGS	
Calories: 94	
Dietary Fiber: 3 g	Carbohydrate: 14 g
Fat: 4 g	Protein: 3 g

LEMON PESTO PASTA
For an Italian-style pasta dish, combine Lemon Pesto Sauce (see right) with grated Parmesan cheese to taste and toss with your favorite pasta.

Fazool

1 cup	white beans	250 mL
1	medium onion, chopped	1
3 tbsp	chopped ginger root	45 mL
¾ tsp	salt	4 mL
3 tbsp	olive oil	45 mL
2 tbsp	balsamic vinegar	25 mL
¼ tsp	hot pepper sauce	1 mL
Pinch	black pepper	Pinch

1. Cover beans with water; let soak overnight. Drain and rinse.
2. In a large saucepan, combine beans, onion, ginger, ½ tsp (2 mL) of the salt and enough water to cover; bring to boil. Reduce heat and simmer, uncovered, until beans are tender, 35 to 40 minutes. Drain well.
3. In a food processor, purée beans with oil, vinegar, hot pepper sauce, remaining salt and pepper. Chill.

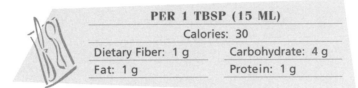

PER 1 TBSP (15 ML)	
Calories: 30	
Dietary Fiber: 1 g	Carbohydrate: 4 g
Fat: 1 g	Protein: 1 g

Makes 2¼ cups (550 mL)

Hans Anderegg, Chef
Cheryl Turnbull-Bruce, Dietitian

This bean spread is great on crackers. Or try it as a substitute for butter or margarine on pita bread or in sandwiches.

TIP
The ginger root, balsamic vinegar and hot pepper sauce in this recipe add loads of flavor without fat.

DIETITIAN'S MESSAGE
Because this tasty spread is lower in fat, it is a healthy alternative to higher-fat spreads.

Lemon Pesto Sauce

1 cup	packed fresh basil leaves (see Tip)	250 mL
1	clove garlic	1
1 tbsp	olive oil	15 mL
1 tbsp	almonds *or* pine nuts	15 mL
4 tsp	lemon juice	20 mL
1 tsp	grated lemon zest	5 mL

1. In a food processor or blender, combine basil, garlic, oil, almonds, lemon juice and zest. Blend until coarsely chopped. Chill or freeze, as desired.

PER 1 TBSP (15 ML)	
Calories: 40	
Dietary Fiber: Trace	Carbohydrate: 2 g
Fat: 4 g	Protein: 1 g

Makes ⅓ cup (75 mL)

Margaret Howard, Dietitian

Keep a supply of this sauce in the freezer as it is used in other recipes in this book.

TIP
When fresh basil is not available, replace with 1 cup (250 mL) fresh parsley leaves and 2 tbsp (25 mL) dried basil.

DIETITIAN'S MESSAGE
Basil contributes to healthy eating because it is a flavor enhancer, which reduces the need for fat and salt.

Makes 1 cup
(250 mL)
....
Margaret Howard,
Dietitian

*Here's an easy-to-make
spread that can be made
with pantry ingredients
and leftover red pepper.
Keep some on hand for
after-school snacks.*

Lemon Pesto Spread

1/3 cup	light mayonnaise	75 mL
1/3 cup	finely chopped red bell pepper	75 mL
3 tbsp	Lemon Pesto Sauce (see recipe, page 75)	45 mL
3 tbsp	grated Parmesan cheese	45 mL
1 1/2 tsp	Dijon mustard	7 mL
	Melba toast, pita bread, crackers	
	Lemon zest	

1. In a bowl, combine mayonnaise, red pepper, Lemon Pesto Sauce, Parmesan cheese and mustard. Serve spread on Melba toast, pita wedges and crackers. Garnish with lemon zest.

PER SERVING (1 TBSP/15 ML)	
Calories: 28	
Dietary Fiber: Trace	Carbohydrate: 1 g
Fat: 3 g	Protein: 1 g

Makes 1 cup
(250 mL)
....
Margaret Howard,
Dietitian

*With a supply of Lemon
Pesto Sauce in the
freezer, you can make
this tasty dip in less than
5 minutes.*

DIETITIAN'S MESSAGE

Served on Melba toast
or crackers or with raw
vegetables, Lemon Pesto
Spread and Lemon Pesto
Dip are lower-fat choices
for an appetizer. They
can make boosting your
vegetable intake easier.

Lemon Pesto Dip

3/4 cup	lower-fat plain yogurt	175 mL
1/4 cup	Lemon Pesto Sauce (see recipe, page 75)	50 mL
	Melba toast, raw vegetables	

1. In a bowl, combine yogurt and Lemon Pesto Sauce. Serve with Melba toast and raw vegetables.

PER SERVING (1 TBSP/15 ML)	
Calories: 17	
Dietary Fiber: 0 g	Carbohydrate: 1 g
Fat: 1 g	Protein: 1 g

Hot Veggies with Garlic Dip

Preheat oven to 400°F (200°C)
Baking sheet, lightly greased

¼ cup	buttermilk	50 mL
2 tbsp	butter *or* margarine, melted	25 mL
2 tbsp	Dijon mustard	25 mL
1 cup	whole-wheat bread crumbs	250 mL
½ cup	grated Parmesan cheese	125 mL
Pinch	freshly ground black pepper	Pinch
1	small eggplant, quartered	1
1	large zucchini	1
1	sweet onion	1
Dip		
1 cup	lower-fat plain yogurt	250 mL
¼ cup	finely chopped green onions	50 mL
1	clove garlic, minced	1
1 tsp	Dijon mustard	5 mL

1. Combine buttermilk, butter and mustard in a shallow bowl.

2. Place bread crumbs, Parmesan cheese and pepper in plastic bag.

3. Cut eggplant and zucchini into ½-inch (1 cm) thick slices. Separate onion into rings. Dip vegetables into liquid, then shake in plastic bag to coat. Arrange vegetables on nonstick or lightly greased baking sheet. Bake in preheated oven for about 6 minutes; turn and bake for 5 minutes or until golden brown.

4. *Dip:* Combine yogurt, onions, garlic and mustard.

PER SERVING	
Calories: 149	
Dietary Fiber: 3 g	Carbohydrate: 19 g
Fat: 6 g	Protein: 7 g

HERBED YOGURT DIP
Use yogurt cheese (see technique, page 154) to whip up a quick dip. In a small bowl and using an electric mixer, blend together ¾ cup (175 mL) yogurt cheese or light sour cream, ¼ cup (50 mL) light mayonnaise, 1 tsp (5 mL) dried basil, ½ tsp (2 mL) minced garlic and ¼ tsp (1 mL) granulated sugar until smooth.

SERVES 8
....
Denise Kilback

Tickle the eye and the appetite with this tasty starter, which can be prepared ahead, then baked at serving time. The hot roasted vegetables and the savory dip are a winning combination.

TIP

Since large eggplants can be bitter, it is a good idea to "sweat" them before using to draw out the bitter juice. Slice, sprinkle with salt and leave in a colander for at least 30 minutes. Rinse well to remove the salt, then pat dry with paper towels.

DIETITIAN'S MESSAGE

Because the vegetables are baked, not fried, this easy-to-prepare appetizer is lower in fat. To complete the meal, serve with Parmesan Herb Baked Fish Fillets (see recipe, page 324), boiled new potatoes and a spinach salad, followed by Peach Cobbler (see recipe, page 403).

Marsha Sharp, Dietitian

This dip will enhance any lazy summer afternoon. For best results, prepare ahead of time and refrigerate.

DIETITIAN'S MESSAGE

Serve this with Creamy Salmon Quiche (see recipe, page 311), raw vegetables, Gib's Gourmet Muffins (see recipe, page 26) and fresh fruit.

To keep the calories low, serve with crudités, such as broccoli, cauliflower, green or red bell peppers, zucchini and carrot sticks.

Cottage Cheese Herb Dip

1 cup	lower-fat cottage cheese	250 mL
½ cup	lower-fat plain yogurt	125 mL
1	green onion, chopped	1
½ tsp	garlic powder	2 mL
½ tsp	celery seed	2 mL
¼ tsp	dry mustard	1 mL
¼ tsp	Worcestershire sauce	1 mL
Pinch	black pepper	Pinch
Dash	hot pepper sauce	Dash

1. In a food processor or blender, cream cottage cheese and yogurt until very smooth. Stir in onion and seasonings. Chill overnight.

PER SERVING (1 TBSP/15 ML)	
Calories: 11	
Dietary Fiber: 0 g	Carbohydrate: 1 g
Fat: 0 g	Protein: 1 g

Grissol

Spread on Melba toast or any dry cracker, this mixture is delicious.

TIP

Try using sodium-reduced soy sauce. Generally, soy sauce labeled "light" has a reduced sodium content, but check the label to be certain.

DIETITIAN'S MESSAGE

Increase fiber by serving this spread with whole-wheat pita bread or with an assortment of fresh vegetables.

Oriental Crab Spread

⅓ cup	light cream cheese	75 mL
1 tbsp	soy sauce	15 mL
1 tsp	granulated sugar	5 mL
Pinch	white pepper	Pinch
1	can (4.2 oz/120 g) crabmeat, drained	1
½ cup	finely chopped water chestnuts	125 mL
⅓ cup	finely chopped red bell pepper	75 mL
1	green onion, thinly sliced	1
2 tbsp	lower-fat plain yogurt	25 mL

1. In a bowl, combine first 4 ingredients. Stir in remaining ingredients. Cover and refrigerate until chilled.

PER SERVING (1 TBSP/15 ML)	
Calories: 15	
Dietary Fiber: 0 g	Carbohydrate: 1 g
Fat: 1 g	Protein: 1 g

Spinach Dip

1	pkg (10 oz/300 g) frozen chopped spinach, thawed and drained	1
½ cup	chopped water chestnuts	125 mL
¼ cup	finely chopped onion	50 mL
¼ cup	chopped red bell pepper	50 mL
1	large clove garlic, mashed	1
1 cup	lower-fat cottage cheese	250 mL
1 cup	lower-fat plain yogurt	250 mL
2 tsp	dried basil	10 mL
¼ tsp	dry mustard	1 mL
¼ tsp	garlic powder	1 mL
	Freshly ground black pepper to taste	
	Round rye or pumpernickel loaf	

1. In a large bowl, combine spinach, water chestnuts, onion, red pepper and garlic. Stir in cottage cheese, yogurt and seasonings. Chill for several hours.

2. To serve, hollow out center of bread. Cut bread into cubes; fill center of bread with dip and surround with bread cubes.

PER SERVING (¼ CUP/50 ML)

Calories: 80	
Dietary Fiber: 1 g	Carbohydrate: 15 g
Fat: 1 g	Protein: 5 g

PITA CRISPS
Cut each of six 5-inch (12.5 cm) pita breads into 12 triangles. Spray triangles lightly with non-aerosol olive oil spray pump or brush lightly with 1 to 2 tsp (5 to 10 mL) olive oil. Bake at 350°F (180°C) for 10 to 15 minutes or until crisp and golden. Cool and store in an airtight container. Makes 72 pita crisps.

SERVES 6
Makes abou
(750 mL)
Alice L

TIPS
For an even more flavorful dip, use 2 tbsp (25 mL) chopped fresh basil instead of the dried basil.

For an attractive presentation, serve party dips in hollowed-out vegetables such as bell peppers or acorn squash halves.

DIETITIAN'S MESSAGE
A fast and easy recipe, this dip has many uses. Stuff leftovers in pita pockets with shredded cheese and lettuce for a fast meal to go or, for a light lunch, serve as an accompaniment to cold meats.

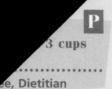

3 cups

·····················

e, Dietitian

TIP

For a fast meal to go, spoon ½ cup (125 mL) salsa into half a pita pocket with shredded cheese and lettuce.

DIETITIAN'S MESSAGE

Eating more meals with beans and corn is one way to increase your intake of fiber and folic acid. Serve this zesty salsa with Pita Crisps (see recipe, page 79) or baked tortilla chips, or as a condiment for any plain grilled or baked meat, fish or chicken.

Black Bean Salsa

1	can (19 oz/540 mL) black beans, drained and rinsed	1
1 cup	drained canned corn kernels	250 mL
1 cup	diced tomatoes	250 mL
1 tbsp	extra-virgin olive oil	15 mL
2 tbsp	lime juice *or* cider vinegar	25 mL
2 tbsp	finely chopped fresh cilantro *or* parsley	25 mL
½ tsp	minced garlic	2 mL
⅛ tsp	black pepper	0.5 mL

1. Combine all ingredients in a medium bowl and gently toss together.

PER ½ CUP (125 ML) SERVING	
Calories: 139	
Dietary Fiber: 5 g	Carbohydrate: 24 g
Fat: 3 g	Protein: 7 g

SERVES 6
Makes about 1½ cups (375 mL)

·····················

Pamela Piotrowski and Shannon Crocker, Dietitians

TIP

Cilantro — also known as fresh coriander or Chinese parsley — has a pungent flavor. Don't confuse it with ground coriander.

DIETITIAN'S MESSAGE

Beans and lentils are protein-rich alternatives to meat. Spread some of this low-fat, high-fiber dip inside a pita pocket and fill with roasted red peppers, grated carrots and shredded lettuce for a delicious and nutritious lunch.

Fiery Verde Dip

1	can (19 oz/540 mL) white kidney *or* cannellini beans, drained and rinsed	1
½ cup	loosely packed fresh cilantro	125 mL
¼ cup	lemon juice *or* lime juice	50 mL
1 tbsp	olive oil	15 mL
1 tsp	minced garlic	5 mL
1 *or* 2	jalapeño peppers, seeded and cut into chunks	1 *or* 2

1. In a food processor or blender, combine beans, cilantro, lemon juice, oil, garlic and peppers; blend until smooth. Chill before serving.

PER ¼ CUP (50 ML) SERVING	
Calories: 98	
Dietary Fiber: 5 g	Carbohydrate: 14 g
Fat: 3 g	Protein: 5 g

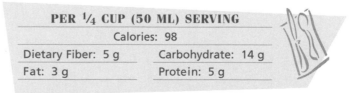

Appetizers and Dips

Honey Mustard Dip

1 cup	yogurt cheese (see technique, page 154) or light sour cream	250 mL
2 tbsp	liquid honey	25 mL
2 tbsp	Dijon mustard	25 mL
3	green onions, chopped	3
1 tbsp	chopped fresh parsley	15 mL
2 tsp	lemon juice	10 mL

1. In a food processor or blender, combine yogurt cheese, honey, mustard, green onions, parsley and lemon juice; blend until smooth. Chill before serving.

PER ¼ CUP (50 ML) SERVING

Calories: 89	
Dietary Fiber: Trace	Carbohydrate: 13 g
Fat: 3 g	Protein: 4 g

SERVES 5
Makes about 1¼ cups (300 mL)
....
Lorraine Fullum-Bouchard, Dietitian

P

Use this for a sandwich spread in place of mustard or mayonnaise. It's also great as a dressing for spinach salad or as a sauce for cold salmon. It will keep for up to 7 days in the refrigerator.

DIETITIAN'S MESSAGE

Serve this dip as part of a lunch box meal. Place in a small leakproof container and pack in an insulated lunch bag with carrot sticks, cucumber slices and a sandwich.

Quick Roasted Red Pepper Dip

3	roasted red bell peppers, skins and seeds removed (see technique, page 127)	3
¾ cup	feta cheese, drained and crumbled (about 6 oz/175 g)	175 mL
½ tsp	minced garlic	2 mL
¼ tsp	hot pepper flakes	1 mL

1. In a food processor or blender, purée peppers, feta cheese, garlic and hot pepper flakes. Chill before serving.

PER ¼ CUP (50 ML) SERVING

Calories: 58	
Dietary Fiber: 1 g	Carbohydrate: 5 g
Fat: 3 g	Protein: 3 g

SERVES 6
Makes 1½ cups (375 mL)
....
Helen Haresign, Dietitian

P

Roasted red peppers are flavorful and offer key nutrients. No wonder they often appear as an ingredient in recipes. You can roast them yourself and freeze them for later use or purchase them already prepared in a jar.

DIETITIAN'S MESSAGE

Red peppers are high in vitamin C, vitamin A and antioxidants. To increase fiber, serve this delicious dip with raw vegetables, whole-wheat pita bread triangles, Pita Crisps (see recipe, page 79) or whole-wheat crackers.

Makes 60
....

Albert Cipryk, Chef
Cynthia Paul, Dietitian

Phyllo dough is available in the freezer section of most supermarkets and makes a delicious wrap for these Greek-style appetizers.

TIPS

Substitute 1 pkg (10 oz/300 g) fresh spinach for frozen and add to onion mixture; stir and cook for 4 to 5 minutes or until wilted. Cool and chop finely.

For best results, defrost phyllo pastry in the refrigerator overnight. This will preserve the quality of the pastry sheets.

DIETITIAN'S MESSAGE

Whether you choose fresh or frozen vegetables, you are essentially getting the same nutrients. In fact, vegetables that have been frozen immediately after harvesting may contain more nutrients than those that must travel to reach you.

Spinach and Goat Cheese in Phyllo

Preheat oven to 425°F (220°C)
Baking sheet

Sauce

¼ cup	lower-fat plain yogurt	50 mL
¼ cup	light sour cream	50 mL
¼ cup	finely diced seeded peeled cucumber	50 mL
1	clove garlic, minced	1

Filling

½ cup	olive oil, divided	125 mL
½ cup	finely chopped onion	125 mL
1	pkg (10 oz/300 g) frozen chopped spinach, thawed and squeezed to remove moisture	1
4 oz	soft crumbled goat cheese	125 g
1 tsp	salt	5 mL
¼ tsp	black pepper	1 mL
¼ tsp	ground nutmeg	1 mL
1 lb	phyllo dough (about 20 sheets)	500 g

1. *Sauce:* In a small bowl, mix yogurt, sour cream, cucumber and garlic. Cover and chill for at least 1 hour before serving.

2. *Filling:* In a small skillet, heat 1 tbsp (15 mL) of the oil; cook onion, stirring, until softened. Remove from heat. Mix in spinach, cheese, salt, pepper and nutmeg until combined.

3. Place 1 sheet of phyllo on work surface, keeping remaining phyllo covered with damp tea towel to prevent drying; brush sheet lightly with some of the oil and top with second sheet; brush with oil.

4. With sharp knife or pizza cutter, cut phyllo lengthwise into 6 equal strips. Place about 1 tsp (5 mL) filling 1 inch (2.5 cm) from bottom end of strip; fold 1 corner to opposite side, forming triangle that covers filling. Continue folding from side to side up entire length of strip. Place seam side down on baking sheet; repeat with remaining phyllo, oil and filling.

5. Brush tops lightly with oil. Cover with plastic wrap and refrigerate for up to 12 hours or freeze in airtight containers.

6. Bake triangles in preheated oven for about 10 minutes or until golden (frozen ones may take a little longer). Serve with sauce.

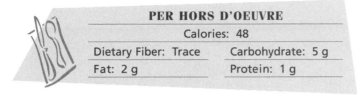

PER HORS D'OEUVRE	
Calories: 48	
Dietary Fiber: Trace	Carbohydrate: 5 g
Fat: 2 g	Protein: 1 g

Eggplant Tapas

Preheat oven to 400°F (200°C)
Baking sheet

1	small eggplant (about ¾ lb/375 g)	1
1	medium green bell pepper	1
1	medium red bell pepper	1
2 tbsp	lemon juice	25 mL
1 tbsp	red wine vinegar	15 mL
1 tsp	olive oil	5 mL
1	clove garlic, minced	1
	Freshly ground black pepper	

1. Place eggplant and peppers on baking sheet. Bake in preheated oven for about 30 minutes or until tender and peppers are charred. (Note: Peppers may be cooked before eggplant.) Remove skin from peppers and eggplant. Cut eggplant into chunks; cut peppers into thin slices.

2. Combine lemon juice, vinegar, oil, garlic, and pepper to taste. Pour over vegetables and stir. Cover and refrigerate for several hours.

PER SERVING	
Calories: 104	
Dietary Fiber: 1 g	Carbohydrate: 4 g
Fat: 1 g	Protein: 0 g

SERVES 6
Makes 2 cups
(500 mL)

Shirley Ann Holmes

Tapas — tasty nibblers served with drinks — originated in Spain, where the practice of meeting friends for appetizers and drinks before dinner is a treasured tradition.

TIP
You can also cook the eggplant and peppers on the barbecue. Roast until charred, then place in a plastic bag to "sweat" before removing skins

DIETITIAN'S MESSAGE

The eggplant and peppers in this tasty appetizer provide an abundance of vitamins, minerals and antioxidants. You can increase the fiber by serving this nibbler with whole-wheat pita bread cut into small wedges or with an assortment of fresh vegetables. Any leftovers can be served as sandwiches, on pita or crusty French bread.

SERVES 6
∙∙∙∙∙∙∙∙∙∙∙∙∙∙∙∙∙∙∙∙∙∙∙∙∙∙∙

**Hans Hartmann, Chef
Donna Antonishak,
Dietitian**

Serve this simple yet elegant appetizer to your most discriminating guests. Not only is it delicious, it is also easy to make.

TIP

One way to clean mushrooms is to brush them with a soft brush to remove any dirt, then wipe gently with a paper towel.

DIETITIAN'S MESSAGE

In this recipe, tofu is a lower-fat alternative to cream cheese. Since tofu is quite bland on its own (it takes on the flavor of ingredients it is combined with), the spinach and walnuts add both taste and fiber to these appetizing treats.

Spinach-Stuffed Mushrooms with Walnuts

*Preheat oven to 375°F (190°C)
13- by 9-inch (3 L) baking dish*

18	jumbo mushrooms	18
2 tbsp	olive oil	25 mL
2 tbsp	lemon juice, divided	25 mL
2 cups	chopped spinach	500 mL
1	small onion, chopped	1
8 oz	tofu	250 g
1	egg	1
1½ tsp	ground cumin	7 mL
¼ tsp	each salt and black pepper	1 mL
18	walnut halves	18

1. Clean mushrooms. Remove stems and chop; set aside. In a skillet over medium heat, heat oil and 1 tbsp (15 mL) of the lemon juice. Add mushroom caps; cover and steam for 2 to 3 minutes, turning once. Drain on paper towels.

2. To pan juices, add chopped mushroom stems, spinach and onion; cook, stirring, for 2 minutes. Drain off excess moisture; cool.

3. In a food processor or blender, purée tofu until smooth. Combine with egg, cumin, salt, pepper, remaining lemon juice and spinach mixture. Spoon into mushroom caps. Place walnut half on top of each. Place in 13- by 9-inch (3 L) baking dish. Bake in preheated oven for 20 to 25 minutes or until heated through. Serve warm.

PER SERVING	
Calories: 147	
Dietary Fiber: 3 g	Carbohydrate: 7 g
Fat: 11 g	Protein: 7 g

Piquant Marinated Vegetables

2 cups	cauliflower florets	500 mL
2 cups	broccoli florets	500 mL
1 cup	fresh button mushrooms	250 mL
½	red bell pepper, cut into strips	½
1 cup	cut-up green beans	250 mL
8	small white pickling onions	8
1	carrot, cut into rounds	1
	Lettuce leaves	
	Cherry tomatoes, chopped fresh parsley	

Marinade

1 cup	red wine vinegar	250 mL
1 tsp	dried oregano	5 mL
1 tsp	dried tarragon	5 mL
½ tsp	granulated sugar	2 mL
½ tsp	salt	2 mL
¼ tsp	freshly ground black pepper	1 mL
¼ cup	olive oil	50 mL

1. In a bowl, combine cauliflower, broccoli, mushrooms, red pepper, green beans, onions and carrot.

2. *Marinade:* In a saucepan, heat vinegar and seasonings; add oil and pour over vegetables. Cool slightly and transfer mixture to a large plastic bag. Refrigerate for 24 hours before serving.

3. Serve in bowl lined with lettuce; garnish with cherry tomatoes and parsley. Provide toothpicks for spearing vegetables.

PER SERVING	
Calories: 53	
Dietary Fiber: 3 g	Carbohydrate: 6 g
Fat: 3 g	Protein: 2 g

SERVES 10   **P**
....
Dietitians of Canada

This intriguing combination of vegetables can be served as a first course salad on leaf lettuce, or as a side salad to a meat entrée as well as an appetizer. Make the entire recipe. It improves with time and keeps very well.

TIP
When purchasing cauliflower or broccoli, take note of the smell. If these vegetables have passed their peak, they will have a strong, unpleasant odor.

DIETITIAN'S MESSAGE
Here's a great way to have a vegetable snack available in the fridge. Cauliflower and broccoli are members of the cruciferous family of vegetables. They contribute antioxidants to our diets, which may help to reduce the incidence of some diseases.

Artichoke Nuggets

*These nuggets freeze
well before they are
baked. Keep a supply in
the freezer and they
will be ready to serve
at a moment's notice.
If frozen, bake for
5 minutes longer than
recipe specifies.*

DIETITIAN'S MESSAGE

When serving an
assortment of appetizers,
keep portions small and
add raw vegetables to
the mix to keep nutrition
high and fat and calories
low. Serve these nuggets
with roasted red peppers
(see technique, page 127)
for extra vitamin C.

Preheat oven to 350°F (180°C)
Baking sheet

1	bottle (6 oz/170 mL) artichoke hearts, drained	1
½ cup	seasoned crouton crumbs (about 1 cup/250 mL croutons)	125 mL
1 tbsp	olive oil	15 mL
1 tbsp	grated Parmesan cheese	15 mL
1	egg, beaten	1
2 tsp	lemon juice	10 mL
1	clove garlic, mashed	1
	Grated Parmesan cheese for coating	

1. In a small bowl, mash artichoke hearts. Stir in crouton crumbs, oil, cheese, egg, lemon juice and garlic. Form into small balls. Roll each ball in additional Parmesan cheese (about ¼ cup/50 mL).

2. Bake on sheet in preheated oven for 10 minutes for small nuggets, 15 minutes for medium.

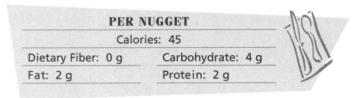

PER NUGGET	
Calories: 45	
Dietary Fiber: 0 g	Carbohydrate: 4 g
Fat: 2 g	Protein: 2 g

Steamed Mussels with Julienne Vegetables

3 lb	fresh mussels	1.5 kg
1 tbsp	olive *or* vegetable oil	15 mL
¼ cup	finely chopped shallots *or* onions	50 mL
¼ cup	julienned red and green bell peppers	50 mL
¼ cup	minced garlic	50 mL
2	medium tomatoes, diced	2
1 cup	beef stock	250 mL
1 cup	dry white wine (optional)	250 mL
Pinch	saffron (optional)	Pinch

1. Wash mussels, cutting off beards and discarding any that are open.

2. In an 8-cup (2 L) saucepan, heat oil over medium heat; cook shallots, red and green peppers, garlic and tomatoes, stirring, for 2 to 3 minutes. Add mussels, stock and, if using, wine and saffron; increase heat to high. Cover and bring to boil; cook for about 5 minutes or until mussels have opened. Discard any that have not opened. Serve in wide soup plates.

PER SERVING	
Calories: 155	
Dietary Fiber: 2 g	Carbohydrate: 12 g
Fat: 6 g	Protein: 14 g

SERVES 4
....

**John Halloran, Chef
Janice Yeaman, Dietitian**

If you enjoy mussels when eating out but have never made them at home, here's your chance to experiment with a fabulous one-pot dish! Serve with crusty French bread to mop up the savory juices.

TIPS
To julienne vegetables, cut them into thin strawlike strips about ⅛ inch (3 mm) thick.

Mussels should be scrubbed and rinsed in several changes of cold water to get rid of the grit. Any beard on the outer shell should be scrubbed off with a hard brush prior to cooking. Discard any with broken shells before you cook. After cooking, toss any that do not open as they are not safe to eat.

DIETITIAN'S MESSAGE
Mussels, served in this tasty sauce, are a good source of protein with little added fat. They make an ideal appetizer for a special meal. For a complete meal, serve with Pasta with Roasted Vegetables and Goat Cheese (see recipe, page 183) and fresh fruit for dessert.

SERVES 8
....
Philippe Guiet, Chef
Dawn Palin, Dietitian

This elegant dish is a unique and memorable starter for a special meal. The pepper coulis and polenta may be prepared ahead, then reheated at serving time.

TIP

Polenta, Italian in origin, is a versatile dish made from cornmeal. Often shredded cheese and fresh herbs are added and its consistency is quite creamy; in this recipe, it is much firmer.

DIETITIAN'S MESSAGE

Follow this substantial appetizer with a lighter main course, such as Warm Thai Chicken Salad (see recipe, page 139).

Scallops with Peppers and Polenta

Preheat oven to 400°F (200°C)
Baking sheet, greased
8- by 4-inch (1.5 L) loaf pan, greased

2	each red and yellow bell peppers	2
12 oz	scallops	375 g
3 tbsp	olive oil	45 mL
¼ cup	chopped fresh dill	50 mL
1	medium onion, chopped	1
1	clove garlic, minced	1
	Salt and black pepper	
8	cherry tomatoes	8
1 tsp	olive oil	5 mL
	Dill sprigs	

Polenta

2 cups	water	500 mL
½ tsp	salt	2 mL
½ cup	cornmeal	125 mL

1. Cut red and yellow peppers in half; remove all stems and seeds. Place cut side down on greased baking sheet. Bake in preheated oven for 30 minutes or until browned. Place in plastic bag and cool for 10 minutes. Remove skins.

2. Marinate scallops in 3 tbsp (45 mL) oil and the dill for 30 minutes.

3. *Polenta:* In a saucepan, bring water and salt to boil; gradually add cornmeal, whisking constantly. Cook over low heat, stirring occasionally, for 15 minutes. Pour into greased 8- by 4-inch (1.5 L) loaf pan. Cool.

4. Reserving scallops, drain oil into small skillet; add onion and garlic and sauté for 5 minutes.

5. In a food processor or blender, purée red peppers. Add half of the onion mixture; blend until smooth. Set aside. Repeat with yellow peppers and remaining onion mixture. Season both mixtures with salt and pepper to taste. Keep warm (or reheat in microwave).

6. Cut tomatoes in half. Place on baking sheet; drizzle with 1 tsp (5 mL) oil. Bake in preheated oven for 10 to 15 minutes or until tender. In a skillet, sauté scallops until golden, 3 to 5 minutes.

7. To serve, cut polenta into 8 servings; place in center of serving plate. Arrange yellow pepper coulis on one side of polenta and red pepper coulis on other side. Place scallops on red pepper coulis and cherry tomatoes on yellow pepper coulis. Garnish with dill sprigs.

PER SERVING	
Calories: 144	
Dietary Fiber: 2 g	Carbohydrate: 14 g
Fat: 6 g	Protein: 9 g

Curried Fish Fillets

SERVES 10 TO 12 P

Maddy Hoogstraten

Preheat oven to 425°F (220°C)
Baking dish

2 lb	fish fillets, cut into pieces	1 kg
1 tsp	each curry powder, ground ginger and salt	5 mL

Marinade

4	onions, sliced	4
¾ cup	raisins	175 mL
1½ cups	water	375 mL
½ cup	vinegar	125 mL
3 tbsp	brown sugar	45 mL
1 tbsp	dry mustard	15 mL
2 tsp	curry powder	10 mL
½ tsp	salt	2 mL
¼ tsp	peppercorns	1 mL
2	bay leaves	2

This recipe stores beautifully — in fact, it is better made several days before serving and keeps well in the refrigerator. Serve cold as a starter on leaf lettuce with cherry tomatoes. Or for a more casual meal, serve in a dish surrounded by crackers and let guests help themselves.

DIETITIAN'S MESSAGE

This delicious and unusual dish is low in fat but rich in protein. Follow it up with a lighter main course that includes vegetables, and complete the meal with Country Apple Berry Crisp (see recipe, page 404). You could also serve this as a light lunch, accompanied by a salad.

1. Sprinkle fish with seasonings. Bake in preheated oven for 10 minutes or until it flakes easily. Transfer to shallow bowl.

2. *Marinade:* In a small saucepan, combine ingredients for marinade. Bring to boil; cook for 3 minutes. Pour over fish; cool slightly. Cover and refrigerate for 3 days; turn daily.

PER SERVING	
Calories: 108	
Dietary Fiber: 1 g	Carbohydrate: 13 g
Fat: 1 g	Protein: 12 g

Shrimp with Dill-Roasted Tomatoes

Preheat oven to 350°F (180°C)
Baking sheet

4	medium plum tomatoes, cored and quartered	4
2 tbsp	olive oil, divided	25 mL
2 tbsp	chopped fresh dill (*or* 1 tsp/5 mL dried)	25 mL
	Salt and black pepper	
12	jumbo tiger shrimp, peeled and deveined (about 8 oz/250 g)	12
2 tbsp	lemon juice	25 mL
⅓ cup	cornmeal	75 mL
4	small green onions, sliced	4
	Grated lemon zest and chopped fresh dill (optional)	

1. In a medium bowl, toss tomatoes with 1 tbsp (15 mL) of the oil, dill, and salt and pepper to taste. Place skin side down on baking sheet. Roast in preheated oven for 10 to 12 minutes or until skins are slightly seared and tomatoes are soft and hot. Set aside and keep warm.

2. Toss shrimp with lemon juice, and salt and pepper to taste; dip into cornmeal to coat. In a medium skillet, heat remaining oil over medium-high heat; cook shrimp for about 1 to 1½ minutes per side or until lightly browned on outside and shrimp are pink.

3. Toss warm tomatoes with green onions. Arrange 4 tomato quarters and 3 shrimp on each of 4 salad plates. Garnish with lemon zest and dill, if using.

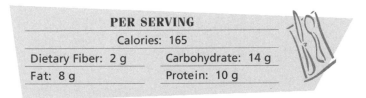

PER SERVING	
Calories: 165	
Dietary Fiber: 2 g	Carbohydrate: 14 g
Fat: 8 g	Protein: 10 g

Vegetarian Pita Pizza

Preheat oven to 400°F (200°C)
Baking sheet

6	whole-wheat pita breads	6
1	can (7½ oz/213 mL) tomato sauce	1
2 tbsp	dried Italian seasoning	25 mL
15	mushrooms, thinly sliced	15
1	green bell pepper, cut into strips	1
1	small onion, coarsely chopped	1
2 cups	shredded mozzarella cheese	500 mL
½ cup	crumbled feta cheese	125 mL
1 tbsp	dried oregano	15 mL

1. Spread pitas evenly with sauce; sprinkle with seasoning.
   Top with vegetables and cheese. Sprinkle with oregano.
   Bake in preheated oven for 10 minutes. Cut into triangles.

PER PITA	
Calories: 312	
Dietary Fiber: 3 g	Carbohydrate: 36 g
Fat: 13 g	Protein: 18 g

SERVES 12

Susie Sziklai

These pizzas can be a tasty appetizer, the focal point for a tasty lunch or a healthy snack.

TIP
Vary the vegetable toppings by using different-colored peppers or other vegetables such as cooked broccoli or spinach.

DIETITIAN'S MESSAGE
These easily prepared pizzas are a nutritious finger food. Add a milk-based chowder, such as Country Vegetable Chowder (see recipe, page 105), a tossed green salad and fresh fruit for a well-balanced, nutritious meal.

Lemon Pesto Pita Pizza

Preheat oven to 450°F (230°C)
Baking Sheet

½ cup	Lemon Pesto Sauce (see recipe, page 75)	125 mL
2 tbsp	grated Parmesan cheese	25 mL
3	whole-wheat pita breads	3
½ cup	chopped red bell pepper	125 mL
1 cup	shredded part-skim mozzarella cheese	250 mL

1. Combine Lemon Pesto Sauce and Parmesan. Spread over
   pitas. Sprinkle with red pepper and mozzarella. Bake in
   preheated oven until cheese melts. Cut into triangles.

PER SERVING	
Calories: 97	
Dietary Fiber: Trace	Carbohydrate: 10 g
Fat: 4 g	Protein: 5 g

SERVES 12

**Margaret Howard,
Dietitian**

Here's another way to use Lemon Pesto Sauce and one more reason for keeping a supply on hand in the freezer.

DIETITIAN'S MESSAGE
Whole-wheat pita breads are a nutritious and versatile convenience food. Use them as a base for pizza or a pouch for sandwich fillings, or cut them into triangles and load them with dips and spreads.

Meatballs are always a popular appetizer, but when fried, they are high in fat. This version lets you use your microwave instead for healthier eating. It's faster, too.

TIP

If you are concerned about sodium intake, try using "low sodium" soy sauce instead of the regular variety.

DIETITIAN'S MESSAGE

Although these pork rolls are substantial for an appetizer, they contribute to healthy eating when balanced with lighter choices for the remainder of the meal. For a healthy dinner, serve these with Pasta with Broccoli Herb Sauce (see recipe, page 190) or Fettuccine with Zucchini and Fresh Tomato Sauce (see recipe, page 185). Finish the meal with fresh fruit for dessert.

Oriental Pork Rolls

Rolls

1 lb	lean ground pork	500 g
1	can (4 oz/113 g) cocktail shrimp, drained	1
½ lb	cooked ham, minced	250 g
½ cup	sliced water chestnuts, finely chopped	125 mL
½ cup	raisins, coarsely chopped	125 mL
4	green onions, chopped	4
2	cloves garlic, crushed	2
2	eggs, lightly beaten	2
2 tbsp	all-purpose flour	25 mL
3 tbsp	soy sauce	45 mL
2 tbsp	chopped fresh cilantro	25 mL
	Cilantro sprigs	

Sauce

½ cup	crushed pineapple, drained	125 mL
½ cup	unsweetened pineapple juice	125 mL
⅓ cup	ketchup	75 mL
¼ cup	vinegar	50 mL
¼ cup	packed brown sugar	50 mL
4 tsp	cornstarch, dissolved in 2 tbsp/25 mL) water	20 mL

1. *Rolls:* Combine ingredients for rolls and shape into 5 rolls 6 inches (15 cm) long and 1 inch (2.5 cm) wide. Wrap in plastic wrap, then in waxed paper.

2. Microwave each roll on High for 5 minutes, rotating after 3 minutes. Allow to cool and cut into 8 slices.

3. *Sauce:* In a saucepan, combine pineapple, juice, ketchup, vinegar and brown sugar. Cook over medium heat for about 5 minutes to dissolve sugar. Add cornstarch mixture and cook, stirring, for 3 minutes or until thickened.

4. To serve, pour sauce onto serving dish; arrange meat slices on top. Garnish with cilantro sprigs.

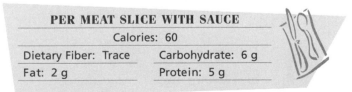

PER MEAT SLICE WITH SAUCE	
Calories: 60	
Dietary Fiber: Trace	Carbohydrate: 6 g
Fat: 2 g	Protein: 5 g

Ham Roulades

1 tbsp	soft margarine	15 mL
1 cup	finely chopped mushrooms	250 mL
¼ cup	chopped green onions	50 mL
4 oz	light cream cheese, softened	125 g
½ cup	chopped fresh parsley	125 mL
2 tsp	Dijon mustard	10 mL
1 tsp	lemon juice	5 mL
Pinch	cayenne pepper	Pinch
6	slices cooked lean ham	6

1. In a skillet, melt margarine over medium heat; cook mushrooms and green onions for 3 to 5 minutes or until tender. Cool.

2. In a bowl, blend together cheese, parsley, mustard, lemon juice and cayenne; stir in mushroom mixture. Spread evenly over ham slices and roll up. Wrap in plastic wrap. Refrigerate for at least 2 hours or until chilled. Cut each roll into 4 pieces. Serve speared with frilled toothpick.

PER HORS D'OEUVRE	
Calories: 29	
Dietary Fiber: Trace	Carbohydrate: 1 g
Fat: 2 g	Protein: 2 g

Makes 24
....
Gerald Philippe, Chef
Debra Reid, Dietitian

These roll-ups are tasty and so easy to make that even young children can assist in their assembly. Kids have a natural affinity for cooking, and your encouragement will boost their self-esteem.

TIP

Try substituting smoked turkey, roast beef or prosciutto for the ham in these tasty nibblers. The filling is also great as a spread for crackers or as a filling for tortillas.

DIETITIAN'S MESSAGE

This easily prepared appetizer can be made ahead of time. Serve these rolls as part of a tray of finger foods, along with roasted red peppers (see technique, page 127) and Artichoke Nuggets (see recipe, page 86).

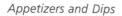

Soups

Along with macaroni and cheese, chocolate chip cookies and Mom's apple pie, soup is one of the original comfort foods. In this chapter, you will find great recipes for soups to suit any occasion or seasonal need: hot soups such as Peppery Potato Soup to warm you up on a cold day, cold soups such as Apple Watercress Vichyssoise to cool you off in the sweltering heat, elegant soups such as Curried Fiddlehead Soup or rustic meal-in-a-bowl soups such as Beef Barley Soup. They are all here, soups to suit any taste and any meal regardless of the occasion or time of year.

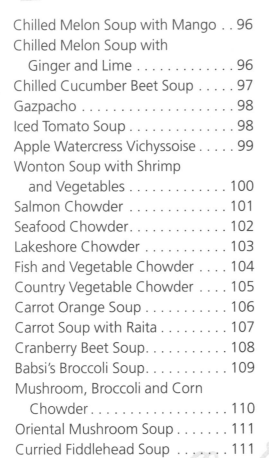

nutrition in a bowl

Soups can make a big difference in your daily nutritional intake and overall health. Many people find it difficult to get the five to 10 daily servings of fruit and vegetables recommended by *Canada's Food Guide to Healthy Eating*. Just ½ cup (125 mL) of vegetable soup counts as one serving from the Vegetables and Fruit group.

Enjoying a great bowl of soup brimming with vegetables and legumes such as peas, lentils or chickpeas will help you to increase your intake of both soluble and insoluble fiber. And soups made with puréed or roasted vegetables — such as squash, pumpkin, carrots, sweet potatoes or red bell peppers — are packed with health-promoting nutrients, not only vitamins and minerals but also phytochemicals (see page 12).

Most soups freeze and reheat well, so they can be made ahead. And soup has the added benefit of being easily transported. When soup is the main component of a meal, be sure to balance it with foods from each of the four food groups.

healthy soup selections

You can make soups from just about anything. Easy and quick, they are a practical way to use up leftover vegetables, meat or poultry. Soups are usually based on beef, chicken, vegetable or fish stock. Some recipes include wine for additional flavor, or dairy products, which add richness and a creamy texture.

Although cream-based soups are delicious, they are higher in calories and fat, so they should be chosen carefully. To maintain the calcium content while reducing the amount of fat, substitute lower-fat milk (1% or 2%), buttermilk or 2% evaporated milk for the cream in any recipe. A creamy texture can be achieved without adding fat by using puréed rice, pasta, legumes or starchy vegetables such as potatoes to thicken soups. Another technique for reducing the fat content of soups is to chill homemade soups thoroughly before serving. Skim off any fat that forms on the surface, then reheat.

You'll always be able to make a quick and delicious soup if you keep your pantry stocked with ingredients such as canned beans and tomatoes, noodles, rice, couscous, dried herbs, and bouillon cubes or canned broth. However, bouillon cubes and canned broths are relatively high in salt. (This is true of canned soup and powdered soup mixes as well.) If you are concerned about salt or sodium intake, check food labels for the presence of sodium or MSG (monosodium glutamate) on the ingredient list. You can also consider making your own homemade stock and freezing it in quantities that are appropriate for your favorite recipes.

These delicious soups are perfect for a hot summer day. They can be the main dish in an elegant lunch or poured into a tall glass for a nutrient-packed cocktail. For an impressive presentation, garnish with edible flower petals.

TIPS
Although these refreshing soups do not freeze well, they will keep for up to 3 days in the refrigerator.

They travel well in a Thermos, so consider them as a centerpiece for a picnic.

Chilled Melon Soup with Mango

2 cups	cubed cantaloupe	500 mL
1 cup	diced mango	250 mL
¾ cup	orange juice	175 mL
½ cup	lower-fat plain yogurt	125 mL
2 tbsp	each lime juice and liquid honey	25 mL
	Chopped fresh mint (optional)	

1. In a food processor or blender, combine fruit; purée until smooth. Add orange juice, yogurt, lime juice and honey. Blend until combined. Chill. Serve sprinkled with mint, if desired.

PER SERVING	
Calories: 131	
Dietary Fiber: 2 g	Carbohydrate: 30 g
Fat: 1 g	Protein: 3 g

TIP
Purée melon in a food processor or blender to make about 4 cups (1 L) when making this recipe.

DIETITIAN'S MESSAGE
Serve either of these soups with Black-Eyed Pea Salad with Cajun Chicken (see recipe, page 136) and crusty bread for a light lunch.

Chilled Melon Soup with Ginger and Lime

2 cups	white wine	500 mL
¼ cup	grated lime zest	50 mL
2 tbsp	each lime juice and liquid honey	25 mL
3 tbsp	grated ginger root	45 mL
1	large honeydew melon, peeled, seeded, cut into chunks and puréed	1

1. In a saucepan, combine wine, lime zest and juice, honey and ginger root; bring to a boil. Reduce heat and simmer, uncovered, until reduced by half. Cool to room temperature. Strain through a fine sieve.

2. Add melon purée to wine mixture. Chill thoroughly.

PER SERVING	
Calories: 97	
Dietary Fiber: 1 g	Carbohydrate: 22 g
Fat: Trace	Protein: 1 g

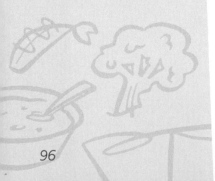

Shrimp with Dill-Roasted ➤
Tomatoes (page 90)

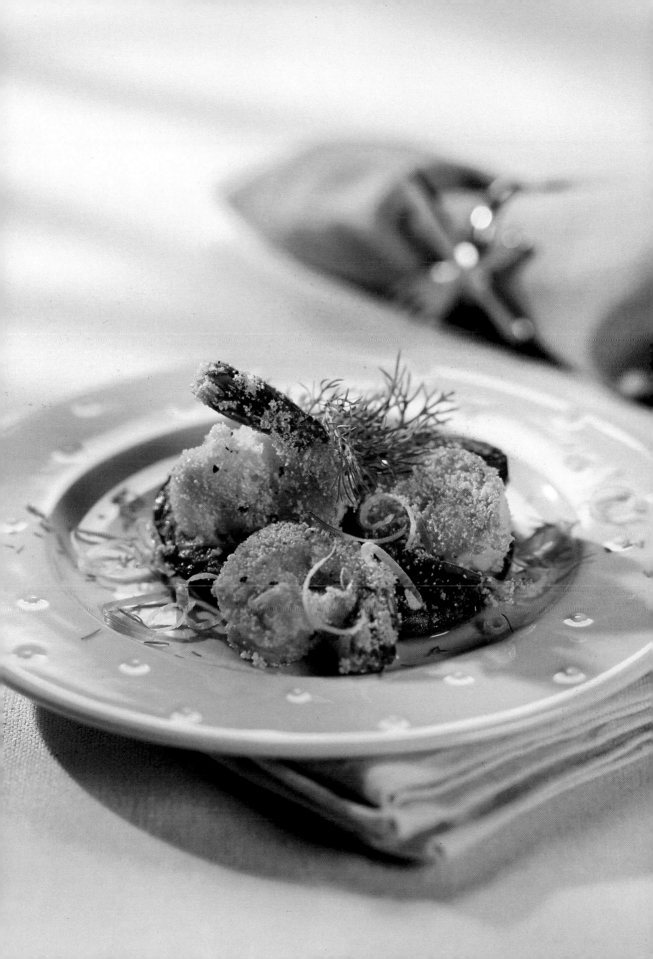

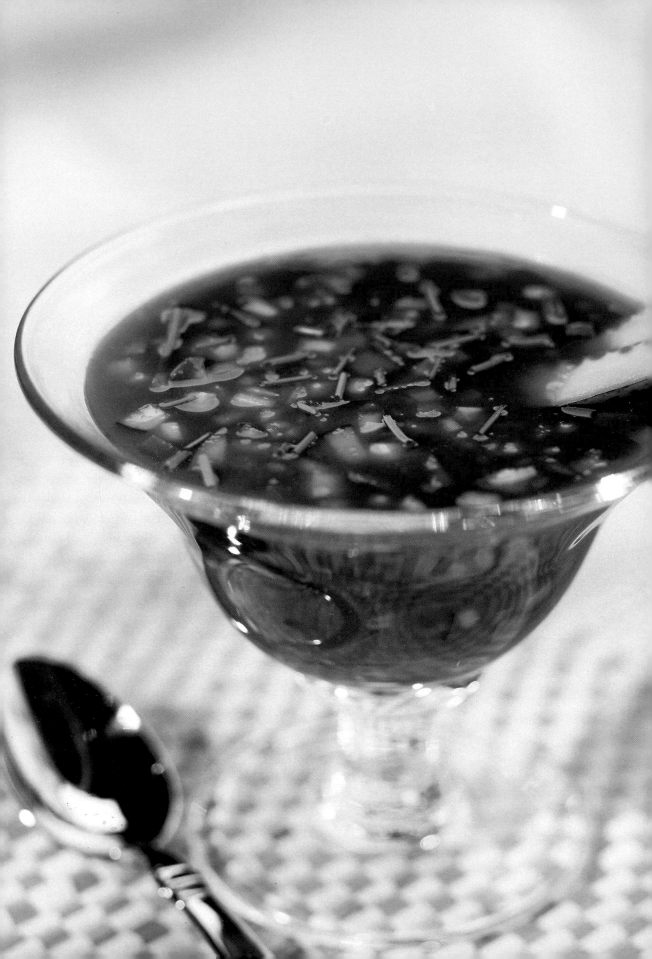

Chilled Cucumber Beet Soup

2	cucumbers	2
1 tsp	salt	5 mL
1 tsp	butter *or* margarine	5 mL
1 tsp	vegetable oil	5 mL
1	large Granny Smith apple, peeled, cored and chopped	1
1	small onion, chopped	1
2½ cups	chicken broth	625 mL
1½ cups	chopped cooked beets (*or* 14-oz/398 mL can, drained)	375 mL
⅓ cup	dry vermouth *or* dry white wine	75 mL
3 tbsp	dry sherry	45 mL
3 cups	shredded Boston lettuce	750 mL
¼ tsp	salt	1 mL
Pinch	white pepper	Pinch
1 cup	light sour cream (*or* ½ cup/125 mL each light sour cream and lower-fat plain yogurt)	250 mL
	Chopped chives	

1. Peel cucumbers and cut in half lengthwise; scoop out seeds. Shred cucumbers and sprinkle with salt; drain in colander for 30 minutes. Squeeze out as much liquid as possible. Set aside.

2. In a large saucepan or Dutch oven, heat butter and oil over medium heat; cook apple and onion, without browning, until softened, about 10 minutes. Add broth, beets, vermouth and sherry; bring to a boil. Add lettuce and cucumbers; cover and simmer for 2 minutes. Cool.

3. In a food processor, purée cold mixture until smooth. Season with salt and pepper. Blend in sour cream. Refrigerate until chilled. Garnish each serving with chopped chives.

PER SERVING	
Calories: 216	
Dietary Fiber: 4 g	Carbohydrate: 25 g
Fat: 6 g	Protein: 10 g

SERVES 4

Bruno Marti, Chef
Laura Cullen, Dietitian

This refreshing soup marries cucumbers and beets for a taste that is delicious and unique.

TIP

If desired, replace the wine or vermouth and sherry in this recipe with chicken stock.

DIETITIAN'S MESSAGE

Using light sour cream does not compromise the taste of this refreshing, colorful soup. Serve this as a prelude to an elegant summer dinner, followed by Grilled Swordfish (see recipe, page 316) and spears of fresh asparagus. Serve Geraldine's Almond Cake (see recipe, page 408) for dessert.

Gazpacho

4 cups	tomato juice	1 L
⅓ cup	red wine vinegar	75 mL
1	each green bell pepper and English cucumber, finely chopped	1
2	medium tomatoes, diced	2
1	small onion, chopped	1
2	cloves garlic, crushed	2
2 tbsp	chopped chives	25 mL
¼ tsp	paprika	1 mL

1. In a large bowl, mix together ingredients. Chill for 3 hours.

PER SERVING	
Calories: 52	
Dietary Fiber: 1 g	Carbohydrate: 12 g
Fat: 0 g	Protein: 2 g

Iced Tomato Soup

1	can (19 oz/540 mL) tomatoes, divided	1
1¼ cups	2% milk	300 mL
1	can (10 oz/284 mL) condensed tomato soup	1
¼ cup	dry vermouth	50 mL
2 tbsp	each chopped green onion and red and green bell pepper, plus additional for garnish	25 mL
1 tbsp	tomato paste	15 mL
1 tbsp	cracked black peppercorns	15 mL
½ tsp	each dried oregano, Italian seasoning and granulated sugar	2 mL

1. In a food processor, combine half of the tomatoes, and the remaining ingredients. Purée until smooth. Add reserved tomatoes and pulse 4 or 5 times. Chill thoroughly. Garnish.

PER SERVING	
Calories: 92	
Dietary Fiber: 1 g	Carbohydrate: 14 g
Fat: 2 g	Protein: 3 g

Soups

Apple Watercress Vichyssoise

2 cups	chicken broth	500 mL
1 cup	unsweetened apple juice	250 mL
2	large potatoes, peeled and chopped	2
2	large leeks (white part only), sliced	2
2	Golden Delicious apples, peeled, cored and chopped	2
¼ tsp	ground cumin	1 mL
½ cup	packed fresh watercress leaves	125 mL
1 cup	2% milk	250 mL
1 cup	light cream *or* 2% milk	250 mL
	Salt and white pepper to taste	
	Watercress sprigs, diced red apple	

1. In a covered saucepan over medium heat, cook chicken broth, apple juice, potatoes, leeks, apples and cumin for about 25 minutes or until all ingredients are soft. Remove from heat; cool slightly.

2. In a blender or food processor, purée potato mixture until smooth. Add watercress leaves and process just until chopped (do not overprocess). Add milk, cream, salt and pepper; mix well. Chill for about 2 hours. Serve garnished with sprigs of watercress and a few apple pieces.

Using Half 2% Milk and Half Cream

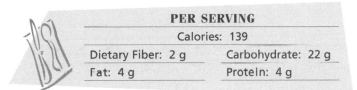

PER SERVING	
Calories: 139	
Dietary Fiber: 2 g	Carbohydrate: 22 g
Fat: 4 g	Protein: 4 g

Using All 2% Milk

PER SERVING	
Calories: 119	
Dietary Fiber: 2 g	Carbohydrate: 22 g
Fat: 2 g	Protein: 4 g

SERVES 8
Makes 6 cups (1.5 L)
Goldie Moraff

Traditional vichyssoise is made with potatoes and leeks and served cold. This version, which adds Golden Delicious apples, apple juice and fresh watercress, is particularly refreshing. Try it hot for a change, garnished with a dollop of Stilton cheese, if desired.

TIPS
Use all milk rather than the combination of milk and cream for lower fat and fewer calories.

Be sure to rinse watercress well as it is often gritty. In this recipe, you can substitute spinach for the watercress, if desired.

DIETITIAN'S MESSAGE
Watercress is a dark green leafy vegetable that contains folic acid and vitamin C. In addition to building bones, calcium, which is contained in milk, contributes to a number of other functions in your body, including nerve functioning and muscle contraction. It also helps with blood clotting.

Alfred Fan, Chef
Leah Hawirko, Dietitian

Here's a Chinese-inspired version of "penicillin in a bowl." The ginger in the wontons adds flavor to this tasty soup.

TIPS

If sodium-reduced soy sauce is unavailable, use regular soy sauce instead and reduce salt when seasoning the soup.

If the soup thickens after standing, add more broth as needed.

DIETITIAN'S MESSAGE

It is the fat rather than the cholesterol content of food that affects blood cholesterol levels the most, so feel free to enjoy this lower-fat soup.

Wonton Soup with Shrimp and Vegetables

½ lb	shrimp, peeled and deveined	250 g
½	can (8 oz/227 mL) sliced water chestnuts, drained	½
1 tbsp	sodium-reduced soy sauce	15 mL
1 to 1½ tsp	grated ginger root	5 to 7 mL
	Salt and black pepper	
42	wonton wrappers	42
5 cups	chicken broth	1.25 L
1 cup	each thinly sliced carrots, leeks and celery	250 mL

1. In a food processor, finely chop shrimp and water chestnuts with soy sauce, ginger root and pinch each of the salt and pepper (or finely chop by hand and mix well).

2. Spoon 1 tsp (5 mL) of the shrimp mixture onto middle of each wonton; bring outer edges of wrapper together over filling and squeeze firmly to form pouch.

3. In an 8-cup (2 L) saucepan, bring chicken broth to boil; add ¼ tsp (1 mL) salt, ⅛ tsp (0.5 mL) pepper, carrots, leeks celery and wontons. Return to boil; cook for 2 minutes. Serve in wide soup bowls.

PER SERVING	
Calories: 242	
Dietary Fiber: 2 g	Carbohydrate: 34 g
Fat: 3 g	Protein: 18 g

Salmon Chowder

1	small onion	1
1	medium potato	1
1	large carrot	1
¼	stalk celery	¼
1	medium green bell pepper, quartered and seeded	1
2 cups	fish *or* chicken broth	500 mL
½ tsp	crumbled dried thyme	2 mL
¼ tsp	crumbled dried basil	1 mL
2 cups	1% milk	500 mL
¼ cup	all-purpose flour	50 mL
4 oz	non-salted hot smoked salmon *or* smoked whitefish	125 g
¾ cup	frozen corn kernels	175 mL
Pinch	salt	Pinch
	Black pepper	

1. Peel and cut onion and potato into ¼-inch (0.5 cm) thick slices. Peel and cut carrot lengthwise into ¼-inch (0.5 cm) thick slices.

2. Place onion, potato, carrot, celery and green pepper on hot barbecue grill or under broiler; cook, turning occasionally, until distinct grill marks are visible and pepper skin is blackened. Place vegetables in plastic bag; seal and let stand for 20 minutes.

3. Peel skins off peppers; dice peppers. Dice remaining roasted vegetables and place in large saucepan. Add 1 cup (250 mL) of the broth, thyme and basil; bring to a boil. Add remaining broth and 1½ cups (375 mL) of the milk; bring just to simmer. Stir flour with remaining milk until smooth; gradually stir into soup. Simmer over low heat for 5 minutes.

4. Remove skin and any bones from fish; cut into ¼-inch (0.5 cm) cubes. Add to soup along with corn; cook for 10 minutes. Season with salt, and pepper to taste. Serve hot.

PER SERVING	
Calories: 169	
Dietary Fiber: 2 g	Carbohydrate: 25 g
Fat: 2 g	Protein: 13 g

SERVES 5

Dean Mitchell, Chef
Suzanne Journault-Hemstock, Dietitian

Impress your guests with this lively smoked salmon chowder, which uses a "hot" smoked salmon that is more strongly flavored. If you can't find "hot" smoked salmon, add crushed chili flakes to taste along with regular smoked salmon. You can also use smoked whitefish or trout.

TIP

"Hot" smoked salmon is smoked at a much higher temperature than cold-smoked salmon. This gives it a fuller, smokier flavor and a firmer texture.

DIETITIAN'S MESSAGE

Roasting the vegetables, rather than softening them in butter or oil, minimizes the fat content. It also concentrates the flavor of the vegetables while retaining their nutritional value. Serve this rich-tasting soup with Fettuccine with Zucchini and Fresh Tomato Sauce (see recipe, page 185) and crusty bread for a delicious lunch.

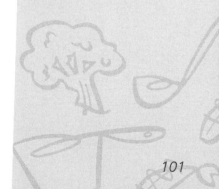

SERVES 8
Makes 8 cups (2 L)
....
Seanna Callaghan

This luscious soup is almost a meal in itself.

TIPS
Substitute any combination of cooked seafood that you prefer for the clams, shrimp and crab. Just make sure that the total amount of seafood is about 3 cups (750 mL).

Although this soup does not freeze well, it can be made up to 2 days ahead, without adding the garnish. Refrigerate until ready to serve.

DIETITIAN'S MESSAGE

Evaporated milk adds a creamy texture and calcium to soups without adding a lot of fat. It can be used in place of cream in many recipes. Serve this chowder with Spicy Bean Salad (see recipe, page 164) and a tossed green salad for a hearty lunch.

Seafood Chowder

2 cups	diced potatoes	500 mL
1 cup	diced carrots	250 mL
½ cup	chopped onions	125 mL
2	cans (each 14 oz/398 mL) 2% evaporated milk	2
1 cup	frozen peas	250 mL
1	can (5 oz/142 g) clams, drained	1
1 cup	chopped cooked shrimp	250 mL
1 cup	chopped cooked crab *or* any type of cooked fish fillets	250 mL
½ tsp	salt	2 mL
	Black pepper	
½ cup	finely chopped green onions *or* chives	125 mL
	Paprika	
1 cup	seasoned croutons	250 mL

1. Place potatoes, carrots and onions in a large saucepan. Add just enough water to cover, about 2 cups (500 mL); bring to a boil. Reduce heat and simmer, uncovered, for 10 to 12 minutes or until tender.

2. Add milk and peas; simmer for 4 to 5 minutes. Add clams, shrimp and crab; simmer for 2 to 3 minutes or until heated through. Season with salt, and pepper to taste.

3. Serve garnished with onions, paprika and croutons.

PER SERVING	
Calories: 225	
Dietary Fiber: 2 g	Carbohydrate: 26 g
Fat: 4 g	Protein: 21 g

Lakeshore Chowder

½ cup	small pasta shells	125 mL
3 cups	boiling water	750 mL
1	large potato, diced	1
1	bay leaf	1
½ tsp	salt	2 mL
¼ tsp	coarsely ground black pepper	1 mL
1	large onion, finely chopped	1
1	stalk celery, finely chopped	1
2 tbsp	butter *or* margarine	25 mL
2 tbsp	all-purpose flour	25 mL
3 cups	2% milk	750 mL
1	can (5 oz/142 mL) baby clams, drained	1
1	can (6.5 oz/184 g) water-packed flaked tuna, drained	1
½ cup	whole kernel corn	125 mL
½ tsp	curry powder	2 mL

1. In a large pot, cook pasta in water for 5 minutes. Add potato, bay leaf, salt and pepper; simmer for about 10 minutes or until potatoes are tender.

2. In a skillet over high heat, cook onion and celery in butter. Add flour; cook, stirring, for about 3 minutes. Stir in milk; cook until thickened and sauce is smooth. Add to potato mixture. Add clams, tuna, corn and curry powder to soup. Reheat to serving temperature; remove bay leaf.

PER SERVING	
Calories: 165	
Dietary Fiber: 1 g	Carbohydrate: 18 g
Fat: 5 g	Protein: 12 g

SERVES 8
Makes 8 cups (2 L)

Kay Miskiw

This easy and nutritious recipe will come in handy for a last-minute supper since it uses foods you are likely to have in your cupboard.

TIP
Omit the curry powder in this recipe if it is not to your taste. Or for a spicier version, substitute (or add) ¼ tsp (1 mL) cayenne pepper.

DIETITIAN'S MESSAGE
Four food groups in one bowl! Serve this comforting chowder with the Healthy Cheese 'n' Herb Bread (see recipe, page 40).

SERVES 6
Makes 6 cups (1.5 L)
••••••••••••••••••••••••••
Elaine Watton

This hearty and flavorful soup is the perfect match for cod, if you are lucky enough to find it. If not, use any firm white fish such as turbot, halibut or haddock.

TIPS

This is a great pantry soup as you can use canned tomatoes and frozen pepper strips, if desired.

Although canned or frozen vegetables usually provide essentially the same nutrients as fresh, canned vegetables may have added salt, making them higher in sodium. If using canned tomatoes, you may need to adjust the seasoning accordingly.

DIETITIAN'S MESSAGE

This soup contains a wonderful assortment of vegetables. Round it out with some whole-wheat bread and Orange Crème Caramel (see recipe, page 423).

Fish and Vegetable Chowder

1	large onion, chopped	1
1	clove garlic, minced	1
2 tbsp	butter *or* margarine	25 mL
1 cup	green bell pepper strips (*or* green and red bell peppers mixed)	250 mL
1 cup	cauliflower florets	250 mL
1 cup	broccoli florets	250 mL
1 cup	chopped tomato	250 mL
½ cup	chopped celery	125 mL
1 tbsp	chopped fresh parsley	15 mL
1 lb	cod fillets, cut into chunks	500 g
2½ cups	hot chicken broth	625 mL
1 tsp	salt	5 mL
¼ tsp	dried thyme	1 mL
¼ tsp	dried basil	1 mL
¼ tsp	freshly ground black pepper	1 mL

1. In a large saucepan over medium heat, cook onion and garlic in butter for 3 minutes. Add pepper strips, cauliflower, broccoli, tomato, celery and parsley; cook for 2 minutes. Add fish; cover and cook for 2 minutes. Add chicken broth and seasonings and simmer for about 5 minutes or until fish flakes with a fork and vegetables are tender-crisp.

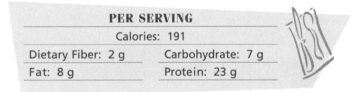

PER SERVING	
Calories: 191	
Dietary Fiber: 2 g	Carbohydrate: 7 g
Fat: 8 g	Protein: 23 g

Country Vegetable Chowder

1 tbsp	margarine	15 mL
1	medium onion, chopped	1
3 cups	vegetable stock *or* water	750 mL
2 cups	cubed peeled potatoes	500 mL
1½ cups	parsnip strips	375 mL
1 cup	turnip strips	250 mL
1 cup	cut-up green beans	250 mL
½ cup	thickly sliced carrots	125 mL
½ tsp	each dried thyme, oregano and salt	2 mL
¼ tsp	white *or* black pepper	1 mL
1	bay leaf	1
2 cups	broccoli florets and sliced peeled stems	500 mL
2 cups	2% milk	500 mL

1. In a 4-quart (4 L) saucepan, melt margarine over medium heat; cook onion, stirring, until softened.

2. Add vegetable stock, potatoes, parsnips, turnips, beans, carrots, thyme, oregano, salt, pepper and bay leaf; bring to a boil. Cover and reduce heat to simmer; cook for 5 to 10 minutes or until vegetables are tender-crisp.

3. Add broccoli; cook until vegetables are tender. Stir in milk; heat until hot but do not boil. Discard bay leaf.

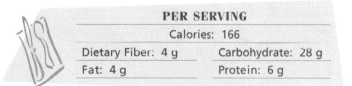

PER SERVING	
Calories: 166	
Dietary Fiber: 4 g	Carbohydrate: 28 g
Fat: 4 g	Protein: 6 g

SERVES 6
....
Yvonne C. Levert, Chef
Nanette Porter-MacDonald, Dietitian

This chowder is lighter than most, but delicious nonetheless. Parsnips and turnips have a long tradition of adding substance and flavor to many dishes. And they taste great alone, whether baked in a gratin, puréed, braised or roasted.

TIP

If desired, substitute green peas for the beans. Add with the broccoli.

DIETITIAN'S MESSAGE

This chowder is an excellent vehicle for adding vegetables to your daily food choices, especially in winter. Served with whole-grain bread, it makes a nutritious lunch that supplies fiber, vitamins and some minerals.

P

Carrot Orange Soup

Oranges and carrots make a delicious flavor combination. Enjoy this soup at home or heat it up and pour it into your Thermos for a healthy hot treat.

TIPS

To make a creamier soup, use evaporated milk instead of regular milk.

A hand-held blender is a convenient tool that allows you to purée the soup right in the saucepan. It also makes cleanup a snap.

DIETITIAN'S MESSAGE

The combination of orange juice and carrots makes this soup a powerhouse of beta-carotene, which is converted into vitamin A in the body.

2 tbsp	butter *or* margarine	25 mL
½ cup	chopped onions	125 mL
4 cups	sliced carrots	1 L
4 cups	chicken stock *or* vegetable stock	1 L
½ cup	orange juice	125 mL
½ tsp	ground nutmeg	2 mL
¼ tsp	white pepper	1 mL
1 cup	milk	250 mL

1. In a large saucepan, heat butter over medium-high heat; add onions and cook for 4 to 5 minutes or until softened. Add carrots and stock; bring to a boil. Reduce heat and simmer for 15 to 20 minutes or until carrots are very soft. Stir in orange juice, nutmeg and pepper.

2. In a food processor or blender, purée carrot mixture in batches until smooth.

3. Return soup to pan; stir in milk. Simmer over very low heat for 2 to 3 minutes or until heated through.

PER SERVING	
Calories: 130	
Dietary Fiber: 2 g	Carbohydrate: 14 g
Fat: 6 g	Protein: 6 g

Carrot Soup with Raita

SERVES 5
....

**James McLean, Chef
Jane Curry, Dietitian**

Raita

1 cup	lower-fat plain yogurt	250 mL
⅔ cup	grated English cucumber	150 mL
¼ cup	minced red onion	50 mL
1 tbsp	lemon juice	15 mL
1 tsp	ground cumin	5 mL

Soup

1 tbsp	olive oil	15 mL
1	medium onion, chopped	1
4 cups	coarsely chopped carrots	1 L
5 cups	vegetable *or* chicken broth	1.25 L
½ tsp	salt	2 mL
¼ tsp	black pepper	1 mL

The sweetness of harvest-fresh carrots permeates this light-tasting soup. The raita suggests exotic India.

TIP

Raita, a sauce made from yogurt and cucumber, is often used as an accompaniment to curry to balance the heat. It is a staple of Indian cuisine. Here, it adds a flavorful and exotic touch to a classically simple soup.

DIETITIAN'S MESSAGE

This colorful soup is rich in vitamin A. For a special meal, serve with Grilled Lamb and Vegetables with Roasted Garlic (see recipe, page 265). End the meal with Apricot Bread Pudding (see recipe, page 424).

1. *Raita:* In a small bowl, mix together yogurt, cucumber, onion, lemon juice and cumin; chill until serving time.

2. *Soup:* In a saucepan, heat oil over medium heat; cook onion, stirring, for 2 to 3 minutes or until softened. Add carrots; cook, stirring, for 1 to 2 minutes. Add broth; bring to a boil. Reduce heat and simmer, uncovered, for 25 to 30 minutes or until carrots are tender.

3. In a blender or food processor, purée soup in batches until smooth. Strain, if desired. Return to saucepan and heat until hot; add salt and pepper. Serve soup in bowls with 2 spoonfuls of raita on top.

PER SERVING	
Calories: 127	
Dietary Fiber: 3 g	Carbohydrate: 18 g
Fat: 5 g	Protein: 5 g

SERVES 5
• • • • • • • • • • • • • • • • • •

Peter Ochitwa, Chef
Susie Langley, Dietitian

You may never have thought of combining beets and cranberries, but the result is a nicely tangy soup with an overlay of fruit.

TIP

For an elegant clear soup, serve without the pulp.

DIETITIAN'S MESSAGE

Cranberries add an unusual and vitamin-rich touch to this soup. Serve this elegant version of borscht with Beef Stroganoff (see recipe, page 250) to continue the Russian theme. Accompany with noodles and steamed green vegetables for color. End the meal with a light dessert such as fresh berries.

Cranberry Beet Soup

3	large beets	3
1½ cups	fresh *or* frozen cranberries	375 mL
⅔ cup	granulated sugar	150 mL
1 tbsp	lemon juice	15 mL
1	cinnamon stick	1
4 tsp	cornstarch	20 mL
2 tbsp	cold water	25 mL
2 tbsp	lower-fat plain yogurt	25 mL

1. Peel beets and shred in a food processor to make about 4 cups (1 L). Finely chop cranberries in food processor; set aside ¼ cup (50 mL) for garnish.

2. In a large saucepan, bring 5 cups (1.25 L) water to boil; remove from heat. Add beets and cranberries; cover and let stand for 20 minutes.

3. Strain into large heatproof bowl, reserving pulp. Return liquid to saucepan. Add sugar, lemon juice and cinnamon stick; bring to a boil. Reduce heat and simmer, uncovered, for 5 minutes.

4. Stir cornstarch with water until smooth; gradually stir into soup until slightly thickened. Return reserved pulp to soup; heat through. Garnish with dollop of yogurt and reserved cranberries.

PER SERVING	
Calories: 139	
Dietary Fiber: 2 g	Carbohydrate: 35 g
Fat: Trace	Protein: 1 g

Babsi's Broccoli Soup

2 cups	chopped broccoli (stems and florets)	500 mL
2 cups	chicken broth	500 mL
1 cup	buttermilk	250 mL
½ tsp	dried basil	2 mL
½ tsp	dried tarragon	2 mL
	Salt and black pepper to taste	
	Small broccoli florets, lower-fat plain yogurt, chives, shredded Cheddar cheese	

1. In a saucepan over medium-high heat, cook broccoli in chicken broth for 10 minutes or until tender. Refrigerate in broth until chilled.

2. In a food processor or blender, purée chilled mixture, buttermilk and seasonings until smooth. Taste and adjust seasonings. Reheat just to serving temperature, or chill and serve as cold soup. Serve garnished with broccoli, yogurt, chives and Cheddar cheese.

PER SERVING	
Calories: 73	
Dietary Fiber: 2 g	Carbohydrate: 7 g
Fat: 2 g	Protein: 7 g

SERVES 6
Makes 3 cups (750 mL)

B.J. Rankin

P

Not only is this soup delicious and nutritious, it is quick and easy to make. It looks elegant when garnished and can be served all year round.

TIP
This is a great way to use leftover broccoli.

DIETITIAN'S MESSAGE

Another delicious way to add a serving of vegetables to your daily plan. Serve this soup with Creamy Salmon Quiche (see recipe, page 311), a tossed green salad and whole-wheat rolls. Finish with a seasonal dessert. Your meal will be abundant in folic acid, vitamins A and C, and calcium.

SERVES 6
Makes 6 cups
(1.5 L)
....

Victoria McKay

A steaming bowl of this comforting chowder on a cold winter night provides a soothing start to any meal.

TIPS

If there is a vegetarian in your family, replace the chicken broth with a vegetable broth.

To reduce the fat content, after making chicken stock, chill the stock until cold. The fat will harden on the surface and can easily be removed with a large spoon.

DIETITIAN'S MESSAGE

Enhance the calcium in this soup by making it the centerpiece of a calcium-rich meal. Serve with Stuffed Pasta Shells (see recipe, page 192) and complete the meal with yogurt.

Mushroom, Broccoli and Corn Chowder

2 cups	chicken broth	500 mL
2	medium stalks broccoli, chopped	2
1 cup	sliced mushrooms	250 mL
½ cup	finely chopped onion	125 mL
2 tbsp	butter *or* margarine	25 mL
2 tbsp	all-purpose flour	25 mL
1½ cups	skim milk	375 mL
2 cups	whole kernel corn	500 mL
1 tbsp	chopped pimiento	15 mL

1. In a large saucepan over medium heat, cook broth and broccoli for 5 minutes; set aside.

2. In a skillet over medium-high heat, cook mushrooms and onion in butter for about 4 minutes or until softened. Blend in flour; cook, stirring, for 2 minutes. Slowly add milk; cook, stirring, until smooth and thickened. Add broccoli mixture, corn and pimiento. Heat to serving temperature or until corn and broccoli are cooked.

PER SERVING	
Calories: 136	
Dietary Fiber: 3 g	Carbohydrate: 20 g
Fat: 4 g	Protein: 7 g

Oriental Mushroom Soup

5 cups	chicken broth	1.25 L
4 tsp	finely chopped ginger root	20 mL
½ lb	sliced mushrooms (shiitake, oyster, portobello *or* a combination), about 2 cups (500 mL)	250 g
2 tbsp	sodium-reduced soy sauce	25 mL
1 tsp	sesame oil	5 mL
8 oz	firm tofu, cut into small cubes	250 g
1	green onion, thinly sliced	1

1. In a saucepan, combine broth, ginger root and mushrooms; bring to a boil. Reduce heat and simmer, uncovered, for 15 minutes. Stir in soy sauce and sesame oil.
2. Place tofu and green onion in individual soup bowls or tureen. Add soup and serve.

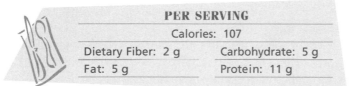

PER SERVING	
Calories: 107	
Dietary Fiber: 2 g	Carbohydrate: 5 g
Fat: 5 g	Protein: 11 g

SERVES 6
....
Samuel Glass, Chef
Rosie Schwartz, Dietitian

For an elegant touch, cut the tofu into stars with cookie cutters.

TIPS
Be sure to use firm tofu in this soup. Otherwise, it won't retain its shape.

Sesame oil is available in large supermarkets and specialty food shops. All you need is a teaspoon (5 mL) to enhance the flavor of this soup.

DIETITIAN'S MESSAGE
The combination of flavors makes this a great-tasting soup. Served with crusty bread for a pleasant light lunch.

Curried Fiddlehead Soup

1 lb	fresh *or* frozen fiddleheads	500 g
2 cups	each chicken broth and 1% milk	500 mL
2 tsp	each margarine and curry powder	10 mL
¼ cup	gin (optional)	50 mL

1. In a large saucepan, cook fiddleheads in chicken broth for 15 to 20 minutes; don't overcook or they will go brown. Remove fiddleheads with slotted spoon and purée in food processor; return to broth. Stir in milk; simmer until hot.
2. In a small skillet, heat margarine over low heat; stir in curry powder and cook, stirring, for 2 to 3 minutes. Add to soup. Stir in gin, if desired.

PER SERVING	
Calories: 91	
Dietary Fiber: Trace	Carbohydrate: 9 g
Fat: 4 g	Protein: 8 g

SERVES 5
....
Darren Meredith, Chef
Johanne Thériault, Dietitian

Fiddleheads, the young shoots of the ostrich fern, are a springtime delicacy. If you have access to a supply, freeze a batch and enjoy this soup year-round.

DIETITIAN'S MESSAGE
Fiddleheads contain vitamin C, which helps the body to absorb iron. Serve this elegant soup followed by Flank Steak Stir-Fry (see recipe, page 249).

Creole Tomato Soup

1 tbsp	vegetable oil	15 mL
1	small onion, chopped	1
1	clove garlic, minced	1
¼ cup	finely sliced celery	50 mL
1	can (19 oz/540 mL) tomatoes, drained and diced	1
2 cups	chicken broth	500 mL
½ tsp	crushed dried thyme	2 mL
¼ tsp	paprika	1 mL
¼ tsp	red pepper flakes	1 mL
¼ tsp	black pepper	1 mL
1 cup	cubed cooked chicken	250 mL
¾ cup	frozen corn kernels	175 mL
⅓ cup	baby pasta shells	75 mL
	Sliced green onions and chopped fresh parsley (optional)	

1. In a saucepan, heat oil over medium heat; cook onion, garlic and celery, stirring often, for 3 to 5 minutes or until softened. Stir in tomatoes, broth, thyme, paprika, red pepper flakes and black pepper; bring to a boil. Cover, reduce heat and simmer for 10 minutes.

2. Stir in chicken, corn and pasta. Simmer, uncovered and stirring occasionally, for about 10 minutes or until pasta is tender. Serve garnished with green onions and parsley, if desired.

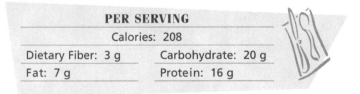

PER SERVING	
Calories: 208	
Dietary Fiber: 3 g	Carbohydrate: 20 g
Fat: 7 g	Protein: 16 g

Creamy Roasted Sweet Pepper Soup

2 tsp	olive oil	10 mL
1	medium onion, chopped	1
1	clove garlic, minced	1
1	each large red, yellow and green bell pepper, roasted and peeled (see technique, page 127)	1
2 cups	chicken broth	500 mL
1	can (10 oz/284 mL) regular *or* seasoned tomatoes, drained	1
2 tbsp	tomato paste	25 mL
1 tsp	ground cumin	5 mL
6 oz	soft tofu	175 g
½ tsp	salt	2 mL
¼ tsp	white pepper	1 mL
	Black sesame seeds *or* toasted white sesame seeds	

1. In a large saucepan, heat oil over medium heat; cook onion and garlic, stirring, for 2 to 3 minutes or until softened. Add peppers, broth, tomatoes, tomato paste and cumin; bring to a boil. Cover, reduce heat and simmer for 30 minutes. Cool slightly.

2. In a blender, purée pepper mixture with tofu in batches. Strain through sieve into saucepan; season with salt and pepper. Reheat over low heat. Garnish with sesame seeds.

PER SERVING	
Calories: 140	
Dietary Fiber: 4 g	Carbohydrate: 17 g
Fat: 6 g	Protein: 8 g

SERVES 4

Margaret Carson, Chef
Pam Lynch, Dietitian
Judy Fraser-Arsenault, Dietitian

This "cream soup", which is lighter in fat, is a great way to add tofu to your diet.

TIPS

Tofu (soybean curd) is a creamy white soy product sold in small blocks. It comes in different forms. Soft or silken is best for blending in shakes, dressings and desserts, whereas the firmer versions hold their shape in soups and main courses.

Save yourself time and money by buying a large quantity of red peppers at the end of the season when they are plentiful. Roast them, remove the skins and freeze in small amounts so they are ready to use throughout the winter.

DIETITIAN'S MESSAGE

The tofu in this recipe gives the soup a creamy texture without the use of cream. Tofu is a good source of protein and is low in fat, relative to some protein sources. Read the label to find tofu with added calcium. Red peppers are high in vitamins A and C and are a great source of antioxidants.

Make this hearty soup when the days are cold and you don't have time to shop as it can be made from ingredients you are likely to have in the larder.

TIP
If desired, substitute 1 or 2 cans (each 10 oz/ 284 mL) condensed beef or vegetable broth for the beef bouillon cube in this recipe. Reduce the quantity of water by 2 cups (500 mL).

DIETITIAN'S MESSAGE
Beans are a great source of vegetable protein and add fiber. Complete this meal with Smoked Turkey Toss (see recipe, page 135) and a dessert such as Winter Fruit Crisp (see recipe, page 405).

Root Vegetable Soup

4 cups	water	1 L
1	beef bouillon cube	1
1 cup	chopped potatoes	250 mL
1 cup	chopped carrots	250 mL
1 cup	chopped turnip	250 mL
1/3 cup	chopped celery	75 mL
1/3 cup	chopped onion	75 mL
1	can (14 oz/398 mL) tomatoes	1
1	can (14 oz/398 mL) kidney beans	1
1/2 tsp	dried oregano	2 mL
1/2 tsp	garlic powder	2 mL
1/2 tsp	paprika	2 mL
	Salt and black pepper to taste	
1/2 cup	cut-up green beans	125 mL

1. In a large stockpot, combine water, bouillon cube, potatoes, carrots, turnip, celery, onion, tomatoes, kidney beans and seasonings; bring to a boil. Reduce heat, cover and simmer for about 1 hour. Add green beans during last 10 minutes of cooking.

PER SERVING	
Calories: 114	
Dietary Fiber: 7 g	Carbohydrate: 23 g
Fat: 1 g	Protein: 6 g

Peppery Potato Soup

SERVES 6
Makes 7 cups
(1.75 L)

F. Vautour, Dietitian

2	large potatoes, cubed	2
2 cups	boiling water	500 mL
1	medium onion, finely chopped	1
1	medium green bell pepper, chopped	1
1	medium red bell pepper, chopped	1
2 tbsp	butter *or* margarine	25 mL
4 oz	cooked ham, cubed	125 g
1 tbsp	mild *or* hot green chilies	15 mL
¼ tsp	white pepper	1 mL
1 cup	chicken broth	250 mL
1	egg yolk, lightly beaten	1
¼ cup	2% milk	50 mL
½ cup	shredded old Cheddar cheese (optional)	125 mL

This flavorful soup is a great way to use leftover ham and boiled potatoes.

TIPS

For this unique potato soup, choose mild or hot green chilies depending on the level of heat you enjoy.

If you prefer a richer broth, cook the potatoes in chicken broth instead of water and add to the soup.

1. In a medium saucepan, cook potatoes in boiling water for about 15 minutes or until tender; drain and reserve liquid.

2. In a skillet, sauté onion and green and red peppers in butter over medium heat for 10 minutes or until softened. Stir in ham, chilies and pepper; set aside.

3. In a food processor or blender, purée cooked potatoes with chicken broth until smooth. Return to saucepan with reserved liquid; add vegetable mixture and reheat.

4. Beat egg yolk with milk; gradually stir into ½ cup (125 mL) hot soup. Return to saucepan. Heat gently but do not boil. Top with Cheddar cheese, if desired.

DIETITIAN'S MESSAGE

This hearty soup is rich in taste as well as vitamins and minerals. Serve with Herb Grain Bread (see recipe, page 39) and Spinach and Grapefruit Salad (see recipe, page 160) and a serving of milk products to feature all the food groups.

PER SERVING	
Calories: 147	
Dietary Fiber: 1 g	Carbohydrate: 15 g
Fat: 7 g	Protein: 7 g

SERVES 6
······················

John Higgins, Chef
Susan Iantorno,
Dietitian

*Colorful, easy to make
and delicious to eat —
what else can you say
about this fabulous soup?*

TIPS
For a variation, use
pumpkin instead
of squash.

Cutting through the
hard exterior of a squash
can be a challenge. One
solution is to heat the
whole squash in the
microwave on High for
2 minutes. It should then
be easy to cut using a
large, sharp knife.

DIETITIAN'S MESSAGE

This simple soup is a
great source of vitamin A.
Serve with Spinach and
Rice Salad (see recipe,
page 167) and a Mixed
Herb Baguette (see
recipe, page 45) and
finish the meal with
Cinnamon Baked Pears
(see recipe, page 385).
You will be adding folic
acid, fiber and other
valuable vitamins and
minerals to your diet.

Curried Squash and Mushroom Soup

1	medium butternut squash, peeled and chopped	1
8 oz	sliced mushrooms	250 g
½ cup	chopped onions	125 mL
2 tbsp	butter *or* margarine	25 mL
2 tbsp	all-purpose flour	25 mL
1 tbsp	curry powder	15 mL
5 cups	chicken broth	1.25 mL
½ cup	dry white wine *or* chicken broth	125 L
1 tbsp	liquid honey	15 mL
Pinch	(approx.) ground nutmeg	Pinch
1 cup	half-and-half (10%) cream *or* 2% milk	250 mL

1. Steam squash until tender; purée in a food processor until smooth.

2. In a saucepan over medium-high heat, cook mushrooms and onions in butter until softened. Add flour and curry powder; cook, stirring, for 5 minutes. Gradually stir in chicken broth and wine; cook until smooth and slightly thickened. Whisk in squash, honey and nutmeg; reduce heat and simmer for 15 minutes.

3. Stir in cream and reheat to serving temperature. Sprinkle with more nutmeg to serve.

Per Serving with Cream

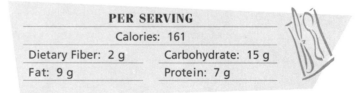

PER SERVING	
Calories: 161	
Dietary Fiber: 2 g	Carbohydrate: 15 g
Fat: 9 g	Protein: 7 g

Per Serving with 2% Milk

PER SERVING	
Calories: 135	
Dietary Fiber: 20 g	Carbohydrate: 15 g
Fat: 6 g	Protein: 7 g

Creamy Squash Soup

2 tbsp	vegetable oil	25 mL
1	large onion, chopped	1
4 cups	coarsely chopped butternut squash	1 L
4 cups	chicken broth	1 L
½ tsp	each salt and black pepper	2 mL
½ cup	whipping cream *or* half-and-half (10%) cream	125 mL

1. In a saucepan, heat oil over medium heat; cook onion, stirring, until softened. Add squash; cook, stirring, for 5 minutes.
2. Add broth and bring to a boil. Reduce heat, cover and simmer until squash is tender. In a food processor, purée in batches; return to saucepan. Add remaining ingredients and heat through.

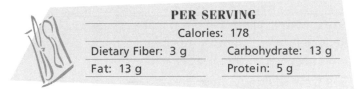

PER SERVING	
Calories: 178	
Dietary Fiber: 3 g	Carbohydrate: 13 g
Fat: 13 g	Protein: 5 g

SERVES 6
Makes 7 cups (1.75 L)

Anne M. Ferraro

Make this soup during the autumn when fresh squash is readily available. Or prepare year-round using frozen mashed squash or canned pumpkin. Mashed cooked pumpkin can also be used.

DIETITIAN'S MESSAGE

The rich orange color of butternut squash indicates that it is a super source of beta-carotene, which is converted into vitamin A in the body.

Tomato and Bean Soup

1	can (19 oz/540 mL) stewed tomatoes	1
1	can (14 oz/398 mL) baked beans in tomato sauce	1
1 cup	water	250 mL
½ cup	chopped onions	125 mL
½ tsp	each dried basil and dried parsley	2 mL
1 cup	shredded Cheddar cheese	250 mL

1. In a saucepan over medium heat, combine all ingredients except cheese; bring to a boil. Reduce heat and simmer, uncovered and stirring occasionally, for 10 to 15 minutes.
2. Top each serving with ¼ cup (50 mL) Cheddar cheese.

PER SERVING	
Calories: 259	
Dietary Fiber: 10 g	Carbohydrate: 33 g
Fat: 10 g	Protein: 14 g

SERVES 4
Makes 4 cups (1 L)

Marylin Cook

This tasty soup can be made in less time than it takes to order from a restaurant.

TIP
If you have fresh basil or parsley, use 1 tbsp (15 mL) or more of each instead of the dried.

DIETITIAN'S MESSAGE
Serve this hearty soup with whole-wheat toast and bagels. Enjoy frozen yogurt or fresh fruit for dessert.

····························

Tyrone Miller, Chef
Karen Jackson, Dietitian

A great make-ahead soup that is practically a meal in itself.

TIPS

In a hurry? Substitute 1 can (19 oz/540 mL) navy or white kidney beans, drained and rinsed, for the dried beans.

Forgot to soak the beans? Use the quick-soak method. Place dried beans in a saucepan with twice their volume of cold water. Cover and bring to a boil over high heat. Boil rapidly for 1 to 2 minutes. Remove from heat and set aside, covered, for at least 1 hour. Drain and rinse.

DIETITIAN'S MESSAGE

Omit the ham and replace the chicken broth with vegetable broth and this soup makes an excellent choice for a vegetarian.

White Bean Soup

1 cup	white (navy) beans	250 mL
1 tbsp	butter *or* margarine	15 mL
2	medium onions, chopped	2
1	large potato, peeled and diced	1
½ cup	chopped celery	125 mL
4 cups	chicken broth	1 L
1	clove garlic, minced	1
1 tsp	crushed dried oregano	5 mL
½ cup	half-and-half (10%) cream	125 mL
½ cup	diced cooked ham	125 mL
¼ tsp	black pepper	1 mL
	Chopped fresh parsley	

1. Cover beans with 2½ cups (625 mL) water; let stand overnight. Drain. In a small saucepan, combine half of the beans with 1¼ cups (300 mL) water; bring to a boil. Reduce heat and simmer, uncovered, for 30 minutes or until softened. Drain and set aside.

2. In a large saucepan, melt butter over medium heat; cook onions, potato and celery for 5 minutes. Add chicken broth, garlic, oregano and remaining beans; bring to a boil. Cover, reduce heat and simmer for about 30 minutes or until beans are softened.

3. In a food processor or blender, purée soup; pass through sieve into saucepan. Add cooked beans, cream, ham and pepper; heat through. Serve garnished with parsley.

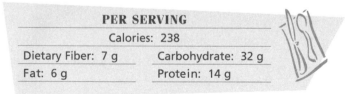

PER SERVING	
Calories: 238	
Dietary Fiber: 7 g	Carbohydrate: 32 g
Fat: 6 g	Protein: 14 g

Cream of Potato and Sausage Soup

3 cups	chicken broth	750 mL
2 cups	diced peeled russet potatoes (2 large)	500 mL
1	large onion, chopped	1
4 oz	diced turkey kielbasa sausage	125 g
1 cup	2% evaporated milk	250 mL
¼ tsp	dried dillweed	1 mL
	White pepper	

1. In an 8-cup (2 L) saucepan, bring chicken broth to a boil. Add potatoes; cook until tender, about 10 minutes. Remove from heat and remove half of the potatoes with slotted spoon; reserve.

2. In a small nonstick skillet, cook onions with sausage, stirring until lightly browned.

3. In a blender or food processor, purée remaining potatoes with broth; return to saucepan. Add reserved potatoes, sausage mixture, milk and dillweed. Heat over medium-low heat until hot but do not boil. Season with pepper to taste.

PER SERVING

Calories: 217

Dietary Fiber: 2 g	Carbohydrate: 29 g
Fat: 5 g	Protein: 15 g

SERVES 4
....

Larry DeVries, Chef
Jackie Kopilas, Dietitian
Rachel Barkley, Dietitian

Here's a contemporary update on a rich and hearty soup. This lighter version uses potatoes as a thickener, 2% evaporated milk for creaminess and turkey sausage, which delivers traditional sausage taste with less fat.

TIP

Use fresh chopped dill to taste instead of the dried, if available. Double the quantity.

DIETITIAN'S MESSAGE

Turkey kielbasa is a good source of protein and a flavorful and lower-fat alternative to traditional kielbasa sausage made from pork.

Raymond Colliver, Chef
Dani Flowerday,
Dietitian

Impress friends and family with your own version of this Chinese classic.

TIP

Use thin green or red chilies or Thai finger chilies in this recipe rather than jalapeño chilies. If using a fresh chili pepper, wash your hands thoroughly after chopping.

DIETITIAN'S MESSAGE

The tofu, chicken and egg whites in this soup combine to make a good source of protein. Serve with "Fire and Ice" Shrimp Salad (see recipe, page 132) to continue the Asian theme.

Hot and Sour Chicken Soup

6	dried Chinese mushrooms	6
5 cups	chicken broth	1.25 L
2 cups	shredded cooked chicken (7 oz/200 g)	500 mL
1 tbsp	finely chopped ginger root	15 mL
1	chili pepper, chopped (*or* ½ tsp/2 mL crushed chili flakes)	1
1 cup	diced firm tofu	250 mL
2 tbsp	white wine vinegar	25 mL
1 tbsp	sodium-reduced soy sauce	15 mL
1 tbsp	dry sherry	15 mL
1 tbsp	cornstarch	15 mL
1 tbsp	cold water	15 mL
3	egg whites, lightly beaten	3
2	shallots, thinly sliced (optional)	2

1. Cover Chinese mushrooms with hot water and soak for 10 minutes. Drain, discard stems and slice caps.

2. In a large saucepan, bring broth to a boil; add mushrooms, chicken, ginger root and chili pepper. Reduce heat and simmer, covered, for 5 minutes. Add tofu, vinegar, soy sauce and sherry; simmer for 2 minutes.

3. Stir cornstarch with water until smooth; gradually stir into soup and simmer for 2 to 3 minutes or until thickened slightly. Remove from heat; immediately swirl egg whites through soup. Garnish with shallots, if desired.

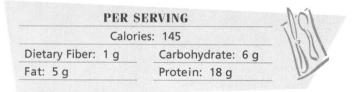

PER SERVING	
Calories: 145	
Dietary Fiber: 1 g	Carbohydrate: 6 g
Fat: 5 g	Protein: 18 g

Asian Turkey and Noodle Soup

SERVES 6
Makes 6 cups (1.5 L)
• •
Joanne Saunders

2 tsp	vegetable oil	10 mL
8 oz	boneless skinless turkey breast, cut into strips	250 g
1 cup	sliced mushrooms	250 mL
2	cans (each 10 oz/284 mL) chicken broth	2
3 cups	water	750 mL
1 tsp	minced garlic	5 mL
1 tsp	grated ginger root	5 mL
1 tbsp	rice wine vinegar *or* lemon juice	15 mL
1 tbsp	soy sauce	15 mL
1 tsp	sesame oil	5 mL
¼ tsp	hot pepper sauce	1 mL
4 oz	fresh chow mein *or* rice noodles	125 g
1½ cups	snow peas, trimmed and cut into 1-inch (2.5 cm) pieces	375 mL
½ cup	chopped green onions	125 mL

1. In a large saucepan, heat oil over medium-high heat. Add turkey and stir-fry for 2 to 3 minutes. Add mushrooms; cook for 2 to 3 minutes. Add broth, water, garlic and ginger root; bring to a boil. Add vinegar, soy sauce, sesame oil, hot pepper sauce and noodles; reduce heat and simmer for 3 to 4 minutes.

2. Add snow peas and green onions; simmer for 1 to 2 minutes. Serve immediately.

PER SERVING

Calories: 165	
Dietary Fiber: 1 g	Carbohydrate: 14 g
Fat: 4 g	Protein: 17 g

This soup tastes great made with fresh turkey breast, but you can also use leftover cooked turkey (about 1 cup/250 mL). If using cooked turkey, don't stir-fry. Add with the broth in Step 1.

TIPS

Sesame oil is made from roasted sesame seeds and is used for flavoring many Asian dishes. The darker the oil, the more intense the flavor. A little goes a long way, so add it sparingly. Keep refrigerated after opening.

Grated ginger root and chopped garlic are sold preserved in jars at most supermarkets. They are great time-savers. You can also preserve your own ginger root. Peel and chop finely; place in a jar and cover with dry sherry or sake. Store, tightly covered, in the refrigerator.

DIETITIAN'S MESSAGE

This hearty soup with an Asian flair can be served as an elegant first course before a lighter meal or as a weekend lunch with a sandwich and a glass of milk.

SERVES 12
Makes 12 cups (3 L)
• •
Paula Worton

This is a hearty, family-style soup. The recipe makes a large quantity, but the soup freezes well.

VARIATIONS
For a more robust meal, add uncooked pasta or barley (about ½ cup/125 mL) to this soup. Add barley with vegetables and cook for 35 minutes. If using pasta, add with zucchini and cook for 10 minutes.

TIP
For variety, replace the kidney beans with about 2 cups (500 mL) of a medley of mixed frozen beans. These assortments usually include chickpeas, kidney, black, romano and white (navy) beans.

DIETITIAN'S MESSAGE
This robust soup is perfect for a cold-weather dinner or après-ski. The addition of pasta or barley (see Variation) makes it a complete meal.

Hamburger Soup

1 lb	lean ground beef	500 g
1	can (28 oz/796 mL) tomatoes	1
1	can (19 oz/540 mL) kidney beans, drained and rinsed	1
1	can (10 oz/284 mL) condensed tomato soup	1
5 cups	water	1.25 L
1	medium onion, chopped	1
1	carrot, chopped	1
½ cup	chopped celery	125 mL
½ cup	sliced mushrooms	125 mL
1 tsp	Worcestershire sauce	5 mL
¼ tsp	hot pepper sauce	1 mL
¼ tsp	freshly ground black pepper	1 mL
2	small zucchini, chopped	2

1. In a large stockpot over medium heat, brown beef until crumbly; drain fat. Add tomatoes, kidney beans, tomato soup, water, onion, carrot, celery, mushrooms and seasonings; bring to a boil. Reduce heat and simmer, covered, for about 35 minutes. Add zucchini. Simmer for 10 minutes longer.

PER SERVING	
Calories: 145	
Dietary Fiber: 4 g	Carbohydrate: 15 g
Fat: 5 g	Protein: 11 g

Beef Barley Soup

3½ cups	water	875 mL
¾ cup	tomato sauce	175 mL
¾ cup	dried soup mix (lentils, split peas, barley)	175 mL
1	beef bouillon cube	1
1	medium carrot, diced	1
1	medium potato, diced	1
2 tsp	dried basil	10 mL
½ tsp	salt	2 mL
¼ tsp	freshly ground black pepper	1 mL
½ cup	cubed cooked lean beef	125 mL

1. In a large stockpot, combine water, tomato sauce, dried soup mix, bouillon cube, carrot, potato and seasonings; bring to a boil. Reduce heat and simmer, covered, for about 1 hour. Add beef. Cook for 30 minutes longer.

PER SERVING	
Calories: 194	
Dietary Fiber: 5 g	Carbohydrate: 33 g
Fat: 2 g	Protein: 13 g

SERVES 4
Makes 4 cups (1 L)

P

Karen Dewar

Here's a delicious rib-sticking soup for a cold winter's day.

TIPS

Dried soup mix is available in bulk or health-food stores as well as in the supermarket. If desired, replace with an equal quantity of barley.

For a more robust broth, eliminate the bouillon cube and substitute 1 can (10 oz/284 mL) condensed beef broth. Reduce the quantity of water to 3 cups (750 mL).

DIETITIAN'S MESSAGE

Barley is a grain grown in northern climates; it adds a delightful nutty flavor and a pleasant chewy texture. It is another way to add both soluble and insoluble fiber to the diet. It is available as polished and pearl barley and both can be used in a variety of dishes, including this recipe.

P

Fleur-Ange Joubert

Here's another hearty stick-to-the-ribs soup that will keep you warm on a winter's day.

TIPS

If you don't have beef stock, substitute 2 cans (each 10 oz/284 mL) beef broth plus 3½ cups (875 mL) water, or substitute 6 beef bouillon cubes or sachets (2 tbsp/25 mL) plus 6 cups (1.5 L) water.

Any 19-oz (540 mL) can of beans can be used in place of the mixed beans. Try kidney, romano or white (navy) beans.

If you don't have any zucchini, substitute an equal amount of frozen peas, green beans or corn.

MAKE AHEAD

This soup keeps for up to 3 days in the refrigerator or 4 months in the freezer.

DIETITIAN'S MESSAGE

This soup is very high in fiber and is packed with many essential nutrients, including folic acid. It's a great choice for women who are trying to add more iron and folic acid to their meals.

Beef, Vegetable and Bean Soup

12 oz	lean ground beef	375 g
2 tsp	minced garlic	10 mL
½ cup	chopped onion	125 mL
1 cup	chopped carrots	250 mL
1 cup	chopped celery *or* fennel	250 mL
1 cup	chopped zucchini	250 mL
1 tsp	dried basil	5 mL
1	bay leaf	1
6 cups	beef stock	1.5 L
1	can (28 oz/796 mL) whole tomatoes	1
½ cup	macaroni (*or* any other small pasta)	125 mL
3 cups	chopped fresh spinach	750 mL
1	can (19 oz/540 mL) mixed beans, drained and rinsed	1

1. In a large saucepan or Dutch oven, brown beef over medium-high heat. Add garlic, onion, carrots, celery and zucchini; cook for 5 minutes. Add basil, bay leaf, stock and tomatoes; bring to a boil. Reduce heat and simmer, covered, for 10 minutes.

2. Add pasta; cook for another 5 to 6 minutes. Add spinach and beans; cook for another 3 to 4 minutes. Remove bay leaf before serving.

PER SERVING	
Calories: 225	
Dietary Fiber: 7 g	Carbohydrate: 24 g
Fat: 7 g	Protein: 17 g

Caribbean Ham and Black Bean Soup

½ cup	chopped onion	125 mL
3 cups	water	750 mL
1	can (19 oz/540 mL) black beans, drained and rinsed	1
1	can (19 oz/540 mL) stewed tomatoes	1
1 cup	diced cooked ham	250 mL
½ cup	frozen corn kernels	125 mL
¼ cup	long-grain rice	50 mL
1 tbsp	lime juice	15 mL
2 tsp	brown sugar	10 mL
1 tsp	hot pepper sauce	5 mL
½ tsp	ground cumin	2 mL
¼ tsp	ground ginger	1 mL

1. In a large saucepan sprayed with vegetable spray, cook onion over medium-high heat for 3 to 4 minutes or until tender. Stir in water, beans, tomatoes, ham, corn, rice, lime juice, brown sugar, hot pepper sauce, cumin and ginger; bring to a boil. Reduce heat and simmer, covered, for 15 to 20 minutes or until rice is tender.

3 ptr

PER SERVING	
Calories: 191	
Dietary Fiber: 5 g	Carbohydrate: 33 g
Fat: 2 g	Protein: 12 g

SERVES 6
Makes 7 cups (1.75 L)

Patricia Mialkowsky

This makes a nice hot meal-to-go. Heat it up in the morning, pop it into a Thermos and enjoy it with your lunch.

TIP

If desired, substitute 1 cup (250 mL) dried black beans, soaked, cooked and rinsed, for the canned beans.

MAKE AHEAD

This soup can be made ahead and kept for up to 3 days in the refrigerator or frozen for up to 4 months. If you are using leftover ham, be sure that it's not more than a day or 2 old.

DIETITIAN'S MESSAGE

This hearty meal in a bowl is simple to make, low in fat and high in fiber. It is also an excellent source of folic acid. To complete the meal, add vegetable sticks, a whole-grain roll and a piece of cheese.

SERVES 6
Makes 6 cups (1.5 L)
....
Lynn Roblin, Dietitian

This super-speedy soup will warm you up on a cold day. The cumin gives the soup a nice flavor, reminiscent of chili. It is very easy for older children or teens to make, so leave the recipe out and encourage whoever arrives home first to get supper started.

TIP

Lentils come in many colors but the most common are red, brown and green. They are available in cans, which makes them easy to add to soups, stews and casseroles. They can also be added cold to salads.

DIETITIAN'S MESSAGE

Lentils, a member of the legume family, are rich in protein and other nutrients. Like beans, they make a valuable contribution to a vegetarian diet.

Chunky Vegetable Lentil Soup

2 cups	water	500 mL
1	vegetable bouillon cube	1
1 cup	chopped carrots	250 mL
1	can (28 oz/796 mL) diced tomatoes	1
1	can (19 oz/540 mL) lentils, drained and rinsed	1
2 tsp	minced garlic	10 mL
1 tsp	dried basil	5 mL
½ tsp	ground thyme	2 mL
½ tsp	ground cumin	2 mL

1. In a large saucepan, bring water to a boil. Add vegetable bouillon cube; stir until dissolved.

2. Add carrots; reduce heat to medium and cook, covered, for 10 minutes.

3. Add tomatoes, lentils, garlic, basil, thyme and cumin; reduce heat to medium-low and cook, stirring often, for 10 minutes or until carrots are tender.

PER SERVING	
Calories: 118	
Dietary Fiber: 5 g	Carbohydrate: 22 g
Fat: 1 g	Protein: 8 g

Southwestern Sweet Potato Soup

1 tbsp	olive oil	15 mL
½ cup	chopped onion	125 mL
2 cups	diced peeled sweet potatoes	500 mL
1 cup	diced peeled baking potatoes	250 mL
4 cups	chicken stock *or* vegetable stock *or* water	1 L
1 cup	fresh *or* frozen corn kernels	250 mL
1	red bell pepper, roasted (see technique below), peeled, seeded and diced	1
1	jalapeño pepper, seeded and chopped	1
	Salt and black pepper	
¼ cup	chopped fresh cilantro *or* green onions *or* parsley	50 mL

1. In a large saucepan, heat oil over medium heat. Add onion and cook for 3 to 4 minutes or until softened but not browned. Add sweet potatoes and baking potatoes; cook for 2 to 3 minutes.

2. Add stock; bring to a boil. Reduce heat and simmer, uncovered, for 12 to 15 minutes or until potatoes are tender.

3. In a blender or food processor, purée potato mixture in batches; return to pan. Add corn, red pepper and jalapeño pepper; cook for 3 to 4 minutes. Season with salt and pepper to taste. Serve soup garnished with cilantro.

PER SERVING	
Calories: 147	
Dietary Fiber: 3 g	Carbohydrate: 24 g
Fat: 4 g	Protein: 5 g

TO ROAST PEPPERS
Heat barbecue or broiler; place peppers on grill or broiling pan and cook until skins turn black. Keep turning peppers until skins are blistered and black. Place roasted peppers in large pot with lid. Steam will make them sweat and skin will be easier to peel off. Let peppers cool. Remove stems, seeds and skin.

SERVES 6
Makes 6 cups (1.5 L)
Claudette Turnbull, Dietitian

Here's a tasty and nutritious soup that capitalizes on the popularity of Southwestern cuisine.

TIP
Make your own roasted red peppers (see technique, below) or substitute ½ cup (125 mL) bottled roasted red peppers.

DIETITIAN'S MESSAGE
Eating dark orange and red vegetables, such as sweet potatoes and red peppers, helps to increase your intake of vitamins A and C and antioxidants. Serve this colorful and tasty soup with whole-wheat pita bread and hummus.

Salads

A salad is great if you're eating alone and perfect for feeding a crowd. It can be a complete meal on its own or a side dish that adds variety and nutrients to the main course. In this chapter, you will find salads that are suitable for every occasion. Most are easy to prepare — in fact, some are simple enough that children can make them on their own.

Southwestern Sweet ➤
Potato Soup (page 127)

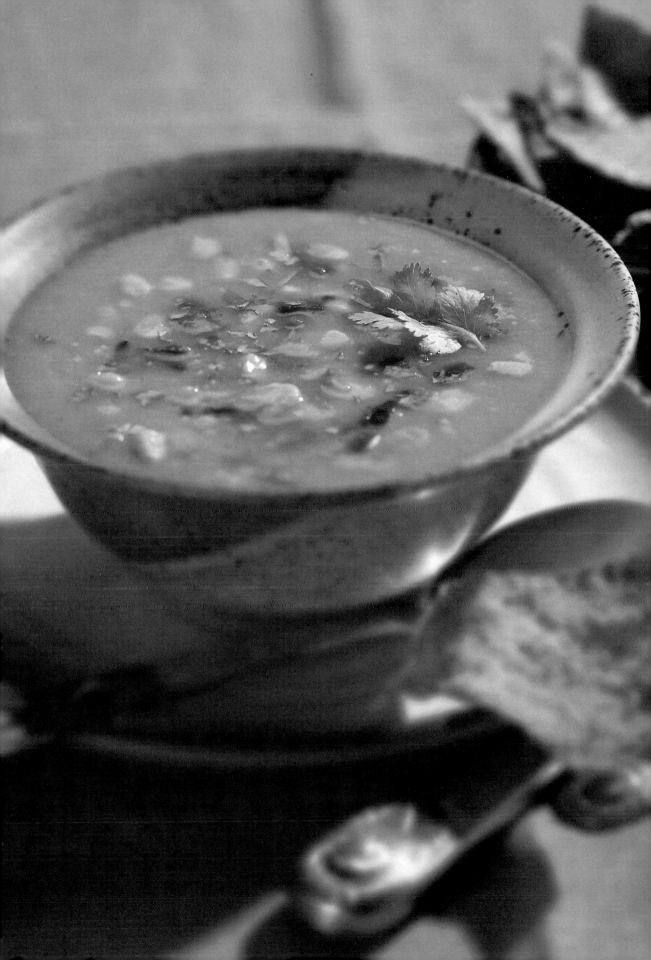

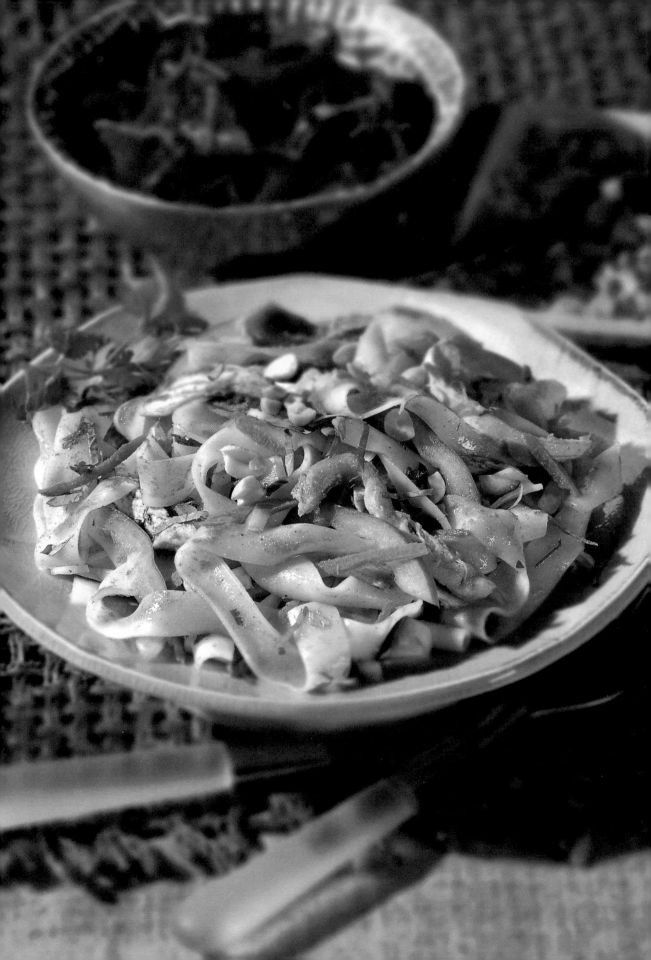

part of a healthy eating plan

Today, we enjoy an overwhelming variety and choice of fresh produce, which makes it easy to serve delicious and interesting salads as part of a regular meal plan. So why is it that a national survey released in 2001 revealed that only 36% of Canadians consume the five to 10 daily servings of vegetables and fruit recommended by *Canada's Food Guide to Healthy Eating*? Perhaps because it seems like a daunting task — particularly if, like many people, you eat most of your vegetables at dinner.

Introducing more salads into your food choices throughout the day is one way to meet this challenge. With a little planning and a well-stocked pantry or crisper, salads are a quick and easy way to help you get your five to 10 servings a day. Pack salad greens in a resealable plastic vegetable bag and dressing in a small container, and enjoy a tasty tossed salad as part of a brown bag lunch. Or make a big salad the focal point of your main meal.

center stage salads

Gone are the days when a salad meant simply mixing lettuce and tomatoes. Today a salad can mean anything from bean, pasta, mixed greens or fruit to lightened-up classics such as potato salad or coleslaw. To transform a simple green salad into a main dish, add some lean grilled chicken strips, eggs, nuts, seeds, beans or tofu, sprinkle with cheese or toss in a lower-fat yogurt dressing. Serve with thick slices of fresh crusty bread or fresh muffins and you've covered all the food groups.

plant power

Remember your mother telling you to "eat your veggies"? Well, she was right. Vegetables — and fruit — contain nutrients and other substances such as phytochemicals (see page 12) that are vital to good health. In fact, eating more vegetables and fruit is an important part of a healthy strategy for decreasing the risk of conditions such as cancer, diabetes, heart disease and stroke.

Not only are vegetables and fruit high in carbohydrates and fiber, they are a powerhouse of essential nutrients. They are particularly rich in vitamins A, C and folic acid. Some even provide small amounts of minerals, such as potassium (bananas, pears and oranges), iron (dried fruit and pumpkin) and calcium (kale, bok choy and mustard greens).

watch the dressing

While most vegetables and fruits are naturally low in fat and calories, their fat content is easily raised with the addition of heavy dressings. Here are a few suggestions for keeping that fat in check

- Add flavor to salads with herbs, lemon juice, flavored vinegars and lower-fat salad dressings.
- Reduce the fat in creamy dressings by mixing dressing with an equal part of lower-fat plain yogurt, yogurt cheese or creamed cottage cheese.
- Reduce the fat in vinaigrette dressings by diluting dressing with fruit juice or a flavored vinegar such as balsamic, rice wine or cider vinegar. Adding a tiny bit of sugar cuts the tartness of the vinegar.
- Make your own dressings to control the amount of oil.

◄ Vietnamese Chicken and
Rice Noodle Salad (page 141)

Erna Braun

Most salad greens perk up with a special dressing that uses interesting vinegars. Raspberry, balsamic and tarragon vinegars all add extra zest to dressings. To make your own raspberry vinegar, add fresh or frozen raspberries to rice or white wine vinegar; let stand at room temperature for several days. Strain and bottle.

TIP
To vary the taste of vinaigrette dressings, try experimenting with the many kinds of vinegar now available, such as balsamic, herb-flavored or rice vinegars.

Raspberry Basil Vinaigrette

½ cup	water	125 mL
2 tbsp	raspberry vinegar	25 mL
1	small clove garlic, crushed	1
1 tsp	cornstarch	5 mL
1 tsp	olive oil	5 mL
1 tsp	chopped fresh basil (or ½ tsp/2 mL dried)	5 mL
½ tsp	poppy seeds	2 mL
¼ tsp	grated lemon *or* orange zest	1 mL
Pinch	salt	Pinch

1. In a small saucepan, cook water, vinegar, garlic and cornstarch for about 2 minutes or until thickened. Cool. In a small bowl, combine oil, basil, poppy seeds, lemon zest and salt. Stir in vinegar mixture; cover and refrigerate for at least 1 hour.

PER SERVING (1 TBSP/15 ML)	
Calories: 8	
Dietary Fiber: 0 g	Carbohydrate: 1 g
Fat: 1 g	Protein: 0 g

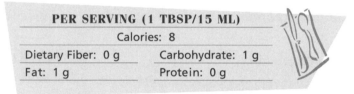

Dietitians of Canada

Enjoy this citrus salad dressing over your favorite greens: Boston lettuce, radicchio or curly or Belgian endive. For variety, add fresh herbs like parsley, dill, oregano or basil, and slivers of Swiss, Cheddar, Muenster or Emmenthal cheese.

Sesame Vinaigrette

¼ cup	lower-fat plain yogurt	50 mL
2 tbsp	grapefruit juice	25 mL
1 tsp	sesame oil	5 mL
¼ tsp	each salt and black pepper	1 mL

1. In a blender, combine yogurt, grapefruit juice, oil and seasonings. Blend on low speed for 30 seconds.

PER SERVING (1 TBSP/15 ML)	
Calories: 18	
Dietary Fiber: 1 g	Carbohydrate: 1 g
Fat: 1 g	Protein: 0 g

Herb Tomato Salad Dressing

1	can (7½ oz/213 mL) tomato sauce	1
2 tbsp	red wine vinegar	25 mL
1 tsp	Worcestershire sauce	5 mL
1 tsp	dried Italian seasoning	5 mL
½ tsp	dried dillweed	2 mL
Pinch	freshly ground black pepper	Pinch
1	green onion, thinly sliced	1

1. In a jar, combine tomato sauce, vinegar and seasonings. Cover and shake well; add green onion. Refrigerate for at least 1 hour for best flavor development.

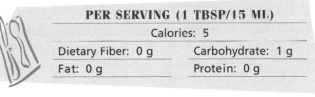

PER SERVING (1 TBSP/15 ML)

Calories: 5

Dietary Fiber: 0 g	Carbohydrate: 1 g
Fat: 0 g	Protein: 0 g

Makes 1 cup (250 mL)

Ellen Vogel, Dietitian

Serve this refreshing no-fat dressing over tasty, crisp greens or drizzled over sliced cucumber.

TIP
If fresh dill is available, substitute 1 tbsp (15 mL) finely chopped for the dried dillweed.

Blue Cheese Salad Dressing

½ cup	lower-fat plain yogurt	125 mL
1 cup	crumbled blue cheese	250 mL
1 tbsp	2% milk	15 mL
1	clove garlic, crushed	1

1. In a food processor or blender, blend yogurt, blue cheese, milk and garlic until smooth. Refrigerate until serving.

PER SERVING (1 TBSP/15 ML)

Calories: 47

Dietary Fiber: 0 g	Carbohydrate: 1 g
Fat: 3 g	Protein: 3 g

Makes ¾ cup (175 mL)

Ann Roberts

Not only will this tangy dressing enhance a tossed green salad or a lettuce wedge, it does double duty as a dip for raw vegetables or fresh fruits.

•••••••••••••••••••••••••••••

David Nicolson, Chef
Leslie Maze, Dietitian

The refreshing combination of chilled orange, lime and mint balances the spark of red chilies in this tasty salad.

TIPS

Look for fish sauce and rice vermicelli in the Asian section of your supermarket.

If you prefer, substitute 1 tsp (5 mL) sambal oelek, a bottled chili paste available in Asian markets, for the crushed chili flakes in this recipe.

DIETITIAN'S MESSAGE

The oranges and lime juice in this recipe provide a surge of vitamin C and folic acid. Combined with the chilies, the citrus juice and fish sauce make a tangy dressing with minimal fat. Serve this salad with crusty whole-wheat or whole-grain bread to add fiber to the meal. Blueberry Semolina Cake (see recipe, page 406) makes a nice finish.

"Fire and Ice" Shrimp Salad

5	medium oranges	5
2 tbsp	lime juice	25 mL
2 tsp	fish sauce	10 mL
2	large cloves garlic, minced	2
1 tsp	crushed chili flakes	5 mL
1 lb	shrimp, peeled, deveined, cooked and cooled	500 g
¼ cup	chopped fresh mint	50 mL
2½ oz	rice vermicelli, soaked and drained (*or* Chinese egg noodles, cooked, drained and chilled)	70 g
	Mint sprigs	

1. With a sharp knife, peel oranges, removing all pith. Cut into segments between membranes, reserving 3 tbsp (45 mL) juice for dressing and discarding any seeds.

2. In a medium bowl, combine reserved orange juice, lime juice, fish sauce, garlic and chili flakes. Add orange segments and shrimp; toss gently. Cover and chill for at least 1 hour or for up to 4 hours.

3. At serving time, stir in chopped mint. Serve over rice vermicelli; garnish with mint sprigs.

PER SERVING (APPETIZER)	
Calories: 123	
Dietary Fiber: 2 g	Carbohydrate: 18 g
Fat: 1 g	Protein: 10 g

LEMON PESTO DRESSING
Here is another reason for keeping a supply of Lemon Pesto Sauce (see recipe, page 75) in the freezer. Margaret Howard combines 3 tbsp (45 mL) Lemon Pesto Sauce with ¼ cup (50 mL) light mayonnaise, and ½ cup (125 mL) buttermilk. She chills it thoroughly, then tosses with her favorite salad greens.

Grilled Tuna with Julienne Vegetables

SERVES 4
....

Trent Breares, Chef
Thomas Hamilton,
Dietitian

Here's a sophisticated and elegant salad that is easy to make.

Dressing

¼ cup	olive oil	50 mL
2 tbsp	Dijon mustard	25 mL
2 tbsp	lemon juice	25 mL
Pinch	black pepper	Pinch

Salad

8 oz	yellowfin *or* other fresh tuna steak	250 g
2	medium carrots, cut into julienne strips	2
1	leek (white part only), cut into julienne strips	1
1	small red onion, cut into julienne strips	1
12	spears asparagus	12

1. *Dressing:* Whisk together oil, mustard, lemon juice and pepper; chill.
2. *Salad:* Grill or broil tuna on greased grill for 3 to 5 minutes per side or until fish flakes easily when tested with fork.
3. Steam or microwave carrots, leek, onion and asparagus just until tender.
4. To serve, divide vegetables among 4 plates. Cut tuna into 4 pieces; place on top of vegetables. Pour 1 tbsp (15 mL) dressing over each salad. Serve warm.

PER SERVING	
Calories: 193	
Dietary Fiber: 2 g	Carbohydrate: 11 g
Fat: 10 g	Protein: 16 g

TIPS

If you can't find fresh tuna, try using swordfish in this tasty salad, or frozen yellowfin tuna, which is available in some supermarkets.

Many recipes call for extra-virgin olive oil, which comes from the first pressing of the olives. This is the most expensive and flavorful of olive oils. It has gone through the least amount of processing. Use extra-virgin olive oil in this recipe, if desired.

DIETITIAN'S MESSAGE

This is a lovely salad, especially when locally grown asparagus is available. Tuna is a lean protein choice and this recipe can be served as a side salad followed by a lighter main meal, or as a meal on its own.

Salmon, Potato and Green Bean Salad

1 lb	small new white potatoes, halved *or* quartered	500 g
1 cup	green beans, cut into 2-inch (5 cm) pieces	250 mL
1	green onion, chopped	1
1 cup	halved cherry tomatoes *or* diced tomatoes	250 mL
2 tbsp	chopped fresh basil (*or* 1 tsp/5 mL dried)	25 mL
⅓ cup	bottled oil-and-vinegar-type dressing	75 mL
2	cans (each 7½ oz/213 g) salmon, drained, bones and skin removed	2
	Salt and black pepper	

1. In a medium saucepan, gently boil potatoes for 10 to 15 minutes or until tender but firm, adding beans during last 4 minutes of cooking time. Drain and transfer vegetables to a large bowl.

2. Add green onion, tomatoes and basil. Add dressing; toss gently to combine. Gently stir in salmon. Season with salt and pepper to taste. Chill until serving.

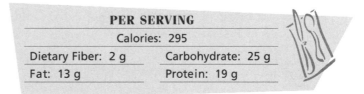

PER SERVING	
Calories: 295	
Dietary Fiber: 2 g	Carbohydrate: 25 g
Fat: 13 g	Protein: 19 g

WHAT'S SPECIAL ABOUT SPECIALTY OILS?
Used in small quantities, specialty oils such as extra-virgin olive oil, walnut oil and sesame oil add distinctive flavors to food.

   If these specialty oils are used in salad dressings, a smaller amount is needed since they enhance the flavor of dressing. Beware: this distinction carries a price tag; these oils are more expensive. And they are not recommended for use in highly seasoned recipes or where their special flavors will be hidden.

Salads

Super Salmon Salad

1 cup	colored fusilli, cooked and drained	250 mL
1½ cups	frozen peas, thawed and drained	375 mL
¼ cup	diced Swiss cheese	50 mL
1	can (3.75 oz/106 g) red salmon, drained and broken into chunks	1
½ cup	grated carrot	125 mL
½ cup	light creamy cucumber dressing	125 mL
	Spinach leaves, stems removed	

1. Combine ingredients except spinach, and toss. Refrigerate, covered. Serve on spinach-lined plates.

PER SERVING

Calories: 286

Dietary Fiber: 3 g	Carbohydrate: 34 g
Fat: 10 g	Protein: 14 g

SERVES 4

Kraft Canada, Inc.

Served on a bed of spinach leaves, this main-course salad is very eye-catching.

DIETITIAN'S MESSAGE

All 4 food groups are represented in this great-tasting and visually appealing salad. Complement it with pumpernickel bread and complete the meal with Buttermilk Oat-Branana Cake (see recipe, page 412).

Smoked Turkey Toss

¼ cup	extra-virgin olive oil	50 mL
2 tbsp	balsamic vinegar	25 mL
1 tbsp	chopped fresh parsley	15 mL
1 tsp	each liquid honey and dried basil	5 mL
Pinch	each salt and black pepper	Pinch
8 cups	thinly sliced romaine lettuce	2 L
4 oz	thinly sliced smoked *or* cooked turkey breast, cut into strips	125 g
4 oz	part-skim mozzarella cheese, cut into cubes	125 g

1. In a small bowl or measuring cup, mix together oil, vinegar, parsley, honey, basil, salt and pepper. Chill.
2. In a large bowl, toss remaining ingredients. Cover and chill. Add dressing and toss.

PER SERVING

Calories: 178

Dietary Fiber: 1 g	Carbohydrate: 4 g
Fat: 14 g	Protein: 10 g

SERVES 6 AS A SIDE SALAD

Alfred Fan, Chef
Leah Hawirko, Dietitian

For best results, make this tasty salad in the summer when fresh basil is abundant, using 1 tbsp (15 mL) chopped fresh basil instead of the dried.

TIP

For variety, replace the romaine lettuce with shredded spinach or red leaf lettuce, or use a combination of lettuces.

DIETITIAN'S MESSAGE

This tasty salad is a good source of protein. To ensure that cheese is lower-fat, look for 20% or less milk fat (M.F.).

SERVES 4
....

Rainer Schindler, Chef
Monica Stanton,
Dietitian

Try this nutritious salad if your taste buds need a little awakening. It is almost a meal in itself.

TIPS

Both black-eyed peas and black beans, popular in Southern-style recipes, are available canned in many supermarkets, as are several brands of Cajun seasoning.

If desired, replace the canned legumes with 1 cup (250 mL) dried black-eyed peas or black beans soaked, cooked, drained and rinsed.

Instead of watercress, use 2 cups (500 mL) shredded spinach or romaine lettuce, if desired.

DIETITIAN'S MESSAGE

This recipe delivers a whopping 7 g of dietary fiber thanks to the legumes (black-eyed peas or black beans), which are a good source of vegetable protein and fiber.

Black-Eyed Pea Salad with Cajun Chicken

1	can (14 oz/398 mL) black-eyed peas *or* black beans	1
3	green onions, chopped	3
1	small bunch watercress	1
1	medium carrot, grated	1
1	medium apple (unpeeled), cored and cubed	1
2/3 cup	bottled no-fat vinaigrette	150 mL
8 oz	boneless skinless chicken breasts	250 g
1 tsp	olive oil	5 mL
1 to 2 tsp	Cajun seasoning	5 to 10 mL
	Russian rye bread (optional)	

1. Drain and rinse peas. In a bowl, combine peas, green onions, watercress, carrot and apple; toss with dressing. Cover and chill for 30 minutes.

2. Slice chicken breasts lengthwise into 8 thin strips. Coat with oil and Cajun seasoning. In a hot skillet, cook chicken until browned and no longer pink inside, about 5 minutes. Serve with salad, and bread, if desired.

PER SERVING	
Calories: 211	
Dietary Fiber: 7 g	Carbohydrate: 27 g
Fat: 3 g	Protein: 21 g

Warm Chicken Salad with Fruit

SERVES 4

Dean Mitchell, Chef
Suzanne Journault-Hemstock, Dietitian

Here it is: a salad dressing with no fat! Use any fresh fruit in this delicious and eye-appealing salad.

TIP

For variety, replace one of the lettuces in this recipe with shredded spinach or red leaf lettuce. Vary the lettuce and the fruit to create a different salad every time you make this recipe.

DIETITIAN'S MESSAGE

Here's a fruit-based no-fat salad dressing that tastes delicious.

Dressing

1 cup	fresh *or* thawed frozen unsweetened raspberries	250 mL
½ tsp	grated orange zest	2 mL
¼ cup	orange juice	50 mL
1 tsp	grated lemon zest	5 mL
1 tbsp	lemon juice	15 mL
1 tbsp	chopped fresh mint	15 mL
1 tsp	liquid honey	5 mL
¼ tsp	salt	1 mL

Salad

4	boneless skinless chicken breasts (3 oz/90 g each)	4
½	each head butter *or* Boston lettuce and romaine	½
½	medium cantaloupe, peeled	½
2 cups	strawberries, hulled and halved	500 mL
1 cup	blueberries *or* blackberries	250 mL

1. *Dressing:* In a food processor or blender, purée raspberries; press through sieve to remove seeds and return to food processor. Add orange zest and juice, lemon zest and juice, mint, honey and salt; process until well blended. Pour into jar; refrigerate for up to 24 hours. Shake well before serving.

2. *Salad:* Broil or barbecue chicken until no longer pink inside. Cut into strips.

3. Meanwhile, tear lettuce and romaine into bite-size pieces; arrange on 4 large plates. Slice cantaloupe into 8 wedges; cut wedges in half crosswise. Arrange on greens along with strawberries and blueberries. Place chicken on top. Drizzle with dressing. Serve immediately.

PER SERVING	
Calories: 192	
Dietary Fiber: 4 g	Carbohydrate: 23 g
Fat: 2 g	Protein: 22 g

This tasty salad is a great way to use leftover chicken. Serve as a main course for a light summer meal.

TIP

Try a variety of other fruits in this salad, such as pineapple or kiwi fruit. Replace the safflower oil with olive oil, if you prefer.

DIETITIAN'S MESSAGE

Vitamin C is plentiful in this tasty salad. Make it the centerpiece of a healthy meal by serving with Healthy Cheese 'n' Herb Bread (see recipe, page 40) and end the meal with frozen yogurt to feature all the food groups.

West Coast Chicken Salad

Dressing

¼ cup	vinegar	50 mL
3 tbsp	liquid honey	45 mL
2 tbsp	lime juice	25 mL
1 tsp	poppy seeds	5 mL
¼ tsp	dry mustard	1 mL
½ cup	safflower oil	125 mL

Salad

3½ cups	cubed cooked chicken	875 mL
	Lettuce leaves	
½	honeydew melon, peeled and cut into wedges *or* balls	½
1	small cantaloupe, peeled and cut into wedges *or* balls	1
1¼ cups	sliced strawberries	300 mL
1 cup	green grapes	250 mL
½ cup	blueberries	125 mL

1. *Dressing:* Whisk together vinegar, honey, lime juice, poppy seeds and dry mustard. Gradually whisk in oil.

2. *Salad:* Place chicken in large bowl. Pour all but ⅓ cup (75 mL) of the dressing over chicken, tossing to mix; reserve remaining dressing. Cover and refrigerate chicken for 1 hour.

3. To serve, arrange lettuce, honeydew and cantaloupe on 6 chilled plates. Spoon chicken mixture into center of each. Toss remaining dressing with strawberries, grapes and blueberries. Spoon fruit mixture on each salad.

PER SERVING	
Calories: 426	
Dietary Fiber: 2 g	Carbohydrate: 31 g
Fat: 24 g	Protein: 24 g

10 pts

Warm Thai Chicken Salad

Marinade

1 cup	lower-fat plain yogurt	250 mL
¼ cup	skim milk	50 mL
1 tbsp	chopped fresh cilantro	15 mL
1 tsp	each curry powder and ground ginger	5 mL
1 tsp	lemon juice	5 mL
	Black pepper to taste	

Salad

6	boneless skinless chicken breasts (about 1½ lb/750 g)	6
6	medium red-skinned potatoes, cooked and quartered	6
6 cups	mixed torn salad greens	1.5 L

Peanut Dressing

⅓ cup	chicken broth	75 mL
¼ cup	light peanut butter	50 mL
¼ cup	sliced green onions	50 mL
3 tbsp	rice vinegar	45 mL
2 tbsp	sesame oil	25 mL
2 tbsp	grated ginger root	25 mL
1 tbsp	each sherry and soy sauce	15 mL
1 tbsp	granulated sugar	15 mL
1	clove garlic, minced	1
¼ tsp	salt	1 mL

1. *Marinade:* In a shallow glass dish, combine ingredients. Add chicken and turn to coat. Cover and refrigerate overnight.

2. *Peanut Dressing:* In a food processor or blender, process ingredients until smooth. Pour into jar; cover and refrigerate.

3. *Salad:* Remove chicken from marinade; grill or broil until no longer pink, adding potatoes for last 6 to 8 minutes.

4. Slice chicken crosswise into strips. Arrange greens on 6 plates; top with chicken and potatoes. Drizzle with dressing.

PER SERVING

Calories: 399	
Dietary Fiber: 4 g	Carbohydrate: 42 g
Fat: 11 g	Protein: 35 g

SERVES 6

John Cordeaux, Chef
Kim Arrey, Dietitian

This delicious salad, which borrows flavorings from Thai cuisine, is partially made the day before, then grilled. Garnish the plates with red onion rings, green onions and cherry tomatoes if desired.

TIP

Always wash your hands, cutting boards, dishes and utensils with hot, soapy water after they come in contact with raw meat, poultry or seafood. To ensure the utmost in food safety, sanitize cutting boards by rinsing in a light bleach solution.

DIETITIAN'S MESSAGE

To increase the nutrient value of this salad, use a variety of salad greens, such as dandelion, spinach or beet greens. Or try mesclun mix, which is available in most supermarkets. Remember, the greener the leaves, the more nutrients they contain. The combination of chicken and peanut butter makes the salad rich in protein. Complete the meal with yogurt to feature all food groups.

This recipe is a great way to use up leftover chicken, but you can also use a small cooked chicken from your grocery store. Pick up a bag of ready-to-use salad greens and you're almost ready for supper.

TIPS

For a change, try substituting black beans or chickpeas for the kidney beans.

If desired, use 1 cup (250 mL) dried beans, soaked, cooked, drained and rinsed, instead of the canned version.

DIETITIAN'S MESSAGE

This protein-rich salad has many uses. For a change, stuff it into a pita pocket or roll it up in a flour tortilla. Add Lemon Sherbet (see recipe, page 399) or Strawberry Sorbet (see recipe, page 398) for dessert.

Chicken and Bean Salad

1	can (14 oz/398 mL) kidney beans, drained and rinsed	1
1 cup	corn kernels, canned *or* frozen	250 mL
1 cup	cubed cooked chicken	250 mL
¾ cup	diced red bell peppers	175 mL
2	green onions, chopped	2
¼ cup	red wine vinegar	50 mL
2 tbsp	vegetable oil	25 mL
½ tsp	minced garlic	2 mL
¼ tsp	salt	1 mL
¼ tsp	black pepper	1 mL
¼ to ½ tsp	hot pepper sauce (optional)	1 to 2 mL

1. In a medium bowl, combine beans, corn, chicken, peppers, onions, vinegar, oil, garlic, salt, pepper and, if using, hot pepper sauce. Toss gently until combined. Chill before serving.

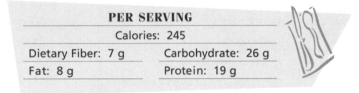

PER SERVING	
Calories: 245	
Dietary Fiber: 7 g	Carbohydrate: 26 g
Fat: 8 g	Protein: 19 g

QUICK MARINATED BEAN SALAD
This salad is great with burgers of any kind. It contains only 1.7 g fat and a whopping 10.2 g fiber per 1-cup (250 mL) serving. Cook 2 cups (500 mL) frozen cut green beans (or fresh, in season) until tender; drain and place in serving bowl. Add 1 can (19 oz/540 mL) marinated bean salad (with liquid), ½ cup (125 mL) sliced red onion, 1 tbsp (15 mL) red wine vinegar, and a little granulated sugar and pepper to taste. Toss.

Vietnamese Chicken and Rice Noodle Salad

SERVES 6
Makes about 8 cups (2 L)
....
Gaitree Peters

3½ oz	wide rice noodles (half a 7-oz/210 g pkg)	99 g
12 oz	shredded cooked chicken	375 g
2 cups	diced cucumbers	500 mL
2 cups	grated carrots	500 mL
1 cup	julienned green bell peppers	250 mL
¼ cup	finely chopped fresh cilantro	50 mL

Dressing

⅓ cup	fish sauce *or* sodium-reduced soy sauce	75 mL
¼ cup	rice wine vinegar	50 mL
2 tbsp	lime juice	25 mL
1 to 2 tbsp	curry paste	15 to 25 mL
2 tsp	granulated sugar	10 mL
1 tsp	minced garlic	5 mL
1 tsp	sesame oil	5 mL
½ cup	chopped peanuts (optional)	125 mL

1. In a large pot of boiling water, cook noodles for 5 to 8 minutes or until barely tender; drain. Rinse under cold water; drain. Transfer to a large bowl. Add chicken, cucumbers, carrots, peppers and cilantro.

2. *Dressing:* In a small bowl, blend together fish sauce, vinegar, lime juice, curry paste, sugar, garlic and sesame oil. Add dressing to noodle mixture; toss to combine. Sprinkle with peanuts, if using.

Here's a tasty salad that capitalizes on 2 culinary trends: Vietnamese food and noodles.

TIP

Vietnamese fish sauce (nuoc mam) is an integral part of Vietnamese cooking. It is a clear, pungent liquid made by fermenting fish with salt. It takes a little getting used to but it is a great flavor enhancer in many dishes. Fish sauce is high in sodium, so use it sparingly. Find it and curry paste in the Asian sections of some supermarkets.

DIETITIAN'S MESSAGE

Rice noodles are an excellent alternative to pasta for people who do not include gluten in their diets. Serve this tasty salad with fruit-flavored yogurt to increase your intake of calcium.

PER SERVING	
Calories: 214	
Dietary Fiber: 2 g	Carbohydrate: 23 g
Fat: 5 g	Protein: 19 g

**John Scott, Chef
Suzanne Journault-
Hemstock, Dietitian**

*This recipe combines
strawberries with mango
and cucumber on top of
crisp salad greens. For an
added flourish, garnish
each plate with a mint leaf
and sliced strawberries.*

TIP

When chopping fresh
herbs, make sure they
are well dried and use
a sharp knife to ensure
clean edges.

DIETITIAN'S MESSAGE

Serve this elegant salad
following a substantial
meal such as Roast Lamb
Loin with Tomato Basil
Linguine (see recipe,
page 206) or Stuffed
Pasta Shells (see recipe,
page 192) and skip
dessert, if you are
so inclined.

Mango, Strawberry and Cucumber Salad

Vinaigrette

⅓ cup	rice wine vinegar	75 mL
3 tbsp	walnut *or* olive oil	45 mL
1 tbsp	granulated sugar	15 mL
1½ tsp	coarsely chopped fresh mint	7 mL
¼ tsp	each salt and black pepper	1 mL

Salad

2 cups	strawberries, sliced	500 mL
1	medium English cucumber, cut into ¼-inch (5 mm) cubes (about 4 cups/1 L)	1
1	large mango, peeled and cut into ¼-inch (5 mm) cubes (about ½ lb/250 g)	1
8 cups	mixed torn greens	2 L

1. *Vinaigrette:* In a large bowl, whisk together vinegar, oil, sugar, mint, salt and pepper. Add strawberries, cucumber and mango; toss gently.

2. *Salad:* Divide greens among 8 plates. Top with strawberry mixture.

PER SERVING	
Calories: 97	
Dietary Fiber: 3 g	Carbohydrate: 12 g
Fat: 6 g	Protein: 2 g

Mandarin Orange Salad with Almonds

8 cups	torn romaine lettuce leaves	2 L
½ cup	sliced celery	125 mL
2	green onions, chopped	2
1	can (10 oz/284 mL) mandarin orange segments, drained	1

Dressing

2 tbsp	vinegar	25 mL
4 tsp	olive oil	20 mL
1 tbsp	chopped fresh parsley (*or* 1 tsp/5 mL dried)	15 mL
2 tsp	granulated sugar	10 mL
¼ tsp	hot pepper sauce	1 mL
¼ tsp	salt	1 mL
	Black pepper	
	Candied almonds (see instructions, below)	

1. In a large bowl, combine lettuce, celery, onions and mandarin oranges. Set aside.
2. *Dressing:* In a small bowl, whisk together vinegar, oil, parsley, sugar, hot pepper sauce and salt. Season with pepper to taste. Pour over salad; toss to coat. Serve sprinkled with candied almonds.

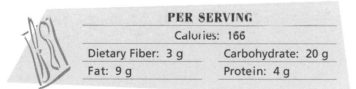

PER SERVING

Calories: 166

Dietary Fiber: 3 g	Carbohydrate: 20 g
Fat: 9 g	Protein: 4 g

TO MAKE CANDIED ALMONDS

In a small nonstick skillet, melt 1 tbsp (15 mL) granulated sugar over low heat. Add ¼ cup (50 mL) slivered almonds and cook, stirring constantly, for 5 to 6 minutes or until almonds are well coated with syrup and lightly browned. Cool; break apart into small pieces.

SERVES 4 **P**

Evelyn Witt

Evelyn serves this salad as part of an Eastern brunch — to rave reviews. But you can serve it at any time, since all of the ingredients are readily available throughout the year.

TIPS

Don't have time to wash salad greens? Plan ahead: instead of washing only the greens you need, wash a whole head of lettuce or a bag of spinach. Toss in a salad spinner to remove extra moisture. Store lettuce in the salad spinner or wrapped in paper towels in a plastic bag until needed.

If desired, replace the canned mandarin orange segments with 2 medium oranges, peeled and sectioned, or 1 cup (250 mL) sliced strawberries in season.

DIETITIAN'S MESSAGE

This salad is a great source of vitamin A, vitamin C and folic acid. Serve with Tuna and Rice Casserole (see recipe, page 222), Brie-Stuffed Breast of Chicken (see recipe, page 276) or Barbecued Stuffed Salmon (see recipe, page 309).

Orange Mushroom Salad

1 tsp	vegetable oil	5 mL
¼ cup	diced onion	50 mL
⅓ cup	frozen orange juice concentrate, thawed	75 mL
¼ cup	lower-fat plain yogurt	50 mL
1 tsp	lemon juice	5 mL
¼ tsp	salt	1 mL
2 cups	quartered fresh mushrooms	500 mL
2	medium oranges	2
	Chopped green onions (optional)	

1. In a small skillet, heat oil over medium heat; cook onion, stirring, for 3 minutes or until tender.

2. In a bowl, combine orange juice concentrate, yogurt, lemon juice and salt; stir in onions. Add mushrooms and toss to coat. Peel oranges and slice thinly crosswise; arrange on 4 salad plates. Top with mushroom mixture. Garnish with green onions, if desired. Serve immediately.

PER SERVING	
Calories: 98	
Dietary Fiber: 2 g	Carbohydrate: 20 g
Fat: 2 g	Protein: 3 g

Beet, Orange and Jicama Salad

SERVES 6
**Makes 3 cups
(750 mL)**
....
Bev Callaghan, Dietitian

1	can (14 oz/398 mL) sliced beets, drained	1
2	large navel oranges, peeled and cut into ¼-inch (5 mm) slices	2
½ cup	thinly sliced sweet white onion	125 mL
½ cup	julienned jicama	125 mL
Dressing		
2 tbsp	balsamic vinegar	25 mL
1 tbsp	orange juice	15 mL
1 tbsp	olive oil	15 mL
⅛ tsp	salt	0.5 mL
	Black pepper to taste	
1 tbsp	chopped fresh parsley (optional)	15 mL

1. In a medium bowl, combine beets, oranges, onion and jicama. Set aside.

2. *Dressing:* In a small bowl, whisk together vinegar, orange juice, olive oil, salt and pepper. Add to beet mixture; toss gently. Chill. Sprinkle with parsley, if using, just before serving.

PER SERVING	
Calories: 71	
Dietary Fiber: 3 g	Carbohydrate: 12 g
Fat: 2 g	Protein: 1 g

Jicama is a crunchy, slightly sweet vegetable that tastes like a cross between a water chestnut and an apple. It adds a delicious crunch to this salad. If you can't find it at your supermarket, substitute an equal quantity of fresh fennel.

DIETITIAN'S MESSAGE

Broaden your culinary horizons — and your nutrient intake — by trying a new vegetable each week. How about jicama, celeriac, rapini, kohlrabi or Swiss chard?

Quick and simple to prepare, this salad can be served with cold or barbecued meats. For a change, replace peach yogurt with other fruit-flavored yogurts.

TIP

Walnuts contain anthocyanins that cause blue discoloration in some foods. Roasting walnuts prior to use prevents discoloration. Spread walnuts in a single layer on a baking sheet and roast in 350°F (180°C) oven for about 7 minutes, stirring or shaking the pan once or twice, or until lightly browned.

DIETITIAN'S MESSAGE

This moist and delicious salad provides fiber and vitamin A, while the yogurt dressing keeps the fat content low.

Carrot and Orange Salad

1½ cups	grated carrot	375 mL
½ cup	orange sections	125 mL
½ cup	raisins	125 mL
⅓ cup	coarsely chopped walnuts	75 mL
¼ cup	lower-fat peach yogurt	50 mL
1 tsp	lemon juice	5 mL
1 tsp	granulated sugar	5 mL
¼ tsp	salt	1 mL
	Lettuce leaves	

1. In a medium bowl, combine carrot and orange sections. Pour boiling water over raisins to cover. Let stand for 5 minutes and drain; add to carrot mixture. Stir in walnuts, yogurt, lemon juice, sugar and salt. To serve, spoon onto lettuce leaves.

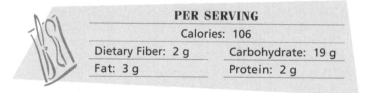

PER SERVING	
Calories: 106	
Dietary Fiber: 2 g	Carbohydrate: 19 g
Fat: 3 g	Protein: 2 g

ORANGE SALAD
Lidia Lingini says her family can't get enough of this delicious salad. Try it as an afternoon snack on a warm summer day. Peel and separate 2 to 3 large thick-skinned oranges. Cut each segment into bite-size pieces. Drizzle with a little olive oil and balsamic vinegar. Add a pinch of salt and pepper, and toss. Serve cold.

Greens with Strawberries

4 cups	assorted lettuce, torn into bite-size pieces	1 L
½ cup	sliced red onion	125 mL
½ cup	alfalfa sprouts	125 mL
Dressing		
¼ cup	orange juice	50 mL
1 tbsp	lemon juice	15 mL
1 tbsp	chopped fresh mint	15 mL
1 tsp	granulated sugar	5 mL
½ tsp	grated orange zest	2 mL
¼ tsp	grated lemon zest	1 mL
1 cup	sliced fresh strawberries	250 mL

1. In a salad bowl, combine lettuce, onion and sprouts; cover and refrigerate.

2. *Dressing:* Combine orange and lemon juices, mint, sugar and orange and lemon zest. Pour over sliced strawberries; cover and refrigerate.

3. Just before serving, pour strawberry mixture over salad greens; toss gently.

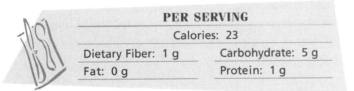

PER SERVING	
Calories: 23	
Dietary Fiber: 1 g	Carbohydrate: 5 g
Fat: 0 g	Protein: 1 g

LIMELIGHT SALAD
Chef Ralph Graham and dietitian Rosanne Maluk suggest this "zingy" dressing for a salad of mixed greens such as Boston and leaf lettuce combined with mixed bell peppers. Try adding a handful of mesclun greens for variety. In a small saucepan, melt 2 tbsp (25 mL) liquid honey with 2 tsp (10 mL) grated ginger root until honey bubbles. (Or microwave on High for 25 seconds.) Stir mixture into 1 cup (250 mL) light mayonnaise along with 3 tbsp (45 mL) lime juice and 1 tsp (5 mL) grated lime zest. Chill thoroughly. (Dressing can be refrigerated for a week.)

SERVES 6

Janice McDowell

Be creative when purchasing greens for this tasty salad. Try different combinations of red leaf lettuce, pungent arugula, peppery watercress and sharp radicchio, as well as Bibb and iceberg lettuce. Or add a handful or 2 of mesclun mix to torn romaine.

TIPS
If desired, replace the strawberries with drained canned mandarin oranges.

In addition to alfalfa and bean sprouts, growers are now sprouting more piquant varieties such as radish and mustard seeds. These sprouts have a hot flavor. Read the label on sprout packages to find the spicy sprouts, then try them in salads or even as a topping for a hot dog or hamburger. When using raw sprouts, rinse and dry thoroughly before using to ensure that any harmful bacteria don't proliferate.

DIETITIAN'S MESSAGE

The strawberries in this recipe are put to an unusual use — in the dressing. Combined with the greens, they are a great source of folic acid and vitamin C.

TIPS

When tomatoes are in season, there's no better way to enjoy them than in this simple but delicious salad with an Italian flair. If desired, substitute fresh or Buffalo mozzarella for the part-skim version, but be aware that the fat content will go up.

To ripen tomatoes, place them in a brown paper bag with an apple or a pear. These fruits give off ethylene dioxide, which causes the tomatoes to ripen.

Tomato Mozzarella Salad

Vinaigrette

¼ cup	vegetable *or* olive oil	50 mL
2 tbsp	vinegar	25 mL
1 tbsp	chopped fresh parsley	15 mL
2 tsp	Dijon mustard	10 mL
1 tsp	granulated sugar	5 mL
2	cloves garlic, minced	2
½ tsp	dried basil	2 mL
½ tsp	black pepper	2 mL
¼ tsp	salt	1 mL
2 tbsp	water	25 mL

Salad

3	large tomatoes, preferably beefsteak	3
16	romaine *or* Boston lettuce leaves	16
½ cup	cubed part-skim mozzarella cheese	125 mL
6	green onions, sliced	6

1. *Vinaigrette:* In a jar with tight-fitting lid, whisk together oil, vinegar, parsley, mustard, sugar, garlic, basil, pepper, salt and water; chill. Shake before using.

2. *Salad:* Cut tomatoes in half; cut each half crosswise into slices. Arrange 2 lettuce leaves on each of 8 salad plates. Arrange tomato slices on lettuce; sprinkle with cheese and green onion.

3. At serving time, pour vinaigrette over each salad.

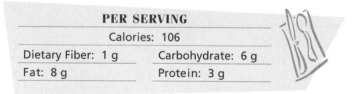

PER SERVING	
Calories: 106	
Dietary Fiber: 1 g	Carbohydrate: 6 g
Fat: 8 g	Protein: 3 g

Basil Marinated Tomatoes

4	medium tomatoes, sliced	4
¼ cup	chopped fresh parsley	50 mL
3 tbsp	olive oil	45 mL
1 tbsp	each white and red wine vinegar	15 mL
1 tbsp	chopped fresh basil	15 mL
¾ tsp	granulated sugar	4 mL
¼ tsp	each salt and black pepper	1 mL

1. Arrange tomatoes on plate. Sprinkle with parsley.
2. Whisk together remaining ingredients and pour over tomatoes. Cover and refrigerate for 1 hour.

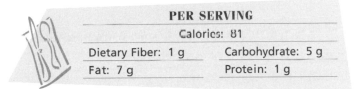

PER SERVING

Calories: 81

Dietary Fiber: 1 g	Carbohydrate: 5 g
Fat: 7 g	Protein: 1 g

SERVES 8

**Barb Armstrong, Chef
Marianna Fiocco,
Dietitian**

Mouthwatering when tomatoes are at their peak, this is a great addition to summer meals.

TIP
For a variation, add sliced fresh mozzarella or crumbled blue cheese, such as Roquefort or Gorgonzola.

DIETITIAN'S MESSAGE
Serve this tasty salad with grilled steak and baked potatoes for a delicious, easy meal.

Roasted Red Pepper Salad

6	roasted red bell peppers (see technique, page 127), each cut into 6 strips	6
1 tbsp	balsamic *or* red wine vinegar	15 mL
2 tsp	olive oil	10 mL
2 tbsp	chopped fresh basil (optional)	25 mL
	Freshly ground black pepper	

1. Arrange peppers in the bottom of a serving dish.
2. In a bowl, whisk together vinegar and olive oil; drizzle over peppers. Sprinkle with basil, if using. Season with pepper to taste. Chill for 1 hour.

PER SERVING

Calories: 48

Dietary Fiber: 2 g	Carbohydrate: 8 g
Fat: 2 g	Protein: 1 g

SERVES 6

Nikola Ajdacic

TIP
Keep roasted red peppers in your freezer and you can make this salad anytime.

DIETITIAN'S MESSAGE
Red peppers are rich in phytochemicals and antioxidants such as beta-carotene and vitamin C. This attractive salad makes a great accompaniment to Barbecued Butterflied Leg of Lamb (see recipe, page 267) or any grilled meat. To complete the meal, add couscous or rice and a milk pudding or Lemon Sherbet (see recipe, page 399).

SERVES 4
Makes 6 cups (1.5 L)
....
Jane Bellman, Dietitian

Here's a simple salad that's sure to please. It's especially good when tomatoes are in season.

TIP

If desired, substitute 1 tbsp (15 mL) chopped fresh basil for the dried.

DIETITIAN'S MESSAGE

This salad is higher in fat so it is best served with lower-fat dishes. If you don't have time to make the dressing, use a bottled oil-and-vinegar-type dressing. Choose a dressing that contains less than 3 g fat per 1 tbsp (15 mL) to help cut the fat.

Fast and Easy Greek Salad

2 cups	diced tomatoes	500 mL
2 cups	diced cucumbers	500 mL
1 cup	cubed feta cheese (about 8 oz/250 g)	250 mL
½ cup	thinly sliced onions	125 mL
¼ cup	sliced black olives (optional)	50 mL
2 tbsp	white wine vinegar	25 mL
2 tbsp	olive oil	25 mL
½ tsp	minced garlic	2 mL
½ tsp	dried basil	2 mL
½ tsp	dried oregano	2 mL
	Black pepper to taste	

1. In a large bowl, combine tomatoes, cucumbers, cheese, onions and, if using, olives. Set aside.

2. In a small bowl or measuring cup, whisk together vinegar, oil, garlic, basil, oregano and pepper. Add to tomato mixture; toss gently to combine. Chill before serving.

PER SERVING	
Calories: 177	
Dietary Fiber: 2 g	Carbohydrate: 9 g
Fat: 14 g	Protein: 6 g

Marinated Vegetable Salad

½ cup	broccoli florets	125 mL
½ cup	cauliflower florets	125 mL
½ cup	sliced carrots	125 mL
½ cup	chopped green bell pepper	125 mL
½ cup	diagonally sliced celery	125 mL
½ cup	coarsely chopped English cucumber	125 mL
¼ cup	diced red *or* Spanish onion	50 mL
1	small tomato, cut into wedges	1

Dressing

3 tbsp	vinegar	45 mL
1 tbsp	olive oil	15 mL
2 tsp	granulated sugar	10 mL
1½ tsp	dried oregano *or* tarragon	7 mL
Pinch	black pepper	Pinch

1. In a large saucepan of boiling water, blanch broccoli, cauliflower and carrots. Drain and plunge into ice water; drain again and place in medium bowl. Add green pepper, celery, cucumber and onion.

2. *Dressing:* In a small bowl or measuring cup, mix together vinegar, oil, sugar, oregano and pepper; pour over vegetables. Marinate at room temperature for 2 to 3 hours, stirring occasionally to ensure vegetables are well coated. Serve garnished with tomato wedges.

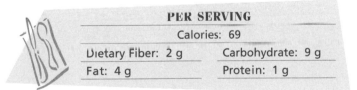

PER SERVING
Calories: 69

Dietary Fiber: 2 g	Carbohydrate: 9 g
Fat: 4 g	Protein: 1 g

HERB VINEGARS

Herb vinegars can add exciting flavors to salads and help reduce the amount of oil needed.

To make your own herb vinegar, pick herbs before they flower; bruise the leaves slightly to help release flavor. Place herbs in clean, sterilized jars. Cover with your choice of good-quality vinegar (red or white wine or rice). The best ratio is ⅔ cup (150 mL) packed fresh herbs to 1 cup (250 mL) vinegar.

Steep for about 2 weeks in a warm, dark place; shake occasionally. Strain and bottle. For a nice touch, add a fresh sprig of the herb used in each bottle. Cork and store in a cool place.

SERVES 4
....

Beth Van Arenthals, Chef
Connie Mallette, Dietitian

Here is a great winter salad to help you get your servings of vegetables. Make this salad more colorful and vary the flavor by using a variety of colored peppers and other vegetables such as snow peas or fennel, if available.

TIPS

Use specialty vinegars such as tarragon, wine, champagne or balsamic to spice up the flavor of this and any salad. Try using white wine vinegar flavored with tarragon instead of the vinegar and tarragon in this recipe.

Blanching enhances the colors of vegetables while maintaining their raw texture. To blanch vegetables, drop them into boiling water. Return to a boil and cook for 2 minutes. Drain and plunge into ice water.

DIETITIAN'S MESSAGE

This medley of vegetables has everything going for it — color, flavor, texture and taste. It is a great way to serve vegetables to your family and guests because you can make it ahead.

Julius Pokomandy, Chef
Leah Hawirko, Dietitian

This simple salad combines fall vegetables with apples tossed in a creamy mustard dressing.

TIP
To vary the taste and appearance of this salad, experiment with the wide selection of apples now available, such as Mutsu, Granny Smith, or even some of the older varieties now being produced by growers.

DIETITIAN'S MESSAGE
This salad is a great way to serve vegetables in winter months. For a great cold-weather dinner, serve with Slow-Cooked Beef Stew (see recipe, page 239) or Almond Chicken Dinner (see recipe, page 294) and finish with Lemon Pudding (see recipe, page 425).

Dilled Winter Salad

3	medium carrots	3
2	medium potatoes, peeled if desired	2
1	medium parsnip	1
¾ cup	frozen peas	175 mL
⅔ cup	diced dill pickle	150 mL
1	medium apple (unpeeled), diced	1
⅓ cup	light mayonnaise	75 mL
⅓ cup	lower-fat plain yogurt	75 mL
2 tbsp	honey mustard	25 mL
¼ tsp	each salt and black pepper	1 mL
	Orange slices	
	Toasted slivered almonds (see technique, page 389)	

1. Dice carrots, potatoes and parsnip into ½-inch (1 cm) cubes. In a saucepan of boiling water or in microwave, cook individually just until tender; drain well. Pour hot water over peas just to thaw; drain well.

2. In a large bowl, combine carrots, potatoes, parsnip, peas, pickle, apple, mayonnaise, yogurt, honey mustard, salt and pepper; cover and refrigerate for about 8 hours before serving. Garnish with orange slices and almonds.

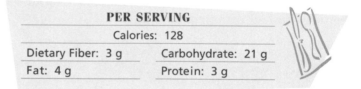

PER SERVING	
Calories: 128	
Dietary Fiber: 3 g	Carbohydrate: 21 g
Fat: 4 g	Protein: 3 g

Winter Vegetable Salad

½ lb	parsnips, cut into ½-inch (1 cm) chunks	250 g
½ lb	carrots, cut into ½-inch (1 cm) chunks	250 g
2	stalks celery, sliced	2
½	small red onion, chopped	½
½ cup	raisins	125 mL
Dressing		
¼ cup	lower-fat plain yogurt	50 mL
1 tbsp	cider vinegar	15 mL
1 tbsp	chili sauce	15 mL
1 tsp	horseradish	5 mL
Pinch	salt	Pinch

1. Steam parsnips and carrots over boiling water until tender-crisp. Rinse under cold water and drain well.

2. In a medium bowl, combine parsnips, carrots, celery, red onion and raisins.

3. *Dressing:* Combine yogurt, vinegar, chili sauce, horseradish and salt. Pour dressing over vegetables; mix until well coated. Cover and refrigerate for at least 1 hour.

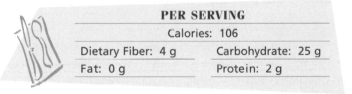

PER SERVING	
Calories: 106	
Dietary Fiber: 4 g	Carbohydrate: 25 g
Fat: 0 g	Protein: 2 g

COTTAGE CHEESE SALAD
Dietitian Susan Close has another great idea for a winter salad that is loaded in protein. Combine 1½ cups (375 mL) 2% cottage cheese, ¾ cup (175 mL) diced English cucumber, ½ cup (125 mL) each grated carrot and zucchini, 1 green onion, chopped, 2 tsp (10 mL) Dijon mustard and ¼ tsp (1 mL) Worcestershire sauce. Serve as a main-course salad on lettuce leaves or as a sandwich filling in a pita pocket, or use as a stuffing for hollowed-out tomatoes.

SERVES 6
....
Betty Jane Humphrey

During the winter months, imported salad greens are often expensive and not of the best quality. This simple alternative to a green salad is easily made from winter vegetables you're likely to have on hand.

TIP
For variety, replace the carrots with sweet potatoes. Substitute chopped dried apricots or dried cranberries for the raisins.

DIETITIAN'S MESSAGE
This unusual salad adds interest to winter vegetables. Dried fruits are a concentrated source of nutrients. A quarter of a cup (50 mL) raisins is the same as 1 serving from the Vegetables and Fruit group.

Cool Cucumber Salad

3 cups	thinly sliced English cucumber unpeeled, about 1 large	750 mL
½ tsp	salt	2 mL
½ cup	yogurt cheese (see technique, below)	125 mL
½ tsp	lemon juice	2 mL
¼ tsp	minced garlic	1 mL
¼ tsp	ground ginger	1 mL

1. Place cucumber slices in a large colander; sprinkle with salt. Let stand for 10 to 15 minutes over a large bowl (or in the sink) to drain. Rinse well under cold water. Pat dry and transfer to a bowl. Set aside.

2. In a separate bowl, blend together yogurt cheese, lemon juice, garlic and ginger. Add mixture to cucumber; toss gently. Chill before serving.

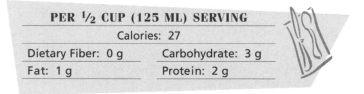

PER ½ CUP (125 ML) SERVING	
Calories: 27	
Dietary Fiber: 0 g	Carbohydrate: 3 g
Fat: 1 g	Protein: 2 g

TO MAKE 1 CUP (250 ML) YOGURT CHEESE
Use 2 cups (500 mL) lower-fat plain yogurt (Balkan-style, not stirred, made without gelatin). Line a sieve with a double thickness of paper towel or cheesecloth. Pour yogurt into the sieve and place over a bowl. Cover well with plastic wrap and refrigerate for at least 2 hours. Discard liquid and keep solids in an airtight container in the refrigerator for up to 1 week.

 If you want to drain the yogurt overnight, use 3 cups (750 mL) yogurt to get 1 cup (250 mL) yogurt cheese. The longer you drain the yogurt, the more tart it becomes.

Raita Cucumber Salad

1	medium English cucumber, thinly sliced	1
1	large tomato, diced	1
1	medium onion, thinly sliced	1
2½ cups	lower-fat plain yogurt	625 mL
1 tbsp	chopped fresh parsley	15 mL
¾ tsp	ground cumin	4 mL
½ tsp	each ground coriander and salt	2 mL
½ tsp	each grated lemon zest and orange zest	2 mL
¼ tsp	hot pepper sauce	1 mL
Pinch	each paprika and black pepper	Pinch

1. In a bowl, combine vegetables. Whisk remaining ingredients together and toss with vegetables. Cover and chill thoroughly.

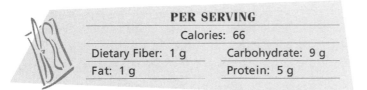

PER SERVING	
Calories: 66	
Dietary Fiber: 1 g	Carbohydrate: 9 g
Fat: 1 g	Protein: 5 g

SERVES 8

**Robert Neil, Chef
Denise Hargrove, Dietitian**

Coriander and cumin are traditionally used in both Middle Eastern and Mexican cuisines. This refreshing salad cools the palate and goes especially well with spicy ethnic dishes such as curries.

TIP
If you prefer a salad with milder flavor, omit the hot pepper sauce.

DIETITIAN'S MESSAGE
The quantity of lower-fat yogurt in this soothing salad will boost your calcium intake.

Heart to Heart Salad

3 tbsp	extra-virgin olive oil	45 mL
1 tbsp	lemon juice	15 mL
1 tbsp	finely diced red or green onion	15 mL
½ tsp	crushed dried thyme	2 mL
1	can (14 oz/398 mL) artichoke hearts, drained and quartered	1
1 tbsp	shredded Gruyère *or* grated Sbrinz cheese	15 mL
1 tbsp	finely chopped fresh parsley	15 mL

1. In a bowl, combine first 4 ingredients. Add artichokes and stir to coat. Cover and chill thoroughly.
2. To serve, sprinkle with cheese and parsley.

PER SERVING	
Calories: 84	
Dietary Fiber: 3 g	Carbohydrate: 7 g
Fat: 6 g	Protein: 3 g

SERVES 4

**Leo Pantel, Chef
Patti Neuman, Dietitian**

Although it takes only minutes to make this salad, for best results marinate overnight.

DIETITIAN'S MESSAGE
Mixing your own salad dressings allows you to control the amount and type of oil used and is less expensive than using store-bought dressings.

SERVES 6

Donna Nadolny, Dietitian

Not only is a vinaigrette-dressed potato salad a refreshing change from the traditional mayonnaise-dressed one, but coarse grainy mustard and tarragon give this old favorite a new and tangy twist.

TIPS

Add sliced radishes just before serving this salad as vinegar removes color from radish skin.

If you have tarragon growing in your garden or on your windowsill, substitute 1 tbsp (15 mL) finely chopped for the dried.

DIETITIAN'S MESSAGE

Cooking potatoes with their skins on preserves nutrients that are close to the skin and helps potatoes to keep their shape. This salad is a lower-fat version of traditional potato salad. The dressing keeps the fat content low. Serve with Italian Broiled Tomatoes (see recipe, page 349) as an accompaniment to Cedar-Baked Salmon (see recipe, page 305). To make the meal a celebration, finish with Light Tiramisu (see recipe, page 422).

Tangy Potato Salad

3	large potatoes (unpeeled)	3
2 tbsp	red wine vinegar	25 mL
1 tbsp	vegetable oil	15 mL
1	small clove garlic, minced	1
2 tsp	dried tarragon	10 mL
1 tsp	coarse grainy mustard	5 mL
½ tsp	horseradish	2 mL
¼ tsp	salt	1 mL
¼ tsp	freshly ground black pepper	1 mL
½ cup	sliced celery	125 mL
¼ cup	sliced green onions	50 mL
¼ cup	chopped yellow bell pepper	50 mL
½ cup	thinly sliced radishes	125 mL
	Celery leaves	

1. Cook potatoes in boiling water until tender; drain and partially cool. Cut into cubes.

2. Whisk together vinegar, oil, garlic and seasonings. Pour dressing over warm potatoes. Cover and refrigerate until cool.

3. Add celery, onions and yellow pepper to potato mixture. Cover and refrigerate for at least 1 hour before serving. Add radishes and garnish with celery leaves to serve.

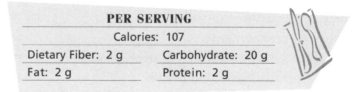

PER SERVING	
Calories: 107	
Dietary Fiber: 2 g	Carbohydrate: 20 g
Fat: 2 g	Protein: 2 g

German Picnic-Style Potato Salad

SERVES 8
Makes 8 cups (2 L)
....
Carol Ermanovics

3 lb	small red new potatoes, halved *or* quartered	1.5 kg
¼ cup	white wine vinegar	50 mL
1 tbsp	granulated sugar	15 mL
½ tsp	salt	2 mL
¼ tsp	celery seed	1 mL
¼ tsp	black pepper	1 mL
6	green onions, chopped	6
2 tbsp	chopped fresh dill (*or* 1 tsp/5 mL dried)	25 mL
¾ cup	light sour cream	175 mL
1 tsp	Dijon mustard	5 mL
4	hard-boiled eggs	4

1. In a large saucepan, gently boil potatoes for 12 to 15 minutes or until tender but firm; drain. Transfer to a large bowl.

2. In a microwave-safe measuring cup, combine vinegar, sugar, salt, celery seed and pepper. Microwave on High for 30 seconds or until very hot; pour over warm potatoes. Stir gently until vinegar is absorbed. Add onions and dill.

3. In the same measuring cup, stir together sour cream and mustard. Fold gently into potato mixture. Chill.

4. Just before serving, cut hard-boiled eggs into quarters. Place 2 quarters on each serving of salad.

PER SERVING

Calories: 196

| Dietary Fiber: 3 g | Carbohydrate: 34 g |
| Fat: 4 g | Protein: 8 g |

Here's a delicious version of an old favorite that will be a welcome addition to any get-together.

TIPS
Foods that sit out for more than 2 hours in the heat — or even at room temperature — should be discarded. In these conditions, bacteria multiply quickly, particularly on high-risk foods such as meats, dairy products, salads and sandwiches.

While the potatoes are cooking, add a large sprig of rosemary, thyme, mint or tarragon to the water to increase their flavor.

MAKE AHEAD
You can prepare the salad through Step 2 up to 1 day ahead. Chill.

DIETITIAN'S MESSAGE
This creamy potato salad contains only 4 g fat per 1-cup (250 mL) serving. Take it along on your next picnic — just be sure to keep it cold in an insulated cooler with lots of ice packs, and keep your cooler in the shade.

Marlyn Ambrose-Chase

This unusual hot cabbage salad has the spicy flavor of Indian curries. If you're fond of curry, you may want to increase the amount of curry powder.

DIETITIAN'S MESSAGE

Cabbage is not only low in calories, it is a source of vitamins A and C, as well as fiber. This delicious salad is also packed with fruit. What a great way to meet the challenge of serving salad in winter!

Hot and Spicy Fruit Slaw

1	small green cabbage	1
1/3 cup	finely chopped green onions	75 mL
1/4 cup	finely chopped celery	50 mL
3 tbsp	butter *or* margarine	45 mL
1 to 2 tsp	curry powder	5 to 10 mL
1 tsp	cornstarch	5 mL
1/4 tsp	salt	1 mL
Pinch	freshly ground black pepper	Pinch
1 cup	orange juice	250 mL
1	carrot, thinly sliced	1
1	red cooking apple, cut into wedges	1
2	oranges, peeled and sectioned	2
1/4 cup	chutney	50 mL

1. Remove 4 to 6 outer cabbage leaves; blanch in boiling water until slightly wilted, about 15 seconds. Rinse under cold water; drain well and set aside. Slice remaining cabbage into very thin strips.

2. In a large skillet over medium-high heat, cook onions and celery in butter for about 3 minutes. Stir in curry powder, cornstarch, salt and pepper; cook, stirring frequently, for 5 minutes. Stir in orange juice, sliced cabbage and carrots. Cover and bring to a boil; reduce heat and cook for 10 minutes. Add apple; cook, stirring, for about 2 minutes. Stir in oranges and chutney; heat thoroughly for about 4 minutes. Serve in large bowl lined with blanched cabbage leaves.

PER SERVING	
Calories: 161	
Dietary Fiber: 5 g	Carbohydrate: 27 g
Fat: 6 g	Protein: 2 g

Coleslaw for a Crowd

8 cups	chopped green savoy cabbage	2 L
2 cups	chopped red apples (crisp *or* tart)	500 mL
1½ cups	grated carrots	375 mL
1½ cups	chopped celery	375 mL
1 cup	chopped green bell peppers	250 mL
½ cup	chopped green onions	125 mL
⅔ cup	light mayonnaise	150 mL
1 tsp	granulated sugar	5 mL
½ tsp	salt	2 mL

1. In a very large bowl, combine cabbage, apples, carrots, celery, green peppers and green onions.

2. In a small bowl or measuring cup, blend together mayonnaise, sugar and salt. Add to cabbage mixture; toss to blend well. Chill for 2 hours or overnight. (Don't worry if salad appears to need more dressing; after chilling, the mixture becomes creamier as the vegetables give off some juice.)

PER SERVING	
Calories: 58	
Dietary Fiber: 2 g	Carbohydrate: 7 g
Fat: 3 g	Protein: 1 g

SERVES 16
Makes 12 cups (3 L)

Betty Walsh

This delicious cabbage salad is equally popular with children and adults. It's great for feeding a crowd and for potluck meals. If you don't have a crowd to feed, just cut the recipe in half.

TIP
Regular cabbage can be used in place of the savoy cabbage. For best results, chop all ingredients by hand; using a food processor will make the salad too wet and mushy.

MAKE AHEAD
You can buy the ingredients for this salad in advance and make it later in the week. Once made, the salad keeps well in the refrigerator for about 3 days.

DIETITIAN'S MESSAGE
Although cabbage has a reasonably long shelf life, it will keep better if it is uncut and unwashed. Store in the crisper drawer of your refrigerator, if possible in a vegetable storage bag with tiny holes that allow vegetables to breathe.

**SERVES 8 AS A
SIDE SALAD**
....

**Stephen Ashton, Chef
Leah Hawirko, Dietitian**

*Segments of grapefruit
with slices of red onion
are a perfect color and
taste contrast to spinach.
Prepare the dressing in
advance, then cover and
refrigerate until ready
to use.*

TIP

Unless your spinach
comes pre-washed, be
sure to wash it thoroughly
to remove all grit. Soak
in a basin of tepid water,
then rinse thoroughly
under cold running water
before using.

DIETITIAN'S MESSAGE

Spinach is high in beta-
carotene and folic acid,
while the grapefruit
provides vitamin C.
Because vitamin C helps
in the absorption of
iron, serve it with
Sesame Steak (see recipe,
page 251).

Spinach and Grapefruit Salad

2 tsp	poppy seeds	10 mL
½	red onion, thinly sliced	½
4	cloves garlic	4
3	medium red grapefruit	3
3 tbsp	olive oil	45 mL
2 tbsp	white wine vinegar	25 mL
2 tbsp	chopped fresh parsley	25 mL
1 tbsp	grainy mustard	15 mL
½ tsp	liquid honey	2 mL
½ tsp	salt	2 mL
¼ tsp	black pepper	1 mL
1	bunch spinach, washed and torn into bite-size pieces	1

1. Heat a small skillet over medium heat; toast poppy seeds for 1 to 2 minutes, stirring constantly. Remove from heat. Set aside.

2. In a small bowl, cover onion with cold water; let stand for 10 minutes, then drain. In a small saucepan, cover garlic with cold water and bring to a boil; simmer for 3 minutes, then drain. Remove skins and white pith from grapefruit; cut fruit into segments, catching juice in small bowl.

3. In a blender or food processor, combine garlic, oil, vinegar, parsley, mustard, honey, salt, pepper and 2 tbsp (25 mL) of the reserved grapefruit juice; blend until creamy.

4. In a large bowl, combine spinach, onion and grapefruit; toss with dressing. Garnish with reserved poppy seeds.

PER SERVING	
Calories: 99	
Dietary Fiber: 3 g	Carbohydrate: 12 g
Fat: 6 g	Protein: 2 g

Beet, Orange and ➤
Jicama Salad (page 145)
Overleaf: Bulgur Salad (page 168)
Tabbouleh (page 169)

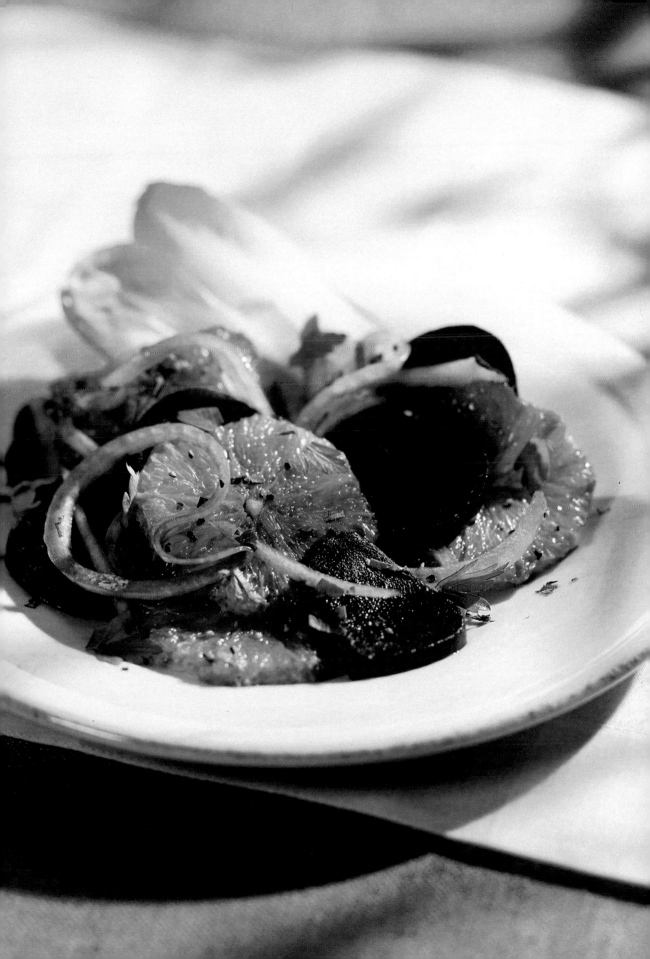

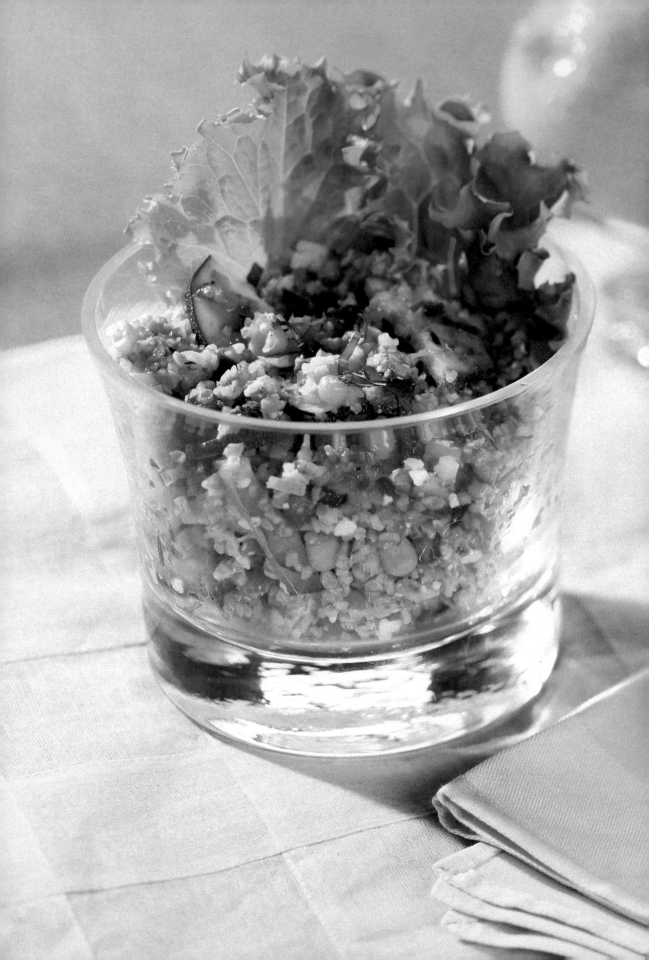

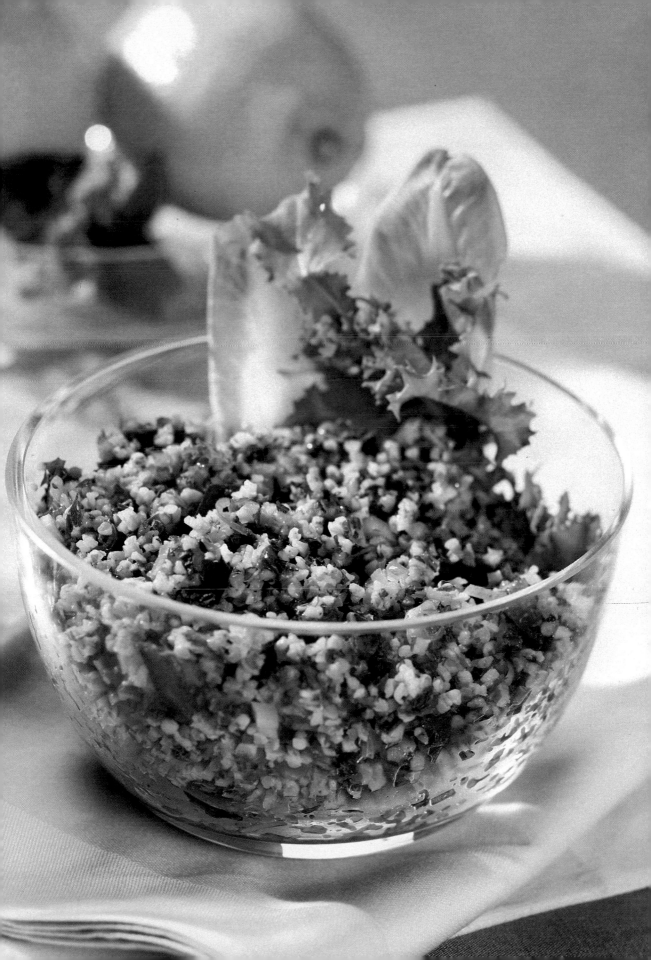

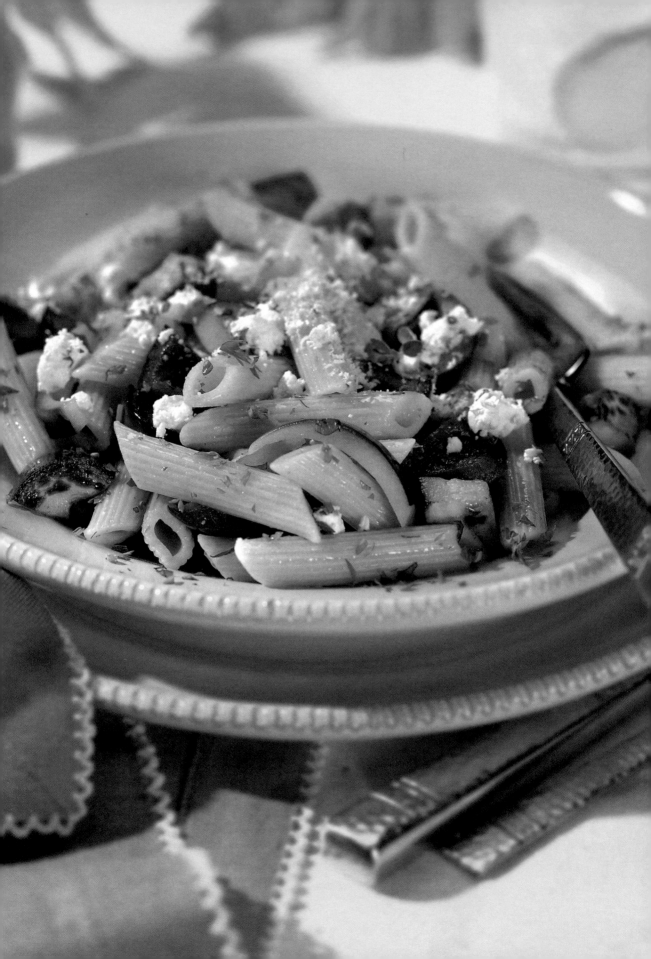

Spinach Salad with Creamy Garlic Dressing

Preheat oven to 350°F (180°C)

1	slice whole-wheat bread	1
10 cups	spinach leaves	2.5 L
1½ cups	sliced mushrooms	375 mL
¼ cup	alfalfa sprouts	50 mL
2 tbsp	grated Parmesan cheese	25 mL
Dressing		
½ cup	lower-fat plain yogurt	125 mL
¼ cup	chopped fresh parsley	50 mL
2 tbsp	light mayonnaise	25 mL
1	large clove garlic, minced	1
Pinch	each salt and black pepper	Pinch

1. Cut bread into cubes; toast in preheated oven for 5 minutes or until crisp and brown.

2. Tear spinach into bite-size pieces. In a large salad bowl, combine toasted bread cubes, spinach, mushrooms, alfalfa sprouts and Parmesan cheese.

3. *Dressing:* Combine yogurt, parsley, mayonnaise, garlic, salt and pepper. Pour dressing over vegetables; toss until well coated.

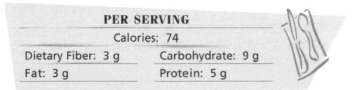

PER SERVING	
Calories: 74	
Dietary Fiber: 3 g	Carbohydrate: 9 g
Fat: 3 g	Protein: 5 g

GOLDEN TREASURE SALAD
Betty Dent suggests this delicious salad as one you can make year-round. Whisk together 1 cup (250 mL) lower-fat plain yogurt, ¼ cup (50 mL) liquid honey and 3 tbsp (45 mL) lemon juice. Toss with 2 cups (500 mL) chopped fresh broccoli, 1 cup (250 mL) grated carrots, 1 cup (250 mL) sunflower seeds, 1 cup (250 mL) raisins and 2 green onions, finely chopped. Cover and chill thoroughly.

SERVES 6

Gail P. Foster

Homemade whole-wheat croutons and yogurt dressing create a light version of this popular salad.

TIPS

For variety, try adding ½ cup (125 mL) chopped red or green bell pepper, tomatoes, red onion, apple or mandarin orange segments to the salad.

It's easy to make your own croutons, and they are a great way to use day-old bread. In a skillet over medium heat, heat 1 to 2 tbsp (15 to 25 mL) oil. Add cubes of bread and sauté until lightly browned. Croutons can be stored in an airtight container for several days.

DIETITIAN'S MESSAGE

This richly flavored salad is low in both fat and calories. For a great meal, serve with Pork Tenderloin with Roasted Potatoes (see recipe, page 263) and finish with Lemon Pudding (see recipe, page 425).

SERVES 6
Makes about 5 cups
(1.25 L)
....
Adeline White

This salad features a delicious dressing — just like the old-fashioned boiled dressings of long ago. Its flavor works particularly well with broccoli. The dressing is also terrific for coleslaw.

MAKE AHEAD
While best made on the day it is to be served, the salad and dressing can be prepared and refrigerated separately up to 1 day ahead. Toss salad with dressing just before serving.

DIETITIAN'S MESSAGE
Cruciferous vegetables such as broccoli, cauliflower, brussels sprouts and rapini are rich in antioxidant vitamins and phytochemicals. Include them often in your diet. This salad is relatively high in fat, so serve it less often.

Creamy Broccoli Salad

Salad

4½ cups	chopped broccoli (about 1 large head)	1.125 L
1 cup	quartered mushrooms	250 mL
4	slices cooked bacon, crumbled	4
½ cup	chopped red onions	125 mL
¼ cup	toasted slivered almonds (see technique, page 389)	50 mL

Dressing

1	egg	1
2 tbsp	white wine vinegar	25 mL
2 tbsp	water	25 mL
2 tbsp	granulated sugar	25 mL
½ tsp	dry mustard	2 mL
½ tsp	cornstarch	2 mL
¼ cup	light mayonnaise	50 mL

1. *Salad:* In a large pot of boiling water, blanch broccoli for no more than 2 minutes. Drain and refresh under cold water; drain again. Transfer to a large bowl. Add mushrooms, bacon, onions and almonds. Chill.

2. *Dressing:* In a microwave-safe bowl, whisk together egg, vinegar, water, sugar, mustard and cornstarch. Microwave on High for 1½ to 2 minutes, stirring at 30-second intervals. Set aside to cool. Blend in mayonnaise. Chill until ready to serve.

3. Just before serving, toss salad with dressing.

PER SERVING	
Calories: 142	
Dietary Fiber: 2 g	Carbohydrate: 12 g
Fat: 9 g	Protein: 6 g

....

SALADE À LA GOUT
Here's a great salad idea from Elaine Gimby. Make a dressing of ⅓ cup (75 mL) lower-fat plain yogurt, 1 tsp (5 mL) lemon juice, 1 tbsp (15 mL) each chopped fresh parsley, chives and dill and 1 large clove of garlic, crushed. Pour over 1 medium head of lettuce, torn into bite-size pieces, 1 can (14 oz/398 mL) drained chickpeas, 1 red bell pepper, quartered and sliced, and ¼ cup (50 mL) sunflower seeds and toss until well coated. Serve with Super Health Bread (see recipe, page 48) for a great light meal.

....

Colorful Bean and Corn Salad

Salad

1	can (19 oz/540 mL) black beans, drained and rinsed	1
1	can (12 oz/341 mL) corn kernels, drained	1
1 cup	chopped tomatoes	250 mL
½ cup	chopped green *or* red bell pepper	125 mL
½ cup	chopped red onion	125 mL
¼ cup	chopped fresh parsley	50 mL

Dressing

2 tbsp	red wine vinegar *or* balsamic vinegar	25 mL
1 tbsp	olive oil	15 mL
½ tsp	ground cumin	2 mL
½ tsp	minced garlic	2 mL
½ tsp	hot pepper sauce (optional)	2 mL
¼ tsp	salt	1 mL
	Black pepper	

1. *Salad:* In a large bowl, combine beans, corn, tomatoes, pepper, onion and parsley. Set aside.
2. *Dressing:* In a small bowl or measuring cup, whisk together vinegar, oil, cumin, garlic, hot pepper sauce, if using, salt, and pepper to taste. Blend well. Pour over salad.

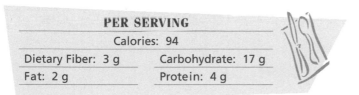

PER SERVING	
Calories: 94	
Dietary Fiber: 3 g	Carbohydrate: 17 g
Fat: 2 g	Protein: 4 g

SERVES 10
Makes 5 cups (1.25 L)

P

Mary Sue Waisman, Dietitian

Let the kids toss some crunchy tortilla chips into the salad just before serving — then watch it disappear!

TIP
If you're in a hurry, give the dressing a pass and add ½ tsp (2 mL) cumin to ¼ cup (50 mL) bottled oil-and-vinegar-type salad dressing.

DIETITIAN'S MESSAGE

This colorful salad is a premium source of folic acid and fiber. For variety, top with crumbled feta cheese and sliced black olives. For a light meal, serve with Healthy Cheese 'n' Herb Bread (see recipe, page 40) and finish with Cranberry Oatmeal Cookies (see recipe, page 432) and sherbet.

Chris Klugman, Chef
Susie Langley, Dietitian

Beans are extremely versatile as they pick up the flavor of herbs and spices in recipes. This zesty salad has a deliciously Eastern flair.

TIPS

Smoking the dried spices — heating them in a pan without oil — intensifies their flavor.

If desired, substitute 1 cup (250 mL) dried beans, cooked and drained, for the canned version.

DIETITIAN'S MESSAGE

Beans are loaded with nutrition and fiber. Although the nutritional benefits vary, all are a rich source of B vitamins, calcium, iron, phosphorous, potassium and zinc. They are also high in folic acid, a B vitamin that plays a role in cell formation. Women of childbearing age should increase their intake through healthy food choices.

Spicy Bean Salad

2 tsp	ground cumin	10 mL
1 tsp	curry powder	5 mL
1	can (14 oz/398 mL) kidney beans, drained and rinsed	1
½	medium Spanish *or* red onion, diced	½
2	tomatoes, chopped	2
2	stalks celery, chopped	2
2	green onions, sliced	2
2 tbsp	lime juice	25 mL
1 tbsp	olive oil	15 mL
¼ cup	chopped fresh cilantro	50 mL

1. In a dry skillet, heat cumin and curry powder over high heat until fragrant. Remove from heat and set aside.

2. In a large bowl, combine vegetables.

3. Mix lime juice and olive oil with roasted spices; pour over bean mixture. Stir in cilantro. Cover and chill thoroughly.

PER SERVING	
Calories: 105	
Dietary Fiber: 6 g	Carbohydrate: 16 g
Fat: 3 g	Protein: 5 g

Triple-Bean Salad with Rice and Artichokes

2 cups	cooked rice *or* quinoa	500 mL
1	can (19 oz/540 mL) marinated bean salad, with liquid	1
1	can (14 oz/398 mL) artichoke hearts, drained and diced	1
1 cup	diced seeded plum tomatoes	250 mL
4	green onions, chopped	4
¼ cup	chopped fresh parsley (optional)	50 mL
1 tbsp	white wine vinegar	15 mL
1 tsp	minced garlic	5 mL
1 tsp	dried oregano	5 mL
½ tsp	black pepper	2 mL

1. In a large bowl, combine rice, bean salad, artichokes, tomatoes, onions and, if using, parsley. Add vinegar, garlic, oregano and pepper; toss to combine. Chill before serving.

PER SERVING	
Calories: 216	
Dietary Fiber: 7 g	Carbohydrate: 37 g
Fat: 5 g	Protein: 8 g

SERVES 6
Makes 6 cups (1.5 L)

Lorraine Fullum-Bouchard, Dietitian

This salad makes a great picnic lunch, on its own or wrapped in a flour tortilla or pita bread.

MAKE AHEAD
For best results, make this salad at least 4 hours, or up to 1 day, ahead to allow the flavors to blend. Once made, it will keep well in the refrigerator for up to 3 days.

TIP
If using quinoa, rinse well before cooking to remove the bitter outer coating.

DIETITIAN'S MESSAGE
Serve this nutritious salad with a glass of cold milk and whole-grain rolls for an easy lunch.

Brown rice, oranges and pineapple are a surprisingly tasty combination. Garnished with whole strawberries, this nutritious salad also has lots of eye appeal.

TIP

If using olives with pits, crush each olive with the flat blade of a chef's knife, then extract the pit. Or purchase an olive pitter; this handy and inexpensive device is available at kitchen stores. It works well with fresh cherries, too.

DIETITIAN'S MESSAGE

Brown rice takes longer to cook than white rice. It is a source of soluble fiber, which helps to keep cholesterol levels in a healthy range. This colorful salad provides vitamin C and B vitamins, as well as fiber.

Brown Rice and Fruit Salad

¾ cup	brown rice	175 mL
2 cups	boiling water	500 mL
¾ cup	sliced celery	175 mL
1	can (10 oz/284 mL) mandarin orange segments, drained	1
½ cup	pineapple chunks	125 mL
12	pitted black olives, sliced	12
2 tbsp	sunflower seeds	25 mL
	Lettuce leaves, whole strawberries, Sunflower seeds	

Dressing

¼ cup	light mayonnaise	50 mL
3 tbsp	orange juice concentrate	45 mL
3 tbsp	vegetable oil	45 mL
1 tbsp	lemon juice	15 mL
1 tbsp	liquid honey	15 mL
¼ tsp	dry mustard	1 mL
⅛ tsp	hot pepper sauce	0.5 mL

1. In a saucepan, add rice to boiling water. Reduce heat, cover and cook for 45 minutes or until tender and water is absorbed. Cool.

2. In a medium bowl, combine rice, celery, orange segments, pineapple, black olives and sunflower seeds.

3. *Dressing:* Combine mayonnaise, orange juice, oil, lemon juice, honey and seasonings. Pour over salad; stir gently to mix. Cover and refrigerate for 1 hour.

4. Line 6 plates with lettuce leaves. Spoon rice mixture onto center; garnish with strawberries and sunflower seeds.

PER SERVING	
Calories: 289	
Dietary Fiber: 2 g	Carbohydrate: 42 g
Fat: 13 g	Protein: 4 g

Spinach and Rice Salad

¾ cup	long-grain white rice	175 mL
2 cups	boiling water	500 mL
¼ cup	olive oil	50 mL
2 tbsp	soy sauce	25 mL
1 cup	bean sprouts	250 mL
1 cup	torn spinach leaves	250 mL
½ cup	chopped green bell pepper	125 mL
¼ cup	raisins	50 mL
2 tbsp	chopped fresh parsley	25 mL
2 tbsp	chopped green onion	25 mL
Dressing		
½ cup	vinegar	125 mL
½ cup	granulated sugar	125 mL
2 tsp	lemon juice	10 mL
1 tsp	chopped fresh parsley	5 mL
1 tsp	dry mustard	5 mL
Pinch	each paprika, cayenne pepper, garlic powder, salt and black pepper	Pinch
1 cup	olive oil	250 mL

1. In a saucepan, add rice to boiling water. Cover and cook over very low heat for 20 minutes or until tender and water is absorbed. Add oil and soy sauce; cool.

2. In a large bowl, combine rice mixture, bean sprouts, spinach, green pepper, raisins, parsley and onion.

3. *Dressing:* Whisk together vinegar, sugar, lemon juice, parsley, mustard and seasonings. Gradually whisk in oil. Pour ¼ cup (50 mL) dressing over salad. Refrigerate remaining dressing for other salads.

PER SERVING	
Calories: 257	
Dietary Fiber: 1 g	Carbohydrate: 29 g
Fat: 15 g	Protein: 3 g

SERVES 6
Makes 1½ cups (375 mL) dressing
....
Gertrude Boudreau

You'll want to keep the dressing on hand for other salads, so make the entire recipe and refrigerate the extra quantity.

TIP
Adding the oil and soy sauce while the rice is still warm keeps the grains of rice separate and ensures that they don't clump together as the rice cools.

DIETITIAN'S MESSAGE
Olive oil, along with canola and peanut oil, is a monounsaturated fat choice that may help to lower cholesterol levels when included as part of healthy eating. The key is to control the total amount of fat you eat, so balance this higher-fat salad with lighter choices. Serve with Broiled Ham Steak with Pineapple Mango Salsa (see recipe, page 264) and complete the meal with Cinnamon Baked Pears (see recipe, page 385).

SERVES 6
....

**Rainer Schindler, Chef
Monica Stanton,
Dietitian**

*This salad has it all: low
calories, low fat, lots of
vegetables — and color
and flavor to spare.*

TIP
In this recipe, using
prepared fat-free Italian
salad dressing adds
flavor without fat.

DIETITIAN'S MESSAGE
Bulgur, or cracked wheat,
is made by steaming
wheat kernels, which are
then dried and crushed.
It is readily available in
larger supermarkets and
specialty food stores.

Bulgur Salad

1 cup	bulgur	250 mL
2 tbsp	finely chopped red *or* Spanish onion	25 mL
1	clove garlic, minced	1
½ cup	cooked corn kernels, cooled	125 mL
1	tomato, seeded and diced	1
½	small zucchini, thinly sliced	½
¼ cup	crumbled feta cheese	50 mL
¼ cup	bottled fat-free Italian dressing	50 mL
Pinch	crushed dried basil	Pinch
	Salt and black pepper	

1. Cover bulgur with 2 cups (500 mL) boiling water; let stand for 30 minutes. Drain.

2. In a bowl, combine bulgur, onion, garlic, corn, tomato and zucchini; stir in cheese, dressing and basil. Season with salt and pepper to taste. Cover and refrigerate for at least 1 hour.

PER SERVING	
Calories: 113	
Dietary Fiber: 5 g	Carbohydrate: 23 g
Fat: 1 g	Protein: 5 g

Tabbouleh

1 cup	medium-grain bulgur	250 mL
1 cup	boiling water	250 mL
5 to 6	green onions	5 to 6
1½ cups	lightly packed sprigs parsley	375 mL
⅓ cup	lightly packed fresh mint leaves	75 mL
2	tomatoes, chopped	2

Dressing

¼ cup	lemon juice	50 mL
3 tbsp	olive oil	45 mL
1	small clove garlic, minced	1
½ tsp	grated lemon zest	2 mL
½ tsp	granulated sugar	2 mL
½ tsp	dry mustard	2 mL
¼ tsp	paprika	1 mL
¼ tsp	salt	1 mL
	Freshly ground black pepper to taste	

1. In a covered saucepan, cook bulgur in boiling water for about 5 minutes or until liquid is absorbed (bulgur should still be crunchy). Spoon into a large bowl; cool.

2. In a food processor, coarsely chop onions, parsley and mint leaves; add to bulgur. Stir in tomatoes.

3. *Dressing:* Whisk together lemon juice, olive oil, garlic, lemon zest, sugar and seasonings. Pour dressing over bulgur mixture; mix together lightly. Cover and refrigerate for several hours or overnight.

PER SERVING	
Calories: 135	
Dietary Fiber: 3 g	Carbohydrate: 20 g
Fat: 5 g	Protein: 3 g

SERVES 8
Makes 6 cups (1.5 L)

Johanne Trudeau, Dietitian

Mint and lemon are the traditional flavors found in this classic Middle Eastern salad. Be sure to serve this with Falafel (see recipe, page 227).

TIP
To keep parsley and mint fresh, store in a tightly covered container in refrigerator.

DIETITIAN'S MESSAGE
Include generous amounts of grains in your diet and experiment with new types. Tomatoes, green onions, parsley and mint help to create a salad that is rich in vitamin C. For a quick lunch and added vitamins and fiber, tuck the Tabbouleh in a whole-wheat pita and serve with raw vegetables.

Penne Salad with Asparagus and Tuna

3 cups	penne (about 10 oz/300 g)	750 mL
3 cups	fresh asparagus, trimmed and cut into bite-size pieces (about 1 lb/500 g)	750 mL
2	cans (each 5.7 oz/170 g) water-packed tuna, drained	2
1 cup	diced red bell peppers	250 mL
2 tbsp	chopped chives *or* green onions	25 mL
2 tbsp	capers, drained (optional)	25 mL
Dressing		
2 tbsp	balsamic vinegar *or* red wine vinegar	25 mL
2 tbsp	olive oil	25 mL
2 tsp	Dijon mustard	10 mL
1 tsp	brown sugar	5 mL
½ tsp	minced garlic	2 mL
½ tsp	minced ginger root	2 mL
	Salt and black pepper	

1. In a large pot of boiling water, cook penne according to package directions or until tender but firm, adding asparagus during last 2 minutes of cooking time; drain. Rinse under cold water; drain. Transfer to a large bowl. Add tuna, red peppers, chives and, if using, capers. Set aside.

2. *Dressing:* In a small bowl or measuring cup, whisk together vinegar, oil, mustard, sugar, garlic and ginger. Season with salt and pepper to taste. Pour over salad; toss gently to combine. Serve immediately.

PER SERVING	
Calories: 223	
Dietary Fiber: 2 g	Carbohydrate: 31 g
Fat: 5 g	Protein: 14 g

Create Your Own Pasta Salad

3 cups	cooked pasta	750 mL
2 cups	diced raw vegetables (any combination of green pepper, radishes, cauliflower, broccoli, carrot, green onions and celery)	500 mL

Dressing

1/3 cup	vinegar *or* cider vinegar	75 mL
1 tsp	prepared mustard	5 mL
1/2 tsp	garlic powder	2 mL
1/2 tsp	dried thyme	2 mL
1/2 tsp	dried oregano	2 mL
Dash	Worcestershire sauce	Dash
3 tbsp	canola *or* safflower oil	45 mL

1. In a large bowl, combine pasta and raw vegetables.
2. *Dressing:* Whisk together vinegar and seasonings. Gradually whisk in oil. Pour over pasta mixture. Cover and refrigerate for 1 hour.

PER SERVING

Calories: 178

Dietary Fiber: 2 g	Carbohydrate: 23 g
Fat: 8 g	Protein: 4 g

SERVES 6 P

Janice Dillman

This delicious pasta salad has many variations. Try rotini, fusilli, elbow macaroni or shells, either plain or colored. To make this into a main-course salad, add cooked chicken, tuna or salmon.

DIETITIAN'S MESSAGE

Use your imagination and make this tasty salad with a variety of vegetables you have in your fridge. Add calcium to complete the meal — a glass of milk, some yogurt or a piece of cheese on the side.

**Antony Nuth, Chef
Lynda Chadwick,
Dietitian**

*Polenta — cornmeal
cooked in water or broth
and often seasoned with
cheese and herbs — is a
staple of Italian cooking.
This zesty version uses
garlic and herbs to
enhance the flavor.*

TIP

If fresh herbs are
available, use them
instead of the dried. Just
double — or triple — the
quantity depending upon
your preference.

DIETITIAN'S MESSAGE

The cornmeal in this
warm salad is a great
source of carbohydrates.
For a special meal, serve
this with a simple fish
dish, such as Quick
Steamed Fish Fillets with
Potatoes and Asparagus
(see recipe, page 325).
Finish with Strawberries
in Phyllo Cups (see recipe,
page 380) or Sumptuous
Fruit Brochettes (see
recipe, page 384).

Warm Polenta Salad with Mushrooms and Herbs

8- by 4-inch (1.5 L) loaf pan, lined with plastic wrap

Herb Polenta

4 cups	chicken *or* vegetable broth	1 L
2	large cloves garlic, minced	2
1 tbsp	dried basil	15 mL
1½ tsp	each crumbled dried rosemary and thyme	7 mL
¼ tsp	each salt and black pepper	1 mL
1 cup	cornmeal	250 mL

Salad

¼ cup	olive oil	50 mL
4 cups	sliced mushrooms (portobello, oyster, chanterelle *or* white)	1 L
4 cups	shredded salad greens (combination of kale, rapini, radicchio, Belgian endive)	1 L
2 tbsp	balsamic vinegar	25 mL
¼ tsp	each salt and black pepper	1 mL

1. *Herb Polenta:* In a large saucepan, bring broth to boil. Add garlic, basil, rosemary, thyme, salt and pepper; gradually add cornmeal, whisking constantly. Cook over low heat, stirring occasionally, for about 15 minutes or until thick and soft. Pour into 8- by 4-inch (1.5 L) loaf pan lined with plastic wrap. Cool. (Refrigerate if preparing ahead of time.)

2. Slice polenta into 8 pieces. Coat with additional cornmeal. In a large skillet sprayed with nonstick cooking spray, brown polenta on both sides. Remove from pan and keep warm.

3. *Salad:* Add 2 tbsp (25 mL) of the oil to skillet; sauté mushrooms for 2 to 3 minutes. Add remaining oil, shredded salad greens, vinegar, salt and pepper; heat through.

4. Divide salad mixture among 8 plates; place polenta on top. Serve immediately.

PER SERVING	
Calories: 160	
Dietary Fiber: 2 g	Carbohydrate: 17 g
Fat: 8 g	Protein: 5 g

Fusilli and Fruit Salad

SERVES 6
Makes 6 cups (1.5 L)
•••••••••••••••••••••••••••
Josie Haresign

1½ cups	fusilli	375 mL
1	can (14 oz/398 mL) pineapple tidbits, drained	1
1	can (10 oz/284 mL) whole mandarin orange segments, drained	1
1 cup	halved red *or* green grapes	250 mL
½ cup	diced red apples (unpeeled)	125 mL
½ cup	yogurt cheese (see technique, page 154) *or* lower-fat thick yogurt	125 mL
2 tbsp	frozen orange juice concentrate, thawed	25 mL
1	small banana, sliced	1

1. In a pot of boiling water, cook pasta until tender but firm; drain. Rinse under cold water; drain. Transfer to a large bowl. Add pineapple, oranges, grapes and apples.

2. In a separate bowl, stir together yogurt cheese and orange juice concentrate. Pour over pasta mixture; toss gently. Chill. Stir in sliced banana just before serving.

PER SERVING	
Calories: 198	
Dietary Fiber: 2 g	Carbohydrate: 43 g
Fat: 1 g	Protein: 5 g

Here's an unusual salad that even the fussiest of kids will enjoy.

TIPS

Try using a variety of different fruits. You will need about 4 cups (1 L) in total.

If you like spice, add 1 tsp (5 mL) curry powder to the yogurt cheese.

MAKE AHEAD

This salad can be made a day ahead. Prepare and refrigerate salad and dressing separately and combine just before serving.

DIETITIAN'S MESSAGE

The unusual combination of ingredients provides folic acid as well as vitamin C. It goes well with cold chicken, so take it on a picnic or pack it for brown baggers.

A new twist on the classic soup — all the zesty flavors of gazpacho prepared as a jellied salad. Loaded with crunch but light on fat, this will fit the bill whenever you are looking for a cool salad.

TIPS

Worcestershire sauce, a flavorful condiment, contains strong-tasting ingredients such as anchovies and tamarind, so use with discretion if these are not to your taste.

If you like spice, you may want to increase the quantity of hot pepper sauce in this recipe.

DIETITIAN'S MESSAGE

This eye-appealing salad is packed with antioxidants, vitamins and minerals. Antioxidants work to neutralize free radicals that are responsible for cell damage throughout the body.

Jellied Gazpacho Salad

6-cup (1.5 L) mold

1 tbsp	unflavored gelatin (1 pkg)	15 mL
1¼ cups	vegetable juice cocktail, divided	300 mL
1 tsp	beef bouillon powder	5 mL
2 tbsp	cider vinegar *or* vinegar	25 mL
1 tsp	Worcestershire sauce	5 mL
Dash	hot pepper sauce	Dash
1	medium tomato, peeled	1
½	large green bell pepper	½
½	large cucumber, peeled and seeded	½
1	small onion	1
1	small clove garlic	1
1	small celery stalk with leaves	1
	Celery leaves	

1. In a medium saucepan, sprinkle gelatin over ¼ cup (50 mL) of the vegetable juice. Stir over low heat for 3 minutes or until gelatin is completely dissolved. Stir in beef bouillon, ¾ cup (175 mL) of the remaining vegetable juice, vinegar, Worcestershire sauce and hot pepper sauce. Refrigerate, stirring occasionally, until mixture is consistency of unbeaten egg whites, about 30 minutes.

2. In a food processor or blender, purée half the tomato, the green pepper, cucumber, onion and garlic with remaining vegetable juice until smooth. Coarsely chop remaining tomato and celery. Stir purée and chopped vegetables into gelatin mixture. Pour into a rinsed 6-cup (1.5 L) mold. Cover and refrigerate until firm, at least 3 hours.

3. To serve, unmold gazpacho onto serving plate. Garnish with celery leaves.

PER SERVING	
Calories: 31	
Dietary Fiber: 1 g	Carbohydrate: 6 g
Fat: 0 g	Protein: 2 g

Hawaiian Cranberry Salad

4-cup (1 L) mold

1 cup	boiling water	250 mL
1	pkg (4-serving size) orange-flavored gelatin	1
1	can (6½ oz/184 mL) whole-cranberry sauce	1
1 cup	crushed pineapple, with juice	250 mL
½ cup	chopped celery	125 mL
	Orange slices and fresh parsley or lettuce leaves	

1. In a small bowl, pour boiling water over gelatin; stir until dissolved. Stir in cranberry sauce, pineapple and celery. Pour into a rinsed 4-cup (1 L) mold; cover and refrigerate until firm, about 3 hours.
2. To serve, unmold onto serving plate; garnish with orange slices and parsley or lettuce.

PER SERVING
Calories: 132

Dietary Fiber: 1 g	Carbohydrate: 33 g
Fat: 0 g	Protein: 2 g

SERVES 6
....
Carol Sage

This molded salad is an excellent accompaniment to a poultry dinner. For a buffet party, the recipe can be doubled.

TIP
Gelatin is made from an animal protein. Some fruits, such as pineapple, kiwi fruit and honeydew melon, contain an enzyme that will attack the gelatin and prevent it from setting. If you wish to use these fruits with gelatin, you must first destroy the enzyme by heating them to a temperature high enough to kill the enzyme (170° to 185°F/77° to 85°C).

DIETITIAN'S MESSAGE
This salad will add oomph and color to a Thanksgiving buffet or a poultry dinner. It will also provide fruits and vegetables in a festive way.

Pasta, Rice and Legumes

In this chapter, you will find a range of dishes using the many varieties of pasta, various kinds of rice, and healthful dried beans and lentils, known as legumes. All are delicious and will add vital nutrients to your plan for healthy eating.

carbohydrate good guys

Did you know that breads, cereals, pasta, rice and nutrients are the body's best fuel source? They are all high in carbohydrates, which are your body's best source of glucose — its major fuel. Carbohydrates should account for over half of the calories you eat every day.

Unfortunately, carbohydrates have acquired a "bad guy" reputation as many popular high-protein, low-carbohydrate diets recommend cutting back on carbo-hydrates to control weight. Although eating a carbohydrate-rich meal does raise blood glucose levels temporarily, there is no evidence that this leads to weight gain in healthy individuals. In fact, a high-carbohydrate diet can make you gain weight only if you consume more calories than your body burns. It is too many calories, not too many carbohydrates, that cause people to gain weight!

folic acid alert

Folic acid is an important B vitamin that helps to prevent neural tube defects, such as spina bifida, in infants. Consequently, women of childbearing age should increase their intake of folic acid through healthy food choices. Half a cup (125 mL) of cooked, drained red kidney beans provides more than 50% of the recommended daily intake of folic acid. Pasta, like many other grain products, is fortified with folic acid, making it a good source of this valuable nutrient. Other sources include legumes, cooked spinach, broccoli, peas and oranges.

grains savvy

Dietitians encourage food choices that emphasize grains, vegetables and fruit balanced with choices from other food groups as a key to healthy eating. Aim for five to 12 daily servings of grain products.

protein power

Although on their own plant sources of protein do not contain the complete array of amino acids you need, you can ensure a full complement of protein each day by combining legumes such as kidney beans, lentils and chickpeas with grains (rice, bread), nuts and seeds. Build your main meals with whole-grain breads, brown rice and enriched pastas, and add lots of brightly colored, antioxidant-rich vegetables to improve your health.

eating vegetarian

More and more, Canadians are trying vegetarian options — a meal at a time, a day at a time, or as an ongoing pattern of eating. However, the more foods you eliminate from your diet, the more challenging healthy eating becomes. Although a well-planned vegetarian diet can meet your nutritional needs, there is more to becoming a vegetarian than eliminating meat from your diet. A haphazard approach to a vegetarian diet can put people at risk of nutritional deficiencies — specifically protein, iron, vitamin B12, calcium, vitamin D and zinc. Children and pregnant and breastfeeding women in particular, need top-notch nutrition. They should pay special attention to food choices and may need supplements to provide necessary nutrients if following a vegetarian diet.

vitamins and dietary fiber

Not only are carbohydrates our body's number one source of energy, grains also provide B vitamins (including folic acid), iron, phytochemicals and fiber. A diet that is abundant with carbohydrate from grains and low in fat has been linked with a reduced risk of heart disease and some types of cancer, as well as fewer digestive problems such as constipation.

Good sources of insoluble fiber include wheat bran, whole-grain products and some vegetables. Grains such as oats and barley, legumes, and other fruit and vegetables are high in soluble fiber. To increase fiber intake and meet dietary recommendations, consider including whole grains, vegetables and fruits at every meal. This may require a different approach to meal planning. Rather than starting with meat, why not consider carbohydrates first? Make rice, pasta, legumes, bread or cereal the core of the meal. Add meat, eggs, cheese, fish or poultry and vegetables for a perfectly balanced meal.

Tip: *When increasing your fiber intake, do so gradually and make sure you drink more fluids.*

tofu and soy products

Soy protein, in simulated meat products and tofu, is a high-quality protein that can be a valuable substitute for animal protein. There are many ways to enjoy tofu. Try adding it to shakes, stir-fries, lasagna, enchiladas — even desserts. For recipes containing tofu, consult the index of this book. When purchasing tofu, read the labels and purchase a variety with added calcium. Similarly, not all soy beverages are created equal. Some are fortified with six nutrients, others contain as many as 15. Check labels to ensure that the product contains all the nutrients you want.

nutritional powerhouses

Legumes include dried peas, beans and lentils. Not only are they an economical food source, they are nutritional powerhouses, serving as the main source of protein for many vegetarians and people in developing countries. In addition to being low in fat, high in protein and an excellent source of soluble fiber, most legumes deliver phytochemicals, folic acid, iron and other B vitamins. Legumes are extremely versatile and can be used in soups, stews, salads, casseroles and even dips. They are also delectable when properly cooked. To get a taste of how delicious legumes can be, try some of the recipes in this chapter, such as Mexican Pie, Vegetarian Chili and Lentil Spaghetti Sauce.

Versatile Tomato Sauce

SERVES 6
....
Brenda Steinmetz

1	medium onion, chopped	1
½ cup	chopped celery	125 mL
½ cup	grated carrot *or* zucchini	125 mL
½ cup	chopped green bell pepper	125 mL
1	clove garlic, chopped	1
1 tsp	vegetable oil	5 mL
1	can (28 oz/796 mL) tomatoes	1
¼ cup	red wine	50 mL
1	bay leaf	1
½ tsp	each dried oregano and dried basil	2 mL
¼ tsp	each salt and black pepper	1 mL
¼ tsp	dried parsley	1 mL
Pinch	ground cinnamon (optional)	Pinch

1. In a large saucepan over medium-high heat, cook onion, celery, carrot, green pepper and garlic in oil, stirring frequently, for about 10 minutes or until tender. Stir in tomatoes, red wine and seasonings.

2. Cook over medium heat, uncovered and stirring often, for about 1 hour or until thickened. Remove bay leaf before serving.

PER ½ CUP (125 ML)
Calories: 48
Dietary Fiber: 2 g | Carbohydrate: 9 g
Fat: 1 g | Protein: 2 g

While bottled and canned pasta sauces are convenient, their flavor can't compete with that of a good homemade sauce. Even better, homemade sauces are lower in sodium than commercially prepared sauces.

TIP
When tomatoes are in season, you can replace the canned tomatoes in this recipe with 8 to 10 peeled ripe tomatoes. You may need to cook the sauce longer, depending on the amount of liquid in the tomatoes. Make 1 batch or several, and freeze for later use.

VARIATIONS
Meat Sauce: Add ½ lb (250 g) lean ground beef, browned, to Versatile Tomato Sauce along with the tomatoes.

Red Clam Sauce: Add 1 can (5 oz/142 g) clams, undrained, to Versatile Tomato Sauce.

Stuffed Peppers: Stuff peppers with cooked rice; bake topped with Versatile Tomato Sauce.

Cabbage Rolls: Pour Versatile Tomato Sauce over cabbage rolls.

Chicken Marengo: Replace red wine in Versatile Tomato Sauce with white wine and add sliced mushrooms. Cook chicken pieces in this sauce.

Meat Loaf: Serve sliced

P

Laurie A. Wadsworth,
Dietitian

Use this sauce when making cannelloni, pizza or lasagna, among other dishes. It is delicious over cooked pasta — use the whole-wheat variety to add fiber to your diet.

TIPS

When tomatoes are in season, you can replace the canned tomatoes in this recipe with 8 to 10 peeled ripe tomatoes.

Plum or roma tomatoes work best in tomato sauces because of their low water content.

For a smoother sauce, substitute canned crushed tomatoes for the diced tomatoes.

Make batches of this sauce and freeze so you will always have a supply on hand.

DIETITIAN'S MESSAGE

Cooked tomatoes are a great source of lycopene, an antioxidant that has been linked to the reduction of heart disease, stroke and certain types of cancer. Although research into the value of lycopene is in the early stages, it does show that our bodies absorb the lycopene in tomatoes more easily when the tomatoes have been cooked.

Piquant Tomato Sauce

2 tbsp	olive oil *or* vegetable oil	25 mL
1 cup	chopped onions	250 mL
2 tsp	minced garlic	10 mL
1	can (28 oz/796 mL) diced tomatoes	1
1	can (14 oz/398 mL) tomato paste, plus 1 can of water	1
2 tsp	brown sugar	10 mL
1 to 2 tsp	crushed red pepper flakes	5 to 10 mL
	Black pepper to taste	

1. In a large saucepan or Dutch oven, heat oil over medium heat. Add onions and garlic; cook for 4 to 5 minutes or until onions are translucent. Do not allow garlic to brown.

2. Add tomatoes and tomato paste. Fill tomato paste can with water and stir to incorporate any remaining paste; add to tomato mixture along with sugar and red pepper flakes. Cover and bring to a boil. Reduce heat and simmer for 2 hours, stirring occasionally. Season with pepper.

PER SERVING	
Calories: 110	
Dietary Fiber: 4 g	Carbohydrate: 18 g
Fat: 4 g	Protein: 3 g

Lentil Spaghetti Sauce

SERVES 6
....

Lise Bélisle

1 tbsp	vegetable oil	15 mL
1	large onion, chopped	1
1	large stalk celery, chopped	1
2	cloves garlic, chopped	2
1 cup	dried red lentils, washed	250 mL
2 cups	beef broth *or* water	500 mL
1	can (5½ oz/156 mL) tomato paste	1
¾ cup	water	175 mL
1 tbsp	chopped fresh parsley	15 mL
½ tsp	dried oregano	2 mL
½ tsp	salt	2 mL
Pinch	cayenne pepper	Pinch
	Grated Parmesan cheese	

1. In a large saucepan, heat oil over medium heat; cook onion, celery and garlic for about 5 minutes or until tender. Add lentils and beef broth; cover and cook over low heat for about 35 minutes or until lentils are tender.

2. Add tomato paste, water and seasonings; cook, covered, for about 15 minutes or until lentils are soft and mushy. Serve over cooked spaghetti; sprinkle with cheese.

PER SERVING

Calories: 154

Dietary Fiber: 5 g	Carbohydrate: 25 g
Fat: 3 g	Protein: 9 g

Whole-wheat, spinach or plain spaghetti or fettuccine — all can be served with this tasty sauce. If you're making this for vegetarians, substitute vegetable broth for the beef broth.

TIP

Lentils come in red, green and brown. Brown and green hold their shape better and are usually used in salads. Red, which break down during cooking, are used here because they dissolve in the sauce.

DIETITIAN'S MESSAGE

Lentils provide an abundance of carbohydrates, protein and fiber and can be the basis for an economical meal. Serve this sauce over the pasta of your choice or use it as sauce for lasagna. The combination of lentils and pasta in this recipe provides complete protein.

**Kenneth Peace, Chef
Maye Musk, Dietitian**

*Farfalle (bow tie pasta)
and soft crumbled goat
cheese, often called
chèvre, are readily
available in supermarkets
and add a sophisticated
note to this elegant recipe.*

TIPS

For even better results,
use finely chopped fresh
basil instead of the dried
— double or triple the
quantity depending on
your preference and
add after the vegetables
are cooked.

When tossing the pasta,
add roasted garlic for an
additional touch.

DIETITIAN'S MESSAGE

Chèvre, soft or unripened
goat cheese, is usually
sold in a roll. It is lower in
sodium than goat cheese
that has been allowed to
ripen. It combines with
the pasta and vegetables
in this recipe to create a
dish that is bursting with
flavor and eye appeal.

Pasta with Goat Cheese, Snow Peas and Tomatoes

Tomato Coulis

½ cup	diced shallots	125 mL
¼ cup	diced celery	50 mL
1	can (28 oz/796 mL) tomatoes	1
2	cloves garlic, minced	2
2 tbsp	chopped fresh parsley	25 mL
1 tbsp	crushed dried basil	15 mL
2 tsp	brown sugar	10 mL
¼ tsp	each salt and black pepper	1 mL

Pasta

1 tbsp	olive oil	15 mL
8 oz	snow peas	250 g
1 tbsp	crushed dried basil	15 mL
4 cups	farfalle (bow tie pasta), cooked and drained	1 L
	Salt and black pepper	
4 oz	soft crumbled goat cheese *or* shredded mozzarella	125 g

1. *Tomato Coulis:* In a skillet, combine shallots, celery and ¼ cup (50 mL) water; cook over medium heat until soft. Add tomatoes, garlic, parsley, basil, sugar, salt and pepper; bring to a boil. Reduce heat and simmer for 10 minutes, stirring occasionally. Purée in a food processor. Keep warm.

2. *Pasta:* In a large skillet, heat olive oil over medium heat; cook snow peas with basil, stirring, for 3 to 5 minutes or until tender. Stir in pasta. Season with salt and pepper to taste.

3. To serve, place Tomato Coulis in a pasta bowl; top with pasta mixture. Sprinkle with goat cheese.

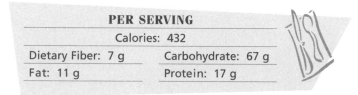

PER SERVING	
Calories: 432	
Dietary Fiber: 7 g	Carbohydrate: 67 g
Fat: 11 g	Protein: 17 g

TO ROAST GARLIC
Place 12 cloves of peeled garlic in foil with 1 tsp (5 mL) olive oil.
Bake in 325°F (160°C) oven until soft, about 20 minutes.

Pasta, Rice and Legumes

Pasta with Roasted Vegetables and Goat Cheese

Preheat oven to 425°F (220°C)
Large rimmed baking sheet, greased

4 cups	cubed zucchini	1 L
2 cups	cubed eggplant	500 mL
2 cups	coarsely chopped red bell peppers	500 mL
1 cup	coarsely chopped sweet white *or* red onions	250 mL
2 tbsp	olive oil	25 mL
1½ tsp	dried Italian seasoning *or* French herbs	7 mL
8 oz	rotini, penne *or* other pasta	250 g
3½ to 4 oz	soft crumbled goat cheese	100 to 125 g
	Grated Parmesan cheese (optional)	

1. Combine zucchini, eggplant, peppers and onions in a large bowl. Add oil and Italian seasoning; toss to coat. Place vegetables in a single layer on prepared baking sheet; roast in preheated oven, stirring occasionally, for 30 to 40 minutes or until vegetables are golden and slightly softened.

2. Meanwhile, in a pot of boiling water, cook pasta according to package directions or until tender but firm; drain.

3. Toss vegetables with pasta. Sprinkle goat cheese over top; toss to combine or leave as is and sprinkle with Parmesan cheese, if desired.

PER SERVING	
Calories: 395	
Dietary Fiber: 6 g	Carbohydrate: 56 g
Fat: 13 g	Protein: 14 g

WHOLE-WHEAT PIZZA WITH ROASTED VEGETABLES
The vegetable mixture in this recipe is equally spectacular on a pizza crust covered with a thin layer of pesto or pizza sauce. Make whole-wheat pizza dough (see recipe, page 49). Spread with sauce and roasted vegetables. Add crumbled goat cheese and grated Parmesan, if desired.

SERVES 4

Renée Crompton, Dietitian

This dish is a great way to increase your vegetable intake. Prepare the recipe with the ingredients here or with any favorite vegetables. Leftovers are delicious served cold or reheated for lunch the next day.

TIP
For best flavor, use fresh herbs rather than dried, but add them at the very end with the cheese. Substitute about 2 tbsp (25 mL) fresh for every 1 tsp (5 mL) dried.

MAKE AHEAD
Vegetables can be roasted up to 1 day in advance. Reheat in a hot oven for 5 to 10 minutes or until piping hot.

DIETITIAN'S MESSAGE
This recipe has cheese, grain and a whopping 4 servings of vegetables. When choosing vegetables for roasting, select those with darker colors of red, orange and green; they are richest in nutrients and phytochemicals.

P

Eric Fergie, Chef
Jane Thornthwaite,
Dietitian

*Here's a simple recipe
that takes advantage of
seasonal vegetables in a
colorful medley. For even
more flavor, use fresh
herbs instead of the dried
— roughly 3 times the
quantity, with the
exception of rosemary
(in this recipe 1 tsp/5 mL
chopped fresh rosemary
would be adequate).*

TIP

For variety, try using
whole-wheat pasta in
this recipe. When
cooking pasta, be sure
to use a large quantity
of boiling water and
leave the pot uncovered
during cooking.

DIETITIAN'S MESSAGE

The selection and
quantity of vegetables in
this recipe will contribute
significant amounts of
vitamins A and C, as
well as antioxidants.
To increase fiber, use
whole-wheat pasta.

Garden Fresh Fettuccine

4 cups	julienned vegetables (peppers, broccoli or cauliflower florets, zucchini, red onion, carrots, celery, sliced mushrooms)	1 L
12 oz	fettuccine *or* penne (3 cups/750 mL)	375 g
	Grated Parmesan cheese	

Sauce

1 cup	vegetable stock *or* water	250 mL
¼ cup	white wine	50 mL
1	clove garlic, minced	1
1 tbsp	chopped fresh parsley	15 mL
1 tbsp	dried basil	15 mL
2 tsp	lemon juice	10 mL
1 tsp	each crushed dried oregano, thyme and tarragon	5 mL
¾ tsp	crumbled dried rosemary	4 mL

1. *Sauce:* In a large skillet, combine stock, wine, garlic, parsley, basil, lemon juice, oregano, thyme, tarragon and rosemary; bring to a boil.

2. Add firmer vegetables; cover and simmer for 5 minutes. Add softer vegetables; simmer for 5 more minutes.

3. Meanwhile, cook fettuccine according to package directions; drain. Toss with vegetables. Garnish with cheese.

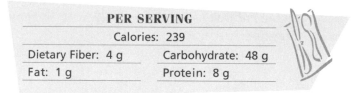

PER SERVING	
Calories: 239	
Dietary Fiber: 4 g	Carbohydrate: 48 g
Fat: 1 g	Protein: 8 g

TO TOAST HAZELNUTS
Spread hazelnuts on baking sheet. Toast in oven at 350°F (180°C) for 10 to 15 minutes or until fragrant. Immediately roll nuts in kitchen towel against work surface to loosen skins. Remove skins with towel and fingers. Crush nuts in food processor.

Fettuccine with Zucchini and Fresh Tomato Sauce

1 cup	finely chopped onion	250 mL
2	cloves garlic, minced	2
2 tbsp	olive oil	25 mL
3 cups	chopped peeled tomatoes	750 mL
3 tbsp	chopped fresh basil (*or* 2 tsp/10 mL dried)	45 mL
1	zucchini, diced	1
8 oz	fettuccine	250 g
	Chopped fresh basil (optional) and grated Parmesan cheese	

1. In a large skillet over medium heat, cook onion and garlic in oil until softened, about 5 minutes. Add tomatoes and basil; simmer for about 10 minutes or until slightly thickened. Add zucchini and cook for 2 minutes.

2. In a large pot of boiling water, cook fettuccine according to package directions or until tender but firm. Drain well.

3. Combine sauce and fettuccine until well coated; sprinkle with chopped fresh basil, if using, and cheese. Serve immediately.

PER SERVING	
Calories: 323	
Dietary Fiber: 5 g	Carbohydrate: 55 g
Fat: 8 g	Protein: 10 g

SERVES 4 P

Kathy Sziklai

Enjoy this light-flavored sauce when garden-fresh zucchini and tomatoes are at their peak.

TIP
When in season, use 1 cup (250 mL) diced red bell peppers (or a mixture of red and yellow peppers) in place of the zucchini.

DIETITIAN'S MESSAGE
This fresh-tasting pasta is a great way to use surplus vegetables from the garden. For a summer dinner, serve with Barbecued Stuffed Salmon (see recipe, page 309) and end the meal with fresh berries and frozen yogurt.

LINGUINE WITH HAZELNUTS AND ROASTED GARLIC
Chef Tim Wood and dietitian Leslie Maze suggest this interesting pasta. Roast 2 heads of garlic (see technique, page 182) and mash with a fork. Toast ¾ cup (175 mL) hazelnuts (see technique, opposite) and crush coarsely. In a large bowl, combine roasted garlic, three-quarters of the hazelnuts, ¼ cup (50 mL) chopped fresh parsley, 2 tbsp (25 mL) balsamic vinegar, and salt and pepper to taste. Add 12 oz (375 g) linguine, cooked and drained, and toss well. Garnish with ⅓ cup (75 mL) grated Parmesan cheese and remaining hazelnuts.

Spaghetti with Zucchini Balls and Tomato Sauce

Preheat oven to 400°F (200°C)
Baking sheet, greased

1 tsp	olive oil	5 mL
1	medium onion, finely chopped	1
1	can (28 oz/796 mL) crushed tomatoes	1
3	cloves garlic, minced	3
1 tsp	crushed dried oregano	5 mL
1 tsp	ground cumin	5 mL
1	stick cinnamon (5 inches/12 cm)	1
¼ tsp	granulated sugar	1 mL
¼ tsp	each salt and black pepper	1 mL
12 oz	spaghetti	375 g
	Grated Parmesan cheese (optional)	

Zucchini Balls

3 cups	grated zucchini (2 medium), drained	750 mL
1 cup	drained chickpeas	250 mL
1	slice whole-wheat bread, crumbled	1
¾ cup	quick-cooking rolled oats	175 mL
½ cup	cornmeal	125 mL
2	cloves garlic, minced	2
1 tsp	ground cumin	5 mL
½ tsp	each ground coriander and ginger	2 mL
½ tsp	each salt and black pepper	2 mL
¼ tsp	cardamom	1 mL
2	eggs, lightly beaten	2

1. In a large skillet, heat oil over medium-high heat; sauté onion for 3 minutes. Add tomatoes, garlic, oregano, cumin, cinnamon stick, sugar, salt and pepper; bring to a boil. Reduce heat and simmer, uncovered, for 30 minutes, stirring occasionally. Remove cinnamon stick.

2. *Zucchini Balls:* Squeeze out excess moisture from zucchini. Purée half of the chickpeas.

3. In a bowl, mix together zucchini, puréed and whole chickpeas, bread, rolled oats, cornmeal, garlic, cumin, coriander, ginger, salt, pepper, cardamom and eggs. Form into 1-inch (2.5 cm) balls; place on greased baking sheet. Bake in preheated oven for 10 to 15 minutes or until lightly browned.

4. Meanwhile, cook spaghetti according to package directions; drain and arrange on 4 plates. Spoon tomato sauce over spaghetti; top with zucchini balls. Serve with Parmesan cheese, if desired.

PER SERVING	
Calories: 632	
Dietary Fiber: 12 g	Carbohydrate: 117 g
Fat: 8 g	Protein: 24 g

Rotini with Vegetable Tomato Sauce

8 oz	rotini *or* fusilli	250 g
3 cups	Piquant Tomato Sauce (see recipe, page 180) *or* commercially prepared pasta sauce	750 mL
1 cup	diced zucchini	250 mL
1 cup	grated carrots	250 mL
½ cup	chopped celery	125 mL
2 tbsp	chopped fresh parsley (optional)	25 mL
¼ cup	grated Parmesan cheese	50 mL

1. In a large pot of boiling water, cook pasta until tender but firm; drain.

2. Meanwhile, in a saucepan over medium-high heat, combine Piquant Tomato Sauce, zucchini, carrots, celery and, if using, parsley; bring to a boil. Reduce heat, cover and simmer for 15 minutes. Serve over pasta. Sprinkle with Parmesan cheese.

PER SERVING	
Calories: 351	
Dietary Fiber: 7 g	Carbohydrate: 62 g
Fat: 7 g	Protein: 13 g

SERVES 4

Laurie A. Wadsworth, Dietitian

The simple sauce used here is perfect for a busy weeknight meal and will help boost your vegetable intake.

TIP
For a heartier version of this dish, add 1 cup (250 mL) cooked lentils or any type of bean and — presto! — you have a protein-rich fagioli or bean sauce.

MAKE AHEAD
Make the Piquant Tomato Sauce ahead of time and freeze in 3-cup (750 mL) portions in airtight containers for up to 3 months.

DIETITIAN'S MESSAGE
When you are in a hurry, bottled or canned pasta sauce makes a good substitute for Piquant Tomato Sauce in this recipe. But you will increase the amount of sodium you consume.

Aphrodite's Pasta

½ cup	2% milk	125 mL
4 tsp	cornstarch	20 mL
1 tsp	each finely minced ginger root and garlic	5 mL
½ cup	lower-fat plain yogurt	125 mL
1	small zucchini, cut into strips	1
3 cups	drained cooked pasta (bow ties, shells *or* fusilli)	750 mL
	Black pepper	
2 tbsp	coarsely chopped fresh parsley	25 mL
½ cup	diced seeded tomatoes	125 mL

1. In a medium saucepan, mix milk and cornstarch until smooth. Add ginger and garlic; bring to a boil, stirring constantly, and cook until thickened.

2. Stir in yogurt and zucchini; simmer for 2 to 3 minutes. Stir in pasta; simmer for 1 to 2 minutes or until hot. Season with pepper to taste. Garnish with parsley and tomatoes.

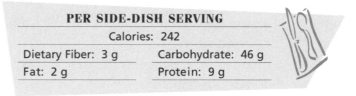

PER SIDE-DISH SERVING	
Calories: 242	
Dietary Fiber: 3 g	Carbohydrate: 46 g
Fat: 2 g	Protein: 9 g

GINGER LINGUINE
Here's an unusual and spicy pasta dish from Paul Howard that is not for the faint of heart. In a skillet over medium heat, melt 2 tbsp (25 mL) butter or margarine. Add 2 tbsp (25 mL) minced ginger root and 3 large cloves of garlic, minced, and cook for about 2 minutes. Stir in 3 finely chopped green onions, 1 tsp (5 mL) hot pepper sauce, and 1 tbsp (15 mL) chopped fresh basil. Cook briefly, then toss with 8 oz (250 g) linguine, cooked and drained. Sprinkle with ¼ cup (50 mL) grated Parmesan cheese and garnish with additional chopped fresh basil.

Penne with Mushrooms and Spicy Tomato Sauce

8 oz	penne	250 g
1 tbsp	olive oil	15 mL
3 cups	sliced mushrooms	750 mL
½ cup	sliced onion	125 mL
¼ cup	red wine	50 mL
3 cups	Piquant Tomato Sauce (see recipe, page 180) *or* commercially prepared pasta sauce	750 mL
½ tsp	hot pepper sauce	2 mL
2 tbsp	chopped fresh parsley	25 mL
¼ cup	grated Parmesan cheese	50 mL

1. In a large pot of boiling water, cook pasta until tender but firm; drain.

2. In a large nonstick skillet, heat oil over medium-high heat. Add mushrooms and onion; cook for 6 to 8 minutes or until softened and moisture has evaporated. Add wine and cook, stirring, until evaporated.

3. Stir in Piquant Tomato Sauce and hot pepper sauce; bring to a boil. Reduce heat and simmer for 1 to 2 minutes. Stir in parsley. Serve over pasta, and sprinkle with Parmesan cheese.

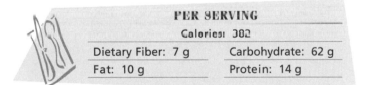

PER SERVING	
Calories: 382	
Dietary Fiber: 7 g	Carbohydrate: 62 g
Fat: 10 g	Protein: 14 g

SERVES 4

Laurie A. Wadsworth, Dietitian

TIP
Use any combination of fresh and dried reconstituted mushrooms to make this delicious sauce. Just be sure that most of the moisture has evaporated before adding the rest of the ingredients.

IF USING DRIED MUSHROOMS
Place mushrooms in a bowl; add enough water to cover by about 1 inch (2.5 cm). Let soak for about 30 minutes; drain. Strain soaking liquid through cheesecloth to remove any grit and use it as a flavoring for soups. Trim stems, slice and use as you would fresh mushrooms.

DIETITIAN'S MESSAGE
If using commercially prepared pasta sauce in this recipe, the sodium content will increase.

*This broccoli sauce is
similar to a basil pesto
sauce and is intended to
be thick. If you prefer
a thinner sauce, add
chicken or vegetable
stock while processing.
Serve over fettuccine,
fusilli or linguine. What
a great way to encourage
kids to eat their broccoli!
Serve as a main course or
an appetizer.*

TIP

As this sauce is thick, like
pesto, it is best served
with a long pasta such as
spaghetti, spaghettini or
fettuccine because it will
cling to the pasta.

DIETITIAN'S MESSAGE

This unusual sauce, made
from puréed broccoli, is
rich in vitamin C, fiber
and folic acid. If serving
as an appetizer, follow
with Yogurt-Marinated
Chicken (see recipe,
page 277) and finish the
meal with fresh fruit.

Pasta with
Broccoli Herb Sauce

2¾ cups	chopped broccoli	675 mL
⅓ cup	olive *or* vegetable oil	75 mL
⅓ cup	grated Parmesan cheese	75 mL
¼ cup	chopped fresh parsley	50 mL
1 tbsp	chopped fresh basil	15 mL
12 oz	pasta	375 g

1. Place broccoli and 2 tbsp (25 mL) water in a 4-cup (1 L) microwave-safe bowl. Microwave, covered, on High for about 5 minutes; drain.

2. In a food processor, purée broccoli, oil, cheese, parsley and basil until broccoli is finely chopped.

3. Cook pasta in boiling water according to package directions or until tender but firm. Drain well and toss with vegetable mixture. Serve immediately.

Main Course

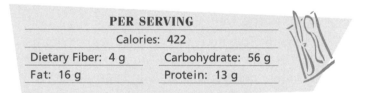

PER SERVING	
Calories: 422	
Dietary Fiber: 4 g	Carbohydrate: 56 g
Fat: 16 g	Protein: 13 g

Appetizer

PER SERVING	
Calories: 211	
Dietary Fiber: 2 g	Carbohydrate: 28 g
Fat: 8 g	Protein: 7 g

Creamy Pasta and Broccoli

12 oz	penne *or* macaroni *or* other pasta	375 g
3 cups	fresh *or* frozen chopped broccoli	750 mL
1 tbsp	butter *or* margarine	15 mL
1 tbsp	all-purpose flour	15 mL
1½ cups	chicken stock *or* vegetable stock	375 mL
1 tsp	minced garlic	5 mL
4 oz	herb-and-garlic-flavored light cream cheese	125 g
	Black pepper	
6 tbsp	grated Parmesan cheese	90 mL

1. In a large pot of boiling water, cook pasta until tender but firm, adding broccoli during last 3 minutes of cooking time; drain. Set aside.

2. Meanwhile, in a medium saucepan, melt butter over medium heat. Add flour and stir until blended. Whisk in stock. Add garlic and cook, stirring constantly, for 4 to 5 minutes or until thickened. Remove from heat; stir in cream cheese until melted. Season with pepper to taste.

3. Toss pasta and broccoli with sauce. Top each serving with 1 tbsp (15 mL) Parmesan cheese.

PER SERVING	
Calories: 334	
Dietary Fiber: 3 g	Carbohydrate: 47 g
Fat: 10 g	Protein: 14 g

SERVES 6

Esther Murphy, Dietitian

This creamy pasta sauce, flavored with cream cheese, may be just the recipe you need to convert your children into broccoli lovers.

DIETITIAN'S MESSAGE

If your children won't eat vegetables, don't force them but don't give up either. Some children prefer the taste and texture of raw vegetables to those that are cooked, so give them a choice. And continue to offer a variety of cooked vegetables in single one-bite servings. Tastes change, and some children take longer to accept certain foods.

John Schroder, Chef
Susie Langley, Dietitian

*In this dish, which is
perfect for entertaining,
jumbo pasta shells are
stuffed with ricotta,
Cheddar-style and
Parmesan cheeses,
sun-dried tomatoes and
herbs, then baked in a
creamy sauce. Make it
the centerpiece of a
delicious meal.*

TIPS

If you don't have fresh
basil on hand, use 2 tsp
(10 mL) dried basil.

For a speedy lunch or
supper, make this recipe
ahead and freeze in
single servings. Omit the
cheese topping until
you're ready to serve.

MAKE AHEAD

This dish can be prepared
up to the baking stage
(complete Step 3), then
covered and refrigerated
for up to 8 hours.

DIETITIAN'S MESSAGE

This meatless dish
features all the food
groups and is almost a
meal in itself. Add a
tossed green salad and
fresh fruit for extra
vitamins and fiber.

Stuffed Pasta Shells

Preheat oven to 350°F (180°C)
13- by 9-inch (3 L) baking dish

2	cloves garlic	2
¼ cup	chopped onion	50 mL
1 tbsp	olive oil	15 mL
1	can (14 oz/398 mL) tomato sauce	1
2 cups	5% ricotta cheese	500 mL
¾ cup	shredded lower-fat medium Cheddar-style cheese, divided	175 mL
½ cup	grated Parmesan cheese, divided	125 mL
¼ cup	diced sun-dried tomatoes	50 mL
2 tbsp	chopped fresh basil	25 mL
3 tbsp	chopped fresh parsley	45 mL
1 tbsp	finely chopped green onions	15 mL
1 tsp	coarsely ground black pepper	5 mL
1	egg, lightly beaten	1
24	jumbo pasta shells, cooked and drained	24
1⅔ cups	2% milk, divided	400 mL
5 tsp	cornstarch	25 mL
½ tsp	salt	2 mL

1. In a saucepan, sauté garlic and onion in oil until tender. Add tomato sauce; simmer over low heat for 8 to 10 minutes or until reduced slightly. Pour into 13- by 9-inch (3 L) baking dish.

2. Combine ricotta, ½ cup (125 mL) of the Cheddar, ¼ cup (50 mL) of the Parmesan, tomatoes, basil, 2 tbsp (25 mL) of the parsley, onions, ½ tsp (2 mL) of the pepper and egg. Spoon into pasta shells and arrange in single layer over sauce.

3. In a saucepan, heat 1½ cups (375 mL) of the milk. Whisk cornstarch into remaining milk; whisk into hot milk and cook, stirring, until sauce thickens and boils. Stir in salt and remaining Parmesan, parsley and pepper; cool for 5 minutes. Pour over prepared shells. Cover with foil.

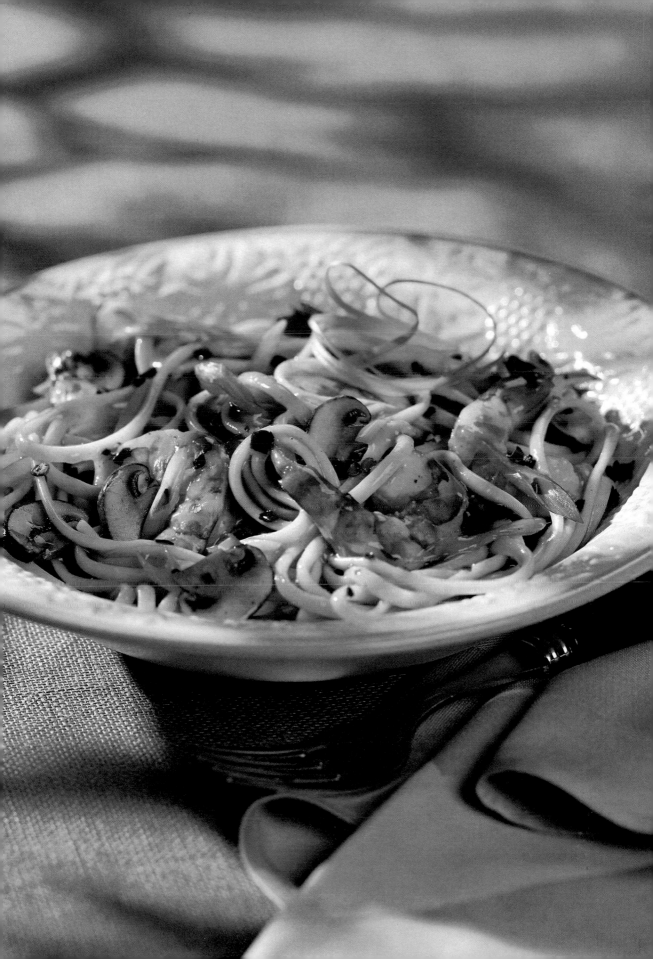

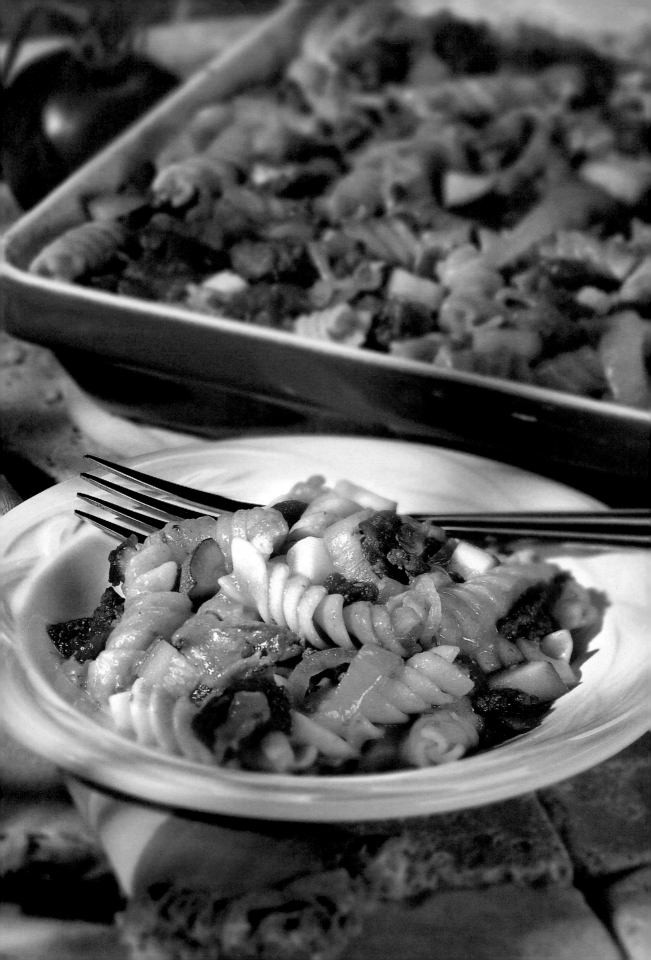

4. Bake in preheated oven for 40 to 45 minutes or until hot and bubbly. Remove foil and sprinkle with remaining Cheddar; bake just until cheese melts.

PER SERVING	
Calories: 309	
Dietary Fiber: 2 g	Carbohydrate: 32 g
Fat: 11 g	Protein: 19 g

Mixed Vegetables with Noodles

2 cups	egg noodles *or* other pasta	500 mL
2	cloves garlic, sliced	2
1	sweet potato, peeled, quartered and cut into ¼-inch (5 mm) thick slices	1
1 cup	broccoli florets	250 mL
1 cup	quartered mushrooms	250 mL
1 cup	shredded mozzarella cheese	250 mL
2 tbsp	sodium-reduced soy sauce	25 mL
¼ tsp	crushed dried thyme	1 mL
¼ tsp	black pepper	1 mL

1. In a large saucepan of boiling water, cook noodles and garlic for 4 minutes. Add sweet potato and cook for 4 minutes. Add broccoli and mushrooms; cook for 2 minutes or until all vegetables are tender. Drain well.

2. In a bowl, toss together noodle mixture, cheese, soy sauce, thyme and pepper until cheese melts.

PER SERVING	
Calories: 207	
Dietary Fiber: 2 g	Carbohydrate: 24 g
Fat: 8 g	Protein: 10 g

SERVES 4

Stephen Ashton, Chef
Leah Hawirko, Dietitian

Packed with flavor, vitamins and minerals, this pasta has an Asian touch.

TIPS
Sodium-reduced soy sauce should be used if sodium intake is a concern.

Use other vegetables (either fresh or frozen) that you have on hand, such as sliced carrots, green beans, cauliflower or peas. Substitute 1 tsp (5 mL) fresh thyme leaves for the dried, if available.

DIETITIAN'S MESSAGE
This one-pot meal is packed with flavor, vitamins and minerals. Including both dark green and orange vegetables, it is a powerhouse of natural antioxidants, which work to rid the body of cell-damaging free radicals.

Liliane Cotton

This macaroni dish provides fewer calories and less fat than conventional macaroni and cheese.

TIP

The sauce will be thin when added to the macaroni but will thicken during the oven baking. If desired, replace Cheddar cheese with Parmesan.

DIETITIAN'S MESSAGE

Serve this lower-fat alternative to macaroni and cheese, which offers a vegetable serving, with a tossed green salad for extra vitamins and fiber and end the meal with Spicy Fruit Compote (see recipe, page 383).

Italian-Style Macaroni

Preheat oven to 375°F (190°C)
6-cup (1.5 L) baking dish

2 cups	tomato juice	500 mL
1 cup	chicken broth	250 mL
2 tbsp	finely chopped onion	25 mL
1	clove garlic, minced	1
1 tsp	dried Italian seasoning	5 mL
Pinch	each salt and black pepper	Pinch
2 cups	cooked elbow macaroni	500 mL
1 cup	shredded old Cheddar cheese	250 mL

1. In a medium saucepan, combine tomato juice, broth, onion, garlic and seasonings. Cook over low heat, uncovered, for about 25 minutes or until reduced by half.

2. Stir tomato sauce into cooked macaroni. Spoon into 6-cup (1.5 L) baking dish. Sprinkle with cheese. Bake in preheated oven for about 25 minutes.

PER SERVING	
Calories: 240	
Dietary Fiber: 1 g	Carbohydrate: 25 g
Fat: 10 g	Protein: 12 g

Turmeric Spaetzle

2	eggs	2
2/3 cup	2% milk	150 mL
1 1/2 cups	all-purpose flour	375 mL
1/2 tsp	turmeric	2 mL
	Salt	
Pinch	ground mace *or* nutmeg	Pinch
1/4 cup	olive oil	50 mL
2	cloves garlic, minced	2
2 tbsp	chopped fresh mint (optional)	25 mL
	Black pepper	

1. In a mixing bowl, beat together eggs and milk. Combine flour, turmeric, 1/4 tsp (1 mL) salt and mace; gradually add to bowl, beating constantly on low speed until smooth and thick.

2. Place colander over a large pot of boiling salted water. With rubber spatula, press the batter, in small batches, through colander, scraping particles off underneath so particles form drops of dough in the water. Boil for 5 minutes. With slotted spoon, remove to large bowl of ice water. Drain and spread on wet tea towel on baking sheet. Cover with another towel. Refrigerate until serving time or for up to several days.

3. In a large skillet, heat olive oil over medium heat; cook garlic and spaetzle, stirring, until hot. Add mint, if using; season with salt and pepper to taste.

PER SERVING	
Calories: 234	
Dietary Fiber: 1 g	Carbohydrate: 26 g
Fat: 12 g	Protein: 6 g

SERVES 6

**Alastair Gray, Chef
Mary Margaret Laing,
Dietitian**

Spaetzle ("little sparrow" in German) is a tiny, light dumpling made from a runny pasta dough. This variation of an Austrian recipe is uniquely flavored — with turmeric, garlic and mint.

TIPS

Transferring spaetzle to ice water after cooking prevents it from sticking together.

Store spaetzle between 2 damp towels in the refrigerator for several days, if desired. Use only as needed.

DIETITIAN'S MESSAGE

Spaetzle is an economical alternative to traditional pasta. It can be served plain or dressed up with herbs and spices. Serve this uniquely flavored spaetzle with Easy Beef Curry (see recipe, page 240), a tossed green salad, and yogurt for calcium.

Lasagna Roll-Ups

Here's a great lasagna recipe for any vegetarians in your family or circle of friends. It adds tofu to the filling for protein.

TIPS

Tofu is a versatile product made from soy milk. Available in a variety of textures, from soft to extra firm, it may also be flavored with herbs and spices. It is found in the produce section of most grocery stores.

Once unpackaged, tofu should be stored in the refrigerator in water to cover. To keep tofu fresh for as long as a week, change the water daily.

DIETITIAN'S MESSAGE

The tofu in this recipe combines with the noodles and the cheese to provide high-quality protein. Serve this lasagna with a tossed green salad and crusty whole-wheat bread for a delicious vegetarian meal.

Preheat oven to 350°F (180°C)
8-inch (2 L) square baking pan

2	large cloves garlic, minced	2
1 tsp	olive oil	5 mL
2 cups	chopped mushrooms	500 mL
½ cup	diced red bell pepper	125 mL
1 tsp	dried thyme	5 mL
1 tsp	fennel seed	5 mL
¼ tsp	salt	1 mL
Pinch	black pepper	Pinch
¼ lb	firm tofu, drained and crumbled	125 g
2 cups	Versatile Tomato Sauce (see recipe, page 179)	500 mL
6	cooked lasagna noodles	6
1 cup	shredded part-skim mozzarella cheese	250 mL

1. In a large skillet over medium-high heat, cook garlic in hot oil for about 2 minutes. Add mushrooms, red pepper and seasonings; cook over high heat, stirring constantly, for about 5 minutes or until liquid evaporates and vegetables are tender. Add tofu.

2. Spoon half of the tomato sauce into bottom of 8-inch (2 L) square baking pan. Spread about ⅓ cup (75 mL) mushroom mixture over each cooked noodle. Divide cheese evenly over filling on each noodle. Roll up, jelly roll–style. Arrange rolls seam side down in baking dish. Spoon remaining tomato sauce over rolls.

3. Cover and bake in preheated oven for 15 minutes; remove cover and bake for about 10 minutes.

PER SERVING	
Calories: 226	
Dietary Fiber: 2 g	Carbohydrate: 30 g
Fat: 7 g	Protein: 13 g

Lazy Lasagna

Preheat oven to 350°F (180°C)
13- by 9-inch (3 L) baking dish, greased

3 cups	penne, rotini *or* other large pasta	750 mL
2 tsp	olive oil	10 mL
12 oz	lean ground beef	375 g
½ cup	chopped onions	125 mL
1 cup	finely chopped *or* grated carrots	250 mL
1	jar (24 to 25 oz/700 to 750 mL) tomato pasta sauce	1
½ tsp	dried Italian seasoning *or* dried oregano *or* basil	2 mL
1	container (17 oz/475 g) light ricotta cheese	1
1	egg	1
1½ cups	shredded part-skim mozzarella cheese	375 mL
¼ cup	grated Parmesan cheese	50 mL

1. In a large pot of boiling water, cook pasta until tender but firm; drain. Toss with olive oil; set aside.

2. In a large skillet, cook beef over medium-high heat until browned. Add onions and carrots; cook for 3 to 4 minutes. Stir in pasta sauce and Italian seasoning. Remove from heat and set aside.

3. In a bowl, combine ricotta cheese, egg and 1 cup (250 mL) of the mozzarella cheese. Set aside.

4. To assemble, spread half of the meat mixture on bottom of greased baking dish. Top with all of the pasta. Spread all of the cheese mixture over pasta. Top with remaining meat mixture. Sprinkle with remaining ½ cup (125 mL) mozzarella cheese and Parmesan cheese.

5. Bake in preheated oven, uncovered, for 35 to 45 minutes or until bubbling and brown on top. Let stand for 10 minutes before serving.

PER SERVING	
Calories: 461	
Dietary Fiber: 4 g	Carbohydrate: 44 g
Fat: 19 g	Protein: 28 g

SERVES 8 P

Bev Callaghan and Lynn Roblin, Dietitians

Here's a quick way to get all the satisfying flavor and texture of lasagna without spending a lot of time in the kitchen.

TIPS

This is a great make-ahead recipe that easily doubles. Make 2 and keep 1 in the freezer for unexpected guests or an easy dinner. It also makes a perfect lunch box treat — just heat it up in the microwave in the morning and pop into a short, wide-mouth Thermos.

If desired, substitute 3 cups (750 mL) Versatile Tomato Sauce (see recipe, page 179) or Piquant Tomato Sauce (see recipe, page 180) for the prepared sauce.

DIETITIAN'S MESSAGE

Lazy Lasagna features all the food groups and is jam-packed with valuable nutrients. For an easy meal, finish with a slice of Blueberry Semolina Cake (see recipe, page 406).

....

Bernard Casavant, Chef
Jane Thornthwaite,
Dietitian

Two simple changes give this lasagna a delicious new flavor — the vegetables are grilled first, and tofu is used as a layer with the cheese, making it rich in calcium.

TIPS

Instead of using traditional noodles as a base, this lasagna uses tofu. For best results, use firm or extra-firm tofu.

For instructions on roasting peppers, see page 127.

DIETITIAN'S MESSAGE

This vegetable lasagna provides an abundance of vitamins and minerals. In addition, the tofu and cheeses add lots of calcium. Serve this with crusty whole-grain bread and a slice of Harvest Raisin Cake (see recipe, page 413) for dessert.

Grilled Vegetable Lasagna

Preheat oven to 350°F (180°C)
13- by 9-inch (3.5 L) baking pan

1	small onion, chopped	1
1 tbsp	vegetable oil	15 mL
3	cloves garlic, chopped	3
1	medium carrot, diced	1
1	stalk celery, diced	1
2 cups	sliced mushrooms	500 mL
1	can (19 oz/540 mL) tomatoes	1
1	can (7½ oz/213 mL) tomato sauce	1
1 tsp	each crushed dried basil and oregano	5 mL
½ tsp	salt	2 mL
¼ tsp	black pepper	1 mL
1½ lb	herb-flavored *or* plain tofu	750 g
2	medium zucchini, sliced lengthwise and grilled	2
½	medium eggplant, sliced and grilled	½
1	red bell pepper, quartered, grilled and peeled	1
1 cup	lower-fat cottage cheese	250 mL
3 cups	shredded part-skim mozzarella cheese	750 mL
⅓ cup	grated Parmesan cheese	75 mL

1. In a Dutch oven, sauté onion in oil until tender. Stir in garlic, carrot, celery and mushrooms; sauté for 5 minutes. Add tomatoes, breaking up with fork; add tomato sauce, basil and oregano. Simmer, uncovered, for 15 to 20 minutes or until thickened and reduced to about 2½ cups (625 mL). Season with salt and pepper.

2. Spray 13- by 9-inch (3.5 L) baking pan with vegetable oil spray. Cut half of the tofu into ¼-inch (5 mm) thick slices; line bottom of pan with slices. Spread with half of the sauce. Cut zucchini, eggplant and red pepper into bite-size pieces; sprinkle half over sauce. Sprinkle with half each of the cottage and mozzarella cheeses.

3. Slice remaining tofu and arrange in layer over cheese. Top with remaining sauce, vegetables and cottage cheese. Blend remaining mozzarella with Parmesan; sprinkle over top. Cover tightly with foil. Bake in preheated oven for 15 minutes. Uncover and bake until hot and golden, 15 to 20 minutes. Let stand for 5 minutes before serving.

PER SERVING	
Calories: 298	
Dietary Fiber: 4 g	Carbohydrate: 16 g
Fat: 15 g	Protein: 27 g

Cumin Shrimp Linguine

8 oz	linguine	250 g
¾ cup	vegetable *or* chicken broth	175 mL
1 tsp	ground cumin	5 mL
¼ to ½ tsp	crushed red chilies	1 to 2 mL
1 cup	sliced mushrooms	250 mL
½ cup	sliced green onions	125 mL
½ lb	large shrimp, peeled and deveined	250 g
1 tbsp	cornstarch	15 mL
1 tbsp	cold water	15 mL

1. Cook linguine according to package directions; drain well.
2. Meanwhile, in a skillet, bring broth, cumin and chilies to a boil. Add mushrooms; simmer for 3 minutes. Add green onions and shrimp; cook until shrimp turn pink. Combine cornstarch and water; stir into skillet until thickened. Divide linguine between 2 plates; top with shrimp sauce.

PER SERVING	
Calories: 552	
Dietary Fiber: 6 g	Carbohydrate: 93 g
Fat: 4 g	Protein: 33 g

SERVES 2

Eric Fergie, Chef
Jane Thornthwaite,
Dietitian

This elegant recipe serves 2 and is ready in a matter of minutes. Feel free to double or triple the quantity, if desired.

TIP
Vary the quantity of crushed red chilies to suit your taste, or substitute a similar quantity of chopped fresh chili pepper, if desired. Since chilies can burn, wear protective gloves when handling or wash your hands thoroughly once you have finished.

DIETITIAN'S MESSAGE

Use this easy recipe to set the stage for a romantic dinner. Add a Spinach and Grapefruit Salad (see recipe, page 160) to sustain the elegance while adding fiber, vitamins and minerals. Finish the meal with a serving of Lemon Mousse (see recipe, page 388).

....

Ron Glover, Chef
Mary Sue Waisman,
Dietitian

*Whole-wheat spaghetti,
dry or fresh, is both
tasty and nutritious and
complements the flavors
of the peppers
and scallops.*

DIETITIAN'S MESSAGE

Pasta is a great meal
planner. Easy on the
budget, it makes more
expensive foods, such as
the scallops in this recipe,
go further. Pasta is
generally low in fat, and
the whole-grain varieties
contribute fiber to your
diet. Serve this interesting
dish with a tossed green
salad for additional
vitamins, minerals and
fiber. Complete the meal
with a fruit dessert.

Whole-Wheat Spaghetti with Scallops

12 oz	whole-wheat spaghetti	375 g
2 tbsp	olive oil	25 mL
1	medium red onion, chopped	1
1	each medium red, green and yellow bell pepper, cut into thin strips	1
12	mushrooms, sliced	12
2	cloves garlic, minced	2
2 tsp	dried basil	10 mL
½ tsp	salt	2 mL
¼ tsp	black pepper	1 mL
Pinch	cayenne pepper	Pinch
1½ lb	scallops	750 g
3	medium tomatoes, seeded and chopped	3
	Chopped fresh parsley and basil	

1. Cook spaghetti according to package directions; drain.
2. Meanwhile, in a large skillet, heat oil over medium-high heat; sauté onion, peppers and mushrooms for 5 to 8 minutes or until tender. Stir in garlic, basil, salt, pepper and cayenne. Add scallops and heat until white but tender, 3 to 5 minutes. Add tomatoes and heat through. Toss with pasta and garnish with chopped parsley and basil.

PER SERVING	
Calories: 382	
Dietary Fiber: 10 g	Carbohydrate: 58 g
Fat: 7 g	Protein: 27 g

Spaghettini with Tuna, Olives and Capers

8 to 12 oz	spaghettini	250 to 375 g
2 tsp	olive oil	10 mL
½ cup	chopped onion	125 mL
5	anchovies (optional)	5
3 cups	Piquant Tomato Sauce (see recipe, page 180) *or* commercially prepared pasta sauce	750 mL
1	can (6 oz/170 g) tuna, drained	1
½ cup	sliced black olives	125 mL
2 tbsp	drained capers	25 mL
¼ cup	chopped fresh basil (*or* 1 tsp/5 mL dried)	50 mL

1. In a large pot of boiling water, cook pasta until tender but firm; drain.

2. In a large nonstick skillet, heat oil over medium-high heat; add onion and sauté for 3 to 4 minutes or until softened. Add anchovies, if using, and cook for 1 to 2 minutes or until dissolved into a paste.

3. Stir in Piquant Tomato Sauce, tuna, olives and capers; bring to a boil. Reduce heat and simmer for 5 minutes. Stir in basil and cook for 1 minute. Serve over pasta.

PER SERVING	
Calories: 390	
Dietary Fiber: 6 g	Carbohydrate: 81 g
Fat: 9 g	Protein: 19 g

SERVES 4
....
Laurie A. Wadsworth, Dietitian

This tasty dish, with a Mediterranean flair, is easy to make and so delicious it is likely to become a kitchen staple.

TIPS

Remember that using commercially prepared pasta sauce in this recipe will increase your sodium intake.

Capers are the pickled flower buds of a bush grown in Mediterranean countries. As they are pleasantly pungent, they are used to add flavor and "bite" to dishes. They go particularly well with fish and seafood.

DIETITIAN'S MESSAGE

This flavorful dish is almost a complete meal. All you need to add is a glass of milk, or yogurt for dessert.

The light sauce, prepared with chicken broth rather than milk or cream, highlights the flavors of the vegetables and tuna.

TIPS

For variety, serve this with whole-wheat spaghetti instead of spaghettini.

You may want to use minced garlic to taste instead of the garlic powder, and 1 tbsp (15 mL) fresh thyme instead of the dried version. Add to the onion-mushroom mixture just before adding the tuna.

DIETITIAN'S MESSAGE

The tuna and vegetables in this recipe provide abundant protein, fiber, vitamins and iron. Serve this nutritious dish with garlic bread and a tossed green salad. End the meal with Cinnamon Baked Pears (see recipe, page 385).

Tuna Garden Pasta

6	large mushrooms, sliced	6
1	small onion, sliced	1
2 tbsp	butter *or* margarine	25 mL
2	cans (each 6½ oz/184 g) water-packed chunk white tuna drained	2
2 cups	chicken broth	500 mL
2 tbsp	all-purpose flour	25 mL
2 tbsp	lemon juice	25 mL
2 tbsp	chopped pimiento	25 mL
1 tsp	grated lemon zest	5 mL
1 tsp	dried thyme	5 mL
¼ tsp	garlic powder	1 mL
Pinch	each salt and black pepper	Pinch
3	medium carrots, sliced	3
2	large bunches broccoli (florets only), chopped	2
8 oz	spaghettini	250 g
	Tomato slices	

1. In a large skillet over medium heat, cook mushrooms and onion in butter for about 5 minutes or until tender. Stir in tuna. Combine chicken broth, flour, lemon juice, pimiento, lemon zest and seasonings. Stir into tuna mixture; cook for about 5 minutes or until slightly thickened.

2. Steam carrots and broccoli over boiling water until tender-crisp. Drain well and add to tuna mixture.

3. In a large pot of boiling water, cook pasta according to package directions or until tender but firm; drain well. Stir tuna and vegetable sauce into pasta; garnish with tomato slices.

PER SERVING	
Calories: 310	
Dietary Fiber: 4 g	Carbohydrate: 39 g
Fat: 5 g	Protein: 30 g

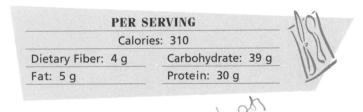

Pasta with White Clam Sauce

SERVES 4
....
Mary Anne Pucovsky

Pasta with clams is an Italian classic and for good reason — it's as good to eat as it is easy to make.

1 tbsp	olive oil	15 mL
¼ cup	chopped onions	50 mL
2 cups	sliced mushrooms	500 mL
2 tsp	all-purpose flour	10 mL
⅓ cup	dry white wine	75 mL
2	cans (each 5 oz/142 g) clams, drained (reserve ¾ cup/ 175 mL clam juice)	2
1 tsp	minced garlic	5 mL
1	can (5½ oz/156 mL) 2% evaporated milk	1
⅛ tsp	ground nutmeg	0.5 mL
8 oz	capellini *or* vermicelli	250 g
2 tbsp	chopped fresh parsley (*or* 2 tsp/10 mL dried)	25 mL
	Black pepper	

TIPS

Fresh clams are superb in this dish. Substitute 2 cups (500 mL) fresh shucked clams for the canned clams. Instead of the reserved clam juice, use ¾ cup (175 mL) fish or vegetable stock.

For a change of color, try making this with red clam sauce: just add 1 cup (250 mL) chopped tomatoes to the sauce at the end of Step 1.

DIETITIAN'S MESSAGE

When recipes call for cream, try replacing it with evaporated milk, which is lower in fat and higher in calcium. Keep some in your pantry so you will always have it on hand.

1. In a large nonstick skillet, heat oil over medium-high heat. Add onions and mushrooms; sauté for 5 to 6 minutes or until softened and moisture has evaporated. Sprinkle with flour; blend well. Add wine, reserved clam juice and garlic; bring to a boil. Reduce heat and simmer for 2 to 3 minutes or until thickened. Stir in clams, evaporated milk and nutmeg; simmer for 1 to 2 minutes or until heated through.

2. Just before serving, cook pasta according to package directions or until tender but firm; drain. Toss with sauce. Sprinkle with parsley. Season with pepper to taste.

PER SERVING	
Calories: 412	
Dietary Fiber: 3 g	Carbohydrate: 54 g
Fat: 7 g	Protein: 30 g

Chicken Vegetable Lasagna

Lasagna is always a popular dish for parties and buffets, and this version, which features chicken and a variety of vegetables instead of ground beef, is both light and satisfying.

TIP

If desired, substitute lean ground turkey for the chicken.

DIETITIAN'S MESSAGE

This is a lower-fat, higher-fiber alternative to traditional lasagna. Chicken, rather than ground beef, provides the protein. Replacing the traditional white sauce or ricotta cheese with vegetables lowers the fat and adds fiber and vitamins.

Preheat oven to 350°F (180°C)
13- by 9-inch (3 L) baking dish

½ lb	lean ground chicken	250 g
½ cup	chopped onion	125 mL
2	cloves garlic, minced	2
1 tbsp	vegetable oil	15 mL
1 tsp	butter *or* margarine	5 mL
1	can (28 oz/796 mL) tomatoes	1
1	can (5½ oz/156 mL) tomato paste	1
¾ cup	water	175 mL
1½ tsp	salt	7 mL
Pinch	black pepper	Pinch
4	medium carrots, diced	4
1	bunch broccoli, chopped	1
½ lb	mushrooms, sliced	250 g
¼ cup	chopped fresh parsley	50 mL
12 oz	lasagna noodles	375 g
1	pkg (6 oz/175 g) sliced part-skim mozzarella cheese	1
	Grated Parmesan cheese	

1. In a saucepan over medium-high heat, cook chicken, onion and garlic in oil and butter until chicken is no longer pink. Add tomatoes, tomato paste, water, salt and pepper. Cook, uncovered, over medium heat for about 15 minutes, stirring occasionally. Add carrots, broccoli, mushrooms and parsley. Cook, covered, over low heat for about 30 minutes or until mixture is thickened.

2. In a large pot of boiling water, cook noodles according to package directions or until tender but firm; drain well.

3. Spoon one-quarter of the sauce into 13- by 9-inch (3 L) baking dish. Place one-third of the lasagna noodles over sauce. Repeat layers twice, ending with sauce. Top with cheese slices; sprinkle lightly with Parmesan cheese. Bake in preheated oven for about 30 minutes. Let stand for 10 minutes before serving.

PER SERVING	
Calories: 348	
Dietary Fiber: 5 g	Carbohydrate: 48 g
Fat: 9 g	Protein: 21 g

Creamy Bow Ties with Chicken, Spinach and Peppers

SERVES 4 **P**

Lisa Wik

12 oz	boneless skinless chicken breasts, cut into strips	375 g
1 tbsp	vegetable oil, divided	15 mL
1 cup	julienned red bell peppers	250 mL
2 cups	shredded fresh spinach	500 mL
2 tsp	lemon juice	10 mL
1 tbsp	all-purpose flour	15 mL
1 tsp	minced garlic	5 mL
2 cups	milk	500 mL
¼ tsp	salt	1 mL
¼ tsp	ground nutmeg	1 mL
¼ tsp	black pepper	1 mL
¾ cup	shredded old white Cheddar cheese	175 mL
6 oz	farfalle (bow tie pasta), cooked and drained	175 g
¼ cup	grated Parmesan cheese	50 mL

1. Spray a large skillet with vegetable spray. Add chicken strips and cook over medium-high heat for 4 to 5 minutes or until browned and juices run clear when chicken is pierced with a fork. Transfer to a plate.

2. In the same skillet, heat 1 tsp (5 mL) of the oil over medium heat. Add peppers and sauté for 3 to 4 minutes or until slightly softened. Stir in spinach and cook until wilted. Stir in lemon juice. Set aside.

3. In a pot, heat remaining oil over medium heat; blend in flour. Add garlic and milk; cook, whisking constantly, until mixture comes to a boil. Reduce heat and simmer for 2 to 3 minutes. Stir in salt, nutmeg and pepper. Remove from heat. Add Cheddar cheese and blend. Stir in pasta, chicken and vegetables. Serve sprinkled with Parmesan cheese.

This attractive dish is perfect for entertaining, but it's so quick and easy you'll want to make it for the family. Kids love it!

TIP
While the old Cheddar adds a wonderfully rich flavor to this dish, other strong-tasting white cheeses, such as Asiago, also work well.

DIETITIAN'S MESSAGE
This recipe is a winner in the balanced meal category as all the food groups are represented. For a special meal, add a green salad and finish with Lemon Tart with Raspberry Coulis (see recipe, page 400).

PER SERVING	
Calories: 478	
Dietary Fiber: 3 g	Carbohydrate: 43 g
Fat: 17 g	Protein: 38 g

Roast Lamb Loin with Tomato Basil Linguine

4 tsp	olive oil	20 mL
1	medium onion, chopped	1
1	medium tomato, chopped	1
½ cup	chopped fresh parsley	125 mL
4 tsp	dried basil	20 mL
1 cup	dry white wine	250 mL
¼ tsp	each salt and black pepper	1 mL
12 oz	tomato basil linguine *or* plain linguine	375 g
4	frozen lamb loins (each 3 oz/90 g), thawed	4
¼ cup	Dijon mustard	50 mL
⅓ cup	(approx.) fine dry bread crumbs	75 mL
	Chopped fresh basil (optional)	

1. In a skillet, heat 3 tsp (15 mL) of the oil over medium heat; cook onion, tomato, parsley and basil for 3 to 5 minutes or until tender. Stir in wine, salt and pepper; bring to a boil, reduce heat and simmer until slightly thickened. Keep warm.

2. Cook linguine according to package directions; drain well.

3. Meanwhile, coat each lamb loin with mustard; roll in bread crumbs to coat well. In a skillet, heat remaining 1 tsp (5 mL) oil over medium-high heat; brown lamb on all sides, about 5 minutes. Slice thinly.

4. Toss linguine with sauce; divide among 4 plates. Top with lamb. Garnish with fresh basil, if using.

PER SERVING	
Calories: 562	
Dietary Fiber: 5 g	Carbohydrate: 76 g
Fat: 13 g	Protein: 31 g

Ham and Mushroom Fettuccine

12 oz	fettuccine	375 g
1 tbsp	olive oil	15 mL
2 cups	sliced mushrooms	500 mL
½ cup	slivered green bell pepper	125 mL
2 tbsp	white wine	25 mL
6 oz	lean ham, cut into thin strips	175 g
2 tbsp	all-purpose flour	25 mL
1½ cups	2% milk	375 mL
½ tsp	dried basil	2 mL
¼ tsp	each salt and white pepper	1 mL
½ cup	chopped green onions	125 mL

1. Cook fettuccine according to package directions. Drain well.

2. Meanwhile, in a large skillet, heat oil over medium-high heat; cook mushrooms and green pepper, stirring, for 3 minutes. Stir in wine; simmer for a few minutes or until reduced. Stir in ham.

3. Dissolve flour in milk; stir into skillet along with basil, salt and pepper. Bring to a boil, stirring constantly. Stir in green onions; cook for 1 minute longer. Stir in fettuccine.

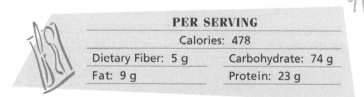

PER SERVING	
Calories: 478	
Dietary Fiber: 5 g	Carbohydrate: 74 g
Fat: 9 g	Protein: 23 g

SERVES 4

Beth Van Arenthals, Chef
Connie Mallette,
Dietitian

This lower-fat version of a dish that is usually higher in fat features ingredients you're likely to have on hand.

TIPS

Substitute 1 tbsp (15 mL) chopped fresh basil for the dried version, if available, and add along with the green onions.

Instead of wine, you can use 2 tbsp (25 mL) water and ½ tsp (2 mL) lemon juice. 1% milk may also be used but the sauce will be thinner than if made with 2% milk.

DIETITIAN'S MESSAGE

Sprinkle with Parmesan cheese to serve. Follow with Basil Marinated Tomatoes (see recipe, page 149) or Roasted Red Pepper Salad (see recipe, page 149) to feature all the food groups.

This delicious dish for pasta lovers combines meat and vegetables in a delectable sauce. For a zestier sauce, add dried or fresh basil, oregano, and rosemary along with the tomatoes.

TIP

Once pasta is cooked, drain but do not rinse and toss immediately with the hot sauce. The coating of starch on pasta helps the sauce to cling to the pasta. For best results, have the sauce ready before cooking the pasta.

DIETITIAN'S MESSAGE

This dish includes all the food groups. Serve with crusty Italian bread and a tossed green salad. Finish with frozen yogurt topped with fresh berries.

Country Club Pasta

2	yellow bell peppers, cut into slices	2
2 tbsp	vegetable oil *or* olive oil	25 mL
1	small onion, chopped	1
1	small carrot, chopped	1
1	stalk celery, chopped	1
1	large clove garlic, minced	1
¼ lb	lean ground beef	125 g
1	can (14 oz/398 mL) tomatoes	1
½ tsp	salt	2 mL
¼ tsp	freshly ground black pepper	1 mL
2 oz	cooked ham, finely chopped	60 g
10 oz	penne	300 g
½ cup	grated Parmesan cheese	125 mL
	Parsley sprigs	

1. In a skillet over medium-high heat, cook peppers in oil for about 3 minutes; set aside.

2. In a medium saucepan, cook onion, carrot, celery, garlic and ground beef until beef is no longer pink; drain fat. Add tomatoes and seasonings. Cook, uncovered, over medium-low heat for 15 minutes. Stir in pepper slices and ham; cook for about 15 minutes or until thickened.

3. In a large pot of boiling water, cook pasta according to package directions or until tender but firm. Drain well. Toss pasta with meat sauce until well coated. Sprinkle with cheese; garnish with parsley. Serve immediately.

PER SERVING	
Calories: 494	
Dietary Fiber: 4 g	Carbohydrate: 66 g
Fat: 15 g	Protein: 23 g

Veggie, Beef and Pasta Bake

Preheat oven to 350°F (180°C)
13- by 9-inch (3 L) baking dish, greased

1 lb	lean ground beef	500 g
1 cup	sliced onions	250 mL
1 cup	diced zucchini	250 mL
2 tsp	minced garlic	10 mL
1	can (28 oz/796 mL) stewed *or* diced tomatoes, with juice	1
2 tbsp	sodium-reduced soy sauce	25 mL
½ tsp	crushed red pepper flakes	2 mL
2 cups	rotini *or* other spiral pasta	500 mL
1½ cups	shredded Cheddar cheese	375 mL

1. In a large nonstick skillet over medium-high heat, combine ground beef, onions, zucchini and garlic; cook for 8 to 10 minutes or until beef is no longer pink and vegetables are softened. Drain fat; pour beef mixture into greased 13- by 9-inch (3 L) baking dish. Set aside.

2. Meanwhile, drain juice from tomatoes into an 8-cup (2 L) microwave-safe measuring cup; add water to make 2 cups (500 mL). Coarsely chop tomatoes; add to measuring cup. Stir in soy sauce and red pepper flakes. Microwave on High for 5 minutes or until very hot. Stir in rotini.

3. Pour tomato-pasta mixture into baking dish and combine with meat mixture. Press pasta down to make sure it is submerged in the liquid. Bake in preheated oven, covered, for 20 minutes. Remove cover; stir gently and sprinkle with cheese. Bake, uncovered, for 15 to 20 minutes or until pasta is tender.

PER SERVING	
Calories: 362	
Dietary Fiber: 3 g	Carbohydrate: 26 g
Fat: 17 g	Protein: 25 g

SERVES 6

Kathyrn Papple

Here's a terrific recipe that makes a complete meal, with something from all the food groups! The pasta does not require any precooking, so you can save preparation and cleanup time.

TIP

If you are concerned about sodium, use sodium-reduced soy sauce instead of the regular variety. One tbsp (15 mL) regular soy sauce contains 1,037 mg sodium; the same amount of sodium-reduced soy sauce contains only 605 mg.

DIETITIAN'S MESSAGE

Crusty bread or a Mixed Herb Baguette (see recipe, page 45) is all that is needed to complement this dish, which includes all the food groups. If desired, add a tossed green salad for additional fiber.

Fettuccine Carbonara

12 oz	fettuccine	375 g
4	eggs	4
1 cup	grated Parmesan cheese	250 mL
¼ cup	chopped fresh parsley (*or* 1 tbsp/15 mL dried)	50 mL
½ tsp	butter	2 mL
½ cup	finely chopped onion	125 mL
¼ cup	chopped cooked ham *or* crumbled cooked bacon	50 mL
⅛ tsp	black pepper	0.5 mL

1. In a large pot of boiling water, cook fettuccine according to package directions or until tender but firm. Drain, reserving about ½ cup (125 mL) pasta cooking water. Return fettuccine to pot.

2. In a medium bowl, whisk together eggs, ¾ cup (175 mL) of the Parmesan cheese and parsley. Set aside.

3. Meanwhile, in a small nonstick skillet, melt butter over medium heat. Add onion and cook until soft and transparent. Stir in ham.

4. Add egg mixture to hot pasta; toss until eggs thicken and coat fettuccine. Stir in onions and ham. If sauce is too thick, add reserved pasta cooking water, a little bit at a time, stirring, until desired consistency is reached. Serve piping hot, sprinkled with remaining Parmesan cheese and pepper.

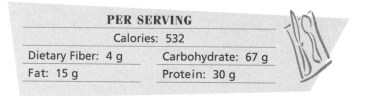

PER SERVING	
Calories: 532	
Dietary Fiber: 4 g	Carbohydrate: 67 g
Fat: 15 g	Protein: 30 g

Rice Soufflé

Preheat oven to 300°F (150°C)
8-cup (2 L) baking dish

½ cup	chopped onion	125 mL
1 tbsp	butter *or* margarine	15 mL
1 tsp	curry powder	5 mL
1	can (10 oz/284 mL) condensed cream of mushroom soup	1
1 cup	shredded old Cheddar cheese	250 mL
6	eggs, separated	6
1½ cups	cooked white rice (½ cup/125 mL uncooked long-grain white rice)	375 mL

1. In a skillet over medium heat, cook onion in butter until softened; stir in curry powder, soup and Cheddar cheese. Heat slowly until cheese melts, stirring occasionally. Beat egg yolks thoroughly and stir into hot soup mixture. Stir in cooked rice.

2. In a large bowl, beat egg whites until stiff but not dry. With spatula, lightly fold egg whites into rice mixture. Turn into an ungreased 8-cup (2 L) baking dish. Bake in preheated oven for about 1 hour or until soufflé is golden brown and knife inserted in center of puff comes out clean. Do not open oven door during first 20 minutes of baking.

PER SERVING	
Calories: 273	
Dietary Fiber: Trace	Carbohydrate: 16 g
Fat: 18 g	Protein: 13 g

SERVES 6
....
Ethel St. Jean

Because they are so glamorous, soufflés are considered difficult to make, but they are actually quite easy. This soufflé uses shortcuts — cooked rice and a can of cream of mushroom soup — but the results are delicious, nonetheless.

TIP
Most people prefer long-grain to short-grain rice because it produces fluffy grains that remain separate when cooked.

DIETITIAN'S MESSAGE
This delicate rice soufflé is rich in complex carbohydrates, protein and calcium. Serve with broccoli spears or a tossed green salad. To add fiber, calcium, vitamin C and folic acid, complete the meal with sliced oranges sprinkled with cinnamon sugar, and yogurt.

P

Rice Pilaf

Mushrooms, almonds and raisins give this savory pilaf an interesting blend of flavors. Use a homemade chicken broth or a low-salt chicken bouillon powder. Since brown rice requires about 45 minutes of cooking time, you may need to watch that it does not boil dry.

TIPS

To get the best flavor and nutrition from mushrooms, rinse and pat them dry just before using. Don't scrub or peel them; it results in a change in texture.

Vary this recipe by using portobello or shiitake mushrooms.

DIETITIAN'S MESSAGE

This recipe provides an appetizing way to make rice the focal point of a meal. The brown rice, raisins and nuts provide fiber. Serve this with Cheesy Salmon Loaf (see recipe, page 312) for protein and calcium and a green vegetable for additional fiber and nutrients.

½ cup	raisins	125 mL
¼ cup	slivered almonds	50 mL
2 tbsp	butter *or* margarine, divided	25 mL
1 cup	brown rice	250 mL
1	small onion, chopped	1
2	cloves garlic, minced	2
2½ cups	chicken broth	625 mL
1	bay leaf	1
2 tbsp	lemon juice	25 mL
1 tsp	grated lemon zest	5 mL
Pinch	freshly ground black pepper	Pinch
1 cup	sliced mushrooms	250 mL

1. In a saucepan over medium heat, cook raisins and almonds in 1 tbsp (15 mL) of the butter of the until golden; reserve.

2. In the same saucepan over medium-high heat, cook rice, onion and garlic in remaining butter for 5 minutes or until light brown. Add chicken broth, bay leaf, lemon juice, lemon zest and pepper. Cover and cook over low heat for 40 minutes. Add mushrooms; cook for 5 minutes. Remove bay leaf. Serve rice sprinkled with reserved raisins and almonds.

PER SERVING	
Calories: 263	
Dietary Fiber: 3 g	Carbohydrate: 42 g
Fat: 8 g	Protein: 7 g

Simple Risotto

4 cups	chicken broth	1 L
¼ cup	finely chopped onion	50 mL
1 tbsp	olive oil	15 mL
1 cup	arborio rice *or* other Italian short-grain rice	250 mL
¼ cup	dry white wine	50 mL
3 tbsp	grated Parmesan cheese	45 mL
	Freshly ground black pepper	

1. In a large covered saucepan, bring chicken broth to a boil.

2. Meanwhile, in a large saucepan over medium heat, cook onion in oil for about 5 minutes or until tender but not browned, stirring frequently. Stir in rice; cook until all grains are coated, about 1 minute. Add wine and cook until almost evaporated. Add ½ cup (125 mL) of the hot chicken broth.

3. Cook, stirring gently with a wooden spoon, until almost all liquid has been absorbed. Continue adding chicken broth in ½-cup (125 mL) amounts until all broth has been used, stirring constantly. This technique will require about 22 minutes total cooking time. The rice will be creamy, moist and tender but firm. Remove from heat; stir in Parmesan cheese. Add freshly ground pepper to taste.

PER SERVING	
Calories: 131	
Dietary Fiber: 1 g	Carbohydrate: 18 g
Fat: 4 g	Protein: 6 g

SERVES 6
Brenda Sledzinski

There are many variations on risotto, a creamy Italian rice dish made with short-grain arborio rice. Risotto can be served as a one-dish main course with the addition of seafood, meat or vegetables, or as a sophisticated side dish.

TIP
While adding the chicken broth, be careful to stir gently so rice kernels do not break up and become mushy. As a timeline guide, when you add the first quantity of chicken broth, set a timer for 22 minutes.

DIETITIAN'S MESSAGE
This risotto makes an excellent accompaniment to such dishes as Poached Beef Tenderloin (see recipe, page 248), Sesame Steak (see recipe, page 251), Cajun-Style Turkey Cutlet with Citrus (see recipe, page 299) and Cedar-Baked Salmon (see recipe, page 305). Start the meal with a soup such as Iced Tomato Soup (see recipe, page 98), serve a tossed green salad, and skip dessert.

Easy Risotto Provençale

2 tbsp	olive oil	25 mL
1	medium onion, chopped	1
1¼ cups	arborio rice	300 mL
2½ cups	water	625 mL
1 tsp	salt	5 mL
Sauce		
1 tbsp	olive oil	15 mL
2	medium shallots (*or* white part of 4 green onions), diced	2
2	cloves garlic, minced	2
½ cup	white wine	125 mL
4	medium tomatoes, peeled and chopped	4
1 cup	quartered mushrooms	250 mL
⅔ cup	diced green, red *or* yellow bell pepper	150 mL
½ cup	diced zucchini	125 mL
1 tbsp	dried basil	15 mL
1 tsp	each crushed dried oregano and thyme	5 mL
Pinch	each salt and black pepper	Pinch
¼ cup	chopped fresh parsley	50 mL
	Grated Parmesan cheese	

1. In a medium saucepan, heat oil over medium heat; cook onion, stirring, for 3 minutes. Add rice; cook, stirring, until golden, about 5 minutes. Add water and salt; bring to a boil. Reduce heat and simmer for 15 to 18 minutes or just until tender but firm.

2. *Sauce:* Meanwhile, in a medium saucepan, heat oil over medium heat; cook shallots and garlic, stirring, for 2 to 3 minutes or until softened. Stir in wine and tomatoes; cook for 5 minutes. Stir in mushrooms, bell pepper, zucchini, basil, oregano and thyme; simmer for 10 to 15 minutes or until thickened slightly. Add salt and pepper.

3. Spoon rice into shape of ring on large warmed serving plate; spoon sauce into middle. Garnish with parsley and grated Parmesan cheese.

PER SERVING	
Calories: 375	
Dietary Fiber: 4 g	Carbohydrate: 62 g
Fat: 11 g	Protein: 6 g

Pasta, Rice and Legumes

Radicchio and Arugula Risotto

2 tsp	olive oil	10 mL
1	small onion, chopped	1
1½ cups	arborio rice	375 mL
3½ cups	shredded radicchio	875 mL
2 cups	shredded arugula	500 mL
3 cups	chicken broth	750 mL
2 tbsp	grated Parmesan cheese	25 mL
	Salt and black pepper	

1. In a large saucepan, heat oil over medium heat; cook onion, stirring, until tender. Stir in rice and cook briefly. Add radicchio and arugula; mix well.

2. Add 1 cup (250 mL) of the broth; cook, stirring constantly, until absorbed. Continue to add broth ½ cup (125 mL) at a time, cooking and stirring constantly until each addition is absorbed before adding next. Total cooking time is 15 to 20 minutes or just until rice is tender. Stir in cheese. Season with salt and pepper to taste. Serve immediately.

PER SERVING	
Calories: 177	
Dietary Fiber: 1 g	Carbohydrate: 32 g
Fat: 2 g	Protein: 6 g

SERVES 8

**Rocco Suriano, Chef
Denise Aucoin, Dietitian**

Usually radicchio and arugula are used to add a distinctive note to salads. In this case, they work their magic on a classically prepared risotto.

TIPS

For a change, replace the radicchio with 3½ cups (875 mL) chopped spinach leaves and the arugula with 1 cup (250 mL) julienned zucchini.

Because arborio rice contains more starch than most other varieties of rice, it absorbs more liquid and the grains stick together. This is the desired result in risotto.

DIETITIAN'S MESSAGE

The bitter-tasting radicchio and tangy arugula add lots of interesting flavor to this dish. Serve with Braised Roasted Veal (see recipe, page 256) and end the meal with fresh fruit.

This rustic dish is a wonderful combination of vegetables, cheese and grains that will appeal to any palate.

TIPS

Since brown rice requires about 45 minutes of cooking time, it is a good idea to cook a larger amount than you require and freeze it for use in recipes such as this. With precooked rice, this side dish can be ready in minutes instead of 1 hour.

Because olives are salty, be cautious when adding them to a recipe if you are concerned about sodium intake. Olives are a good source of monosaturated fat.

DIETITIAN'S MESSAGE

The nutty-tasting brown rice used in this recipe is an appetizing way to add fiber to your diet. The cheese adds calcium. To extend the meal, start with a hearty appetizer such as Curried Fish Fillets (see recipe, page 89) and serve with a side salad and fruit for dessert.

Cheesy Rice Casserole

Preheat oven to 350°F (180°C)
8-cup (2 L) baking dish

3¾ cups	water, divided	925 mL
1 cup	brown rice	250 mL
1 cup	sliced celery	250 mL
½ cup	chopped onion	125 mL
2 tbsp	vegetable oil	25 mL
1	can (19 oz/540 mL) tomatoes	1
⅔ cup	chopped ripe olives	150 mL
2 tbsp	all-purpose flour	25 mL
2 tsp	chili powder	10 mL
1 tsp	salt	5 mL
¼ tsp	garlic powder	1 mL
1 cup	frozen peas	250 mL
⅔ cup	shredded Cheddar cheese	150 mL

1. In a saucepan, bring 3 cups (750 mL) of the water to a boil. Add rice. Cook, covered, for 45 minutes or until rice is tender and water is absorbed.

2. Meanwhile, in a medium saucepan over high heat, cook celery and onion in oil for about 5 minutes or until tender. Add tomatoes and olives; bring to a boil. Mix flour, seasonings and remaining water; stir into hot mixture. Cook for about 3 minutes or until thickened. Stir in frozen peas.

3. Pour half of the sauce mixture into an 8-cup (2 L) baking dish. Top with cooked rice and remaining sauce. Sprinkle with cheese. Bake in preheated oven for about 20 minutes or until heated through.

PER SERVING	
Calories: 294	
Dietary Fiber: 5 g	Carbohydrate: 40 g
Fat: 12 g	Protein: 9 g

Wild Rice and Apple Pancakes

1 cup	water	250 mL
	Salt	
⅓ cup	wild rice	75 mL
1 tbsp	butter *or* margarine	15 mL
4	green onions, chopped	4
3	medium Granny Smith apples, peeled and diced	3
1¼ cups	all-purpose flour	300 mL
1 cup	whole-wheat flour	250 mL
¾ cup	cornmeal	175 mL
2 tbsp	baking powder	25 mL
1½ tsp	brown sugar	7 mL
1 tsp	ground cinnamon	5 mL
4	eggs	4
2½ cups	2% milk	625 mL
2 tbsp	butter *or* margarine, melted	25 mL

1. In a small saucepan, bring water and pinch of salt to a boil. Rinse rice under running water in strainer; add to pan and bring to a boil. Cover, reduce heat and simmer for 45 minutes or until tender but not mushy. Drain off excess liquid. Cool.

2. In a skillet, melt 1 tbsp (15 mL) butter over medium heat; cook green onions and apples for 3 minutes. Cool.

3. In a large bowl, mix together all-purpose and whole-wheat flours, cornmeal, baking powder, sugar, 1 tsp (5 mL) salt and cinnamon. In another bowl, lightly beat eggs; blend in milk and melted butter. Stir into dry ingredients just until blended. Fold in rice and apple mixtures.

4. In a lightly greased skillet or on griddle and using ⅓ cup (75 mL) batter for each pancake, cook pancakes until browned and bubbles form on surface. Turn and brown other side. Makes about 18 pancakes.

PER 3 PANCAKES

Calories: 459

Dietary Fiber: 7 g	Carbohydrate: 73 g
Fat: 12 g	Protein: 16 g

SERVES 6
. . . .
Tim Wood, Chef
Leslie Maze, Dietitian

Although North Americans tend to eat pancakes for breakfast, in other countries, pancakes often grace the main course of a dinner. The best known of these are bao bing, the Chinese pancakes that accompany Peking duck, and potato pancakes such as latkes, which are a staple of Eastern European cuisine. Unlike traditional batter pancakes, these wild rice pancakes are a perfect side dish for meat or poultry. To speed up preparation time, cook the wild rice the day before. Serve with maple syrup.

TIP
Pancake batter may be prepared ahead and chilled for up to 24 hours, but do not add baking powder until the last minute. The temperature of the griddle is critical to pancake lightness — a water drop will dance across the surface of the griddle when the heat is perfect.

DIETITIAN'S MESSAGE
Traditional potato latkes are often served with sour cream. This alternative packs a wallop of flavor as well as a healthy dose of fiber and is delicious served with maple syrup.

*Wild rice is actually a
cereal that grows in
water. It is often
harvested by Native
people using canoes and,
as a result, is much more
expensive than regular
rice. It has a smoky taste
and a chewy texture that
complements the
mushrooms and back
bacon in this recipe.*

DIETITIAN'S MESSAGE

Not only is back bacon
delicious, it offers a lower-
fat alternative to side
bacon. Serve this dish
with a piece of warm
bannock (see recipes,
page 37) for a dish that
reflects the traditions of
Native peoples.

Wild Rice with Bacon and Mushrooms

2½ cups	water	625 mL
1 cup	wild rice	250 mL
½ tsp	salt	2 mL
½ cup	diced back bacon	125 mL
½ cup	chopped onion	125 mL
½ cup	diced celery	125 mL
½ cup	thinly sliced mushrooms	125 mL
2 tbsp	chopped fresh parsley	25 mL
½ cup	chicken stock (optional)	125 mL

1. In a saucepan, bring water to a boil; rinse rice under running water in strainer, then add to water with salt. Reduce heat, cover and simmer for 45 minutes or until rice is tender. Drain off excess liquid.

2. Meanwhile, in a skillet, cook bacon over medium heat until cooked through. Add onion, celery and mushrooms; cook, stirring, until tender. Stir into cooked rice along with parsley. Moisten with chicken stock, if desired.

PER SERVING	
Calories: 121	
Dietary Fiber: 2 g	Carbohydrate: 22 g
Fat: 1 g	Protein: 6 g

2 pts

Wild Rice and Kernel Corn

2¼ cups	water	550 mL
	Salt	
¾ cup	wild rice	175 mL
1 tbsp	butter	15 mL
1	large onion, chopped	1
½ cup	diced celery	125 mL
1 cup	chopped mushrooms	250 mL
1 tbsp	chopped garlic	15 mL
1¾ cups	frozen corn kernels, thawed	425 mL
¼ cup	shelled sunflower seeds	50 mL
	Black pepper	

1. In a saucepan, bring water and ½ tsp (2 mL) salt to a boil. Rinse rice under running water in strainer; add to pan and bring to a boil. Cover and simmer over low heat for 45 minutes or until tender but not mushy. Drain off excess liquid.

2. In a large skillet, melt butter over medium heat; cook onion and celery, stirring, for 2 minutes. Add mushrooms and garlic; cook for 2 to 3 minutes. Add rice, corn, sunflower seeds and ¼ tsp (1 mL) each salt and pepper; heat through.

PER SERVING
Calories: 131
Dietary Fiber: 3 g	Carbohydrate: 22 g
Fat: 4 g	Protein: 5 g

SERVES 8
....

Guy Blain, Chef
Debra Reid, Dietitian

The surprise ingredient in this tasty and colorful dish, which showcases grains and vegetables, is sunflower seeds — which add fiber and crunch.

TIPS

If fresh corn is in season, substitute fresh cooked kernels for the frozen.

Store sunflower seeds in the refrigerator to prevent rancidity.

DIETITIAN'S MESSAGE

Serve this tasty dish with Grilled Chicken Breast with Dried Fruit Salsa (see recipe, page 272) and a green salad. Complete the meal with a serving from the Milk Products group.

SERVES 4
••••••••••••••••••••••••
Karen Quinn

This classic chicken casserole is easy to make and a favorite with all family members. For ease of cleanup and to speed preparation time, you can make it in the microwave, using only 1 dish. For added flavor, use hot chicken or vegetable broth instead of the water.

TIP

If desired, use 1 cup (250 mL) fresh mushrooms, sliced. Cook them with the onion and celery if using the oven method. Increase water to 2½ cups (625 mL).

DIETITIAN'S MESSAGE

This is a hearty dish that is easy to prepare and economical to boot. Serve with Healthy Cheese 'n' Herb Bread (see recipe, page 40) and Icy Yogurt Pops (see recipe, page 67) for dessert.

Easy Chicken 'n' Rice Casserole

Preheat oven to 350°F (180°C)
8-cup (2 L) baking dish

½ cup	chopped onion	125 mL
½ cup	chopped celery	125 mL
2 tbsp	butter *or* margarine	25 mL
2 cups	cooked bite-size chicken pieces	500 mL
1¾ cups	hot water	425 mL
⅔ cup	long-grain white rice	150 mL
1	can (10 oz/284 mL) mushrooms, with liquid	1
1 cup	frozen peas and carrots	250 mL
½ tsp	dried thyme	2 mL
½ tsp	dried rosemary	2 mL

Microwave Method

1. Combine onion, celery and butter in an 8-cup (2 L) microwave-safe dish. Microwave, covered, on High for 5 minutes. Stir in chicken, water, rice, mushrooms, peas, carrots and seasonings. Microwave on High for 6 minutes, then microwave on Medium for 10 to 12 minutes or until rice is tender and most of the water has been absorbed. Let stand for 10 minutes before serving.

Oven Method

1. In a skillet, cook onion and celery in butter until soft. Stir in remaining ingredients. Bake in covered 8-cup (2 L) baking dish in preheated oven for about 30 minutes or until rice is cooked.

PER SERVING	
Calories: 285	
Dietary Fiber: 3 g	Carbohydrate: 24 g
Fat: 11 g	Protein: 23 g

California Casserole

Preheat oven to 350°F (180°C)
6-cup (1.5 L) baking dish, lightly greased

2 cups	water	500 mL
¾ cup	long-grain white rice	175 mL
1 cup	light sour cream	250 mL
1 cup	shredded medium Cheddar cheese	250 mL
½ cup	lower-fat cottage cheese	125 mL
½ cup	chopped onion	125 mL
¼ cup	chopped mushrooms	50 mL
¼ cup	chopped green bell pepper	50 mL
½ tsp	salt	2 mL
¼ tsp	freshly ground black pepper	1 mL

1. In a large saucepan, bring water to a boil; add rice. Cover and cook on low for about 20 minutes or until rice is tender and water is absorbed. Let stand for 5 minutes.

2. Combine hot rice, sour cream, Cheddar and cottage cheese, onion, mushrooms, green pepper and seasonings. Pour into a lightly greased 6-cup (1.5 L) baking dish. Bake, uncovered, in preheated oven for about 25 minutes.

PER SERVING	
Calories: 220	
Dietary Fiber: 1 g	Carbohydrate: 23 g
Fat: 9 g	Protein: 10 g

Here's a recipe that will satisfy even the pickiest vegetarians in your family. For added flavor, substitute vegetable broth for the water and add a small handful of fresh mixed herbs along with the vegetables.

TIP

If desired, substitute brown rice for the long-grain white rice. Increase the quantity of boiling water by ½ cup (125 mL) and the cooking time to 45 minutes.

DIETITIAN'S MESSAGE

Using brown rice in this recipe will increase the fiber content. Start the meal with Carrot Orange Soup (see recipe, page 106) and serve stir-fried vegetables along with the casserole. End the meal with Blueberry Flan (see recipe, page 417) for a meal that offers an abundance of vitamins and minerals as well as some antioxidants.

Here's a delicious change from the usual tuna noodle casserole — and it takes less than 10 minutes to prepare! It's easy enough for older children and teens to make on their own; younger children can help by shredding the cheese and getting the salad ready.

TIP

Replace the cream of mushroom soup with a reduced-fat variety. For a change, try a cream of wild mushroom soup.

DIETITIAN'S MESSAGE

Buying tuna packed in water rather than oil is one way of minimizing fat intake. Accompany this casserole with a green salad and finish with fresh fruit and yogurt for an easy and delicious meal that the whole family will enjoy.

Tuna and Rice Casserole

Preheat oven to 350°F (180°C)
8-inch (2 L) square baking dish, greased

1	can (10 oz/284 mL) condensed cream of mushroom soup	1
1¼ cups	instant rice	300 mL
1 cup	milk	250 mL
½ cup	water	125 mL
1	can (6 oz/170g) water-packed tuna, drained	1
1 cup	frozen peas	250 mL
¼ cup	finely chopped onion	50 mL
1 tsp	lemon juice	5 mL
	Black pepper to taste	
½ cup	shredded Cheddar cheese	125 mL
	Paprika to taste	

1. In a large bowl, stir together soup, rice, milk, water, tuna, peas, onion, lemon juice and pepper. Pour into a greased 8-inch (2 L) square baking dish. Sprinkle with cheese and paprika. Bake in preheated oven for 30 to 35 minutes or until bubbling and rice is tender.

PER SERVING	
Calories: 330	
Dietary Fiber: 2 g	Carbohydrate: 35 g
Fat: 12 g	Protein: 19 g

Cassoulet

Preheat oven to 275°F (140°C)

2½ cups	white (navy) beans, soaked (see Tip, at right)	625 mL
2 tbsp	olive oil	25 mL
8 oz	boneless skinless chicken *or* pheasant breast, cut into large pieces	250 g
8 oz	well-trimmed pork loin, cut into large pieces	250 g
4 oz	well-trimmed boneless lamb, cut into large pieces	125 g
4 oz	chicken livers	125 g
1	large onion, sliced	1
2	cloves garlic, minced	2
1	can (5½ oz/156 mL) tomato paste	1
½ cup	maple syrup	125 mL
½ cup	dry white wine	125 mL
1 tbsp	dry mustard	15 mL
1 tsp	each dried thyme and salt	5 mL
½ tsp	black pepper	2 mL
1	bay leaf	1

1. Cover beans with fresh water; bring to a boil. Simmer for 30 minutes. Drain, reserving cooking water.

2. In a large ovenproof saucepan or Dutch oven, heat oil over medium heat; brown chicken, pork, lamb and chicken livers all over. Remove and set aside. Place half of the beans, half of the onion and half of the garlic in bottom of pan; layer meats on top. Add remaining beans, onion and garlic.

3. Mix together tomato paste, maple syrup, wine, mustard, thyme, salt and pepper; pour over beans. Cover beans with reserved cooking water; nestle bay leaf in beans.

4. Cover and bake in preheated oven for 2 hours; uncover, stir and increase temperature to 325°F (160°C). Cook, uncovered, for about 2 hours or until thickened and beans are tender. Discard bay leaf.

PER SERVING	
Calories: 557	
Dietary Fiber: 15 g	Carbohydrate: 72 g
Fat: 12 g	Protein: 42 g

SERVES 6

Alain Mercier, Chef
Fabiola Masri, Dietitian

Cassoulet is a French country casserole that's made with beans and a variety of meats and poultry, then traditionally slow-cooked. This version, which uses maple syrup, has a Quebec flair. Although it's a lot of work, it is rich and delicious.

TIP

To soak beans, cover with plenty of cold water and leave for 8 hours or overnight. Quick-soak method: Cover beans with water and bring to a boil for 2 minutes. Remove from heat and let stand for 1 hour. With either method, drain beans, rinse and proceed as directed.

DIETITIAN'S MESSAGE

This filling and robustly flavored dish is perfect as the centerpiece of a winter buffet or after a day in the outdoors. It is packed with protein and fiber as well as many other nutrients. Since it has all the calories you need for a meal, choose light accompaniments such as Lemon Pesto Dip (see recipe, page 76) with vegetable crudités to start and fresh fruit or yogurt for dessert.

Prepare this recipe ahead and freeze or refrigerate for après-ski or a busy Saturday evening meal. To turn up the heat, add a finely chopped jalapeño pepper along with the tomatoes.

TIP

If desired, use 1 cup (250 mL) dried kidney beans, soaked, cooked and drained, instead of the canned.

DIETITIAN'S MESSAGE

The beans, cornmeal, cheese, milk and eggs combine to provide high-quality protein in the absence of meat. To add extra fiber, serve with a spinach salad and a multigrain roll. Finish with Spicy Fruit Compote (see recipe, page 383), a great ending to a meal that will provide calcium, iron and vitamins A and C.

Mexican Pie

Preheat oven to 350°F (180°C)
13- by 9-inch (3 L) baking dish

1	medium onion, chopped	1
1 tbsp	vegetable oil	15 mL
1	can (19 oz/540 mL) tomatoes, coarsely chopped	1
1	can (14 oz/398 mL) kidney beans, drained and rinsed	1
1	can (12 oz/341 mL) whole kernel corn	1
1 tbsp	chili powder	15 mL
¾ cup	cornmeal	175 mL
1 cup	2% milk	250 mL
2	eggs	2
1½ cups	shredded cheese (old Cheddar, Swiss, mozzarella *or* a mixture of all 3)	375 mL

1. In a large skillet over medium-high heat, cook onion in oil until transparent. Add tomatoes, kidney beans, corn and chili powder to skillet. Cook over low heat, uncovered, for about 1 hour or until slightly thickened, stirring occasionally. Pour mixture into 13- by 9-inch (3 L) baking dish. Sprinkle cornmeal evenly over surface.

2. In a bowl, beat together milk and eggs; pour evenly over cornmeal. Sprinkle with cheese. Bake in preheated oven for 50 to 55 minutes. Cut into squares to serve.

PER SERVING	
Calories: 350	
Dietary Fiber: 7 g	Carbohydrate: 42g
Fat: 14 g	Protein: 18 g

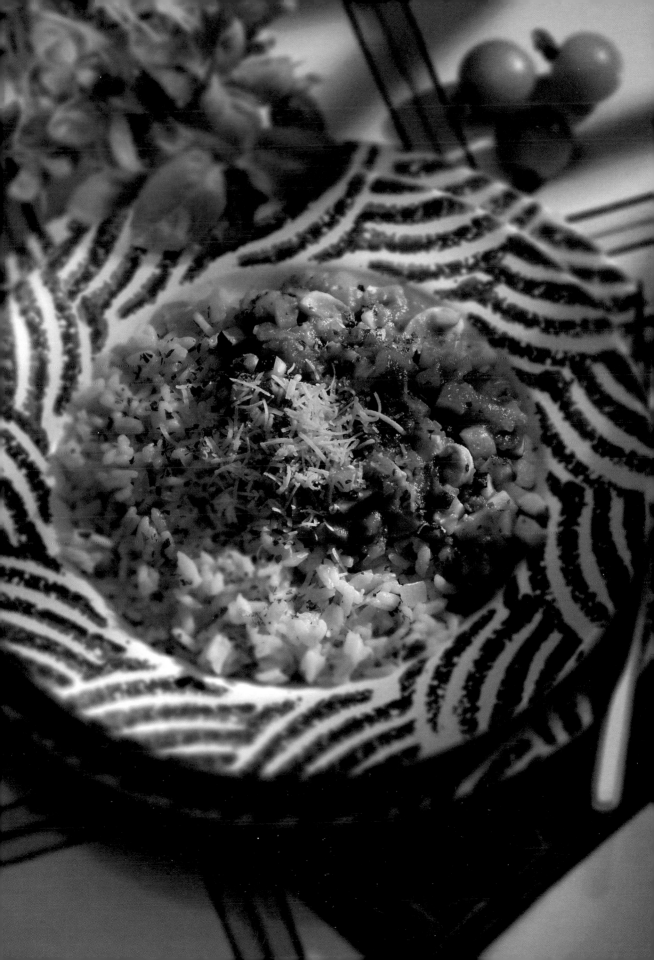

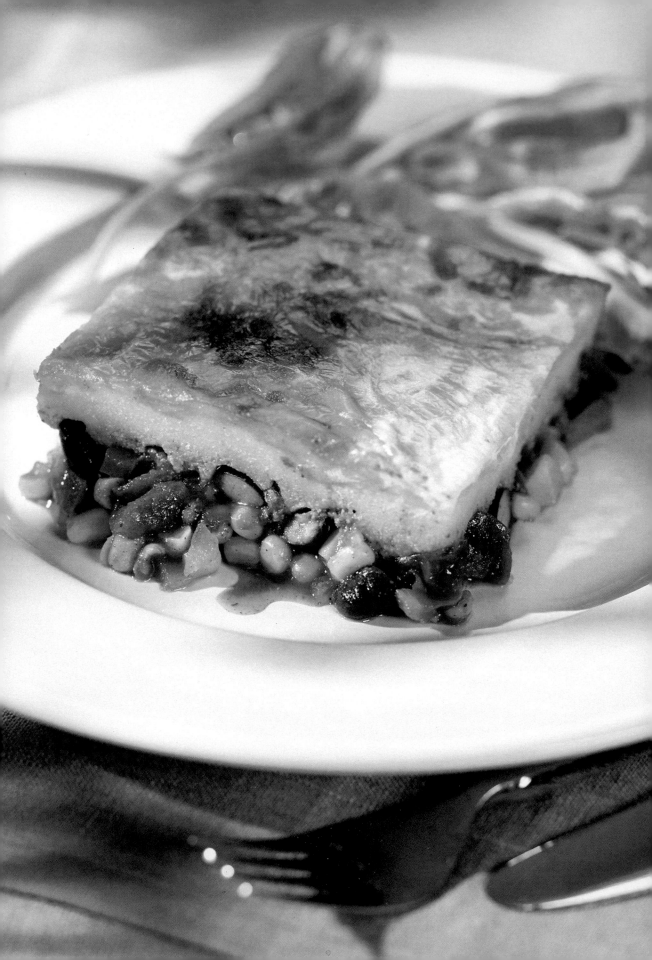

Egg and Mushroom Fried Rice

4	eggs	4
2 tsp	vegetable oil	10 mL
1 cup	sliced mushrooms	250 mL
1 tsp	minced garlic	5 mL
1 tsp	minced ginger root (or ½ tsp/2 mL ground ginger)	5 mL
3 cups	cooked rice	750 mL
½ cup	frozen peas	125 mL
½ cup	chopped green onions	125 mL
⅓ cup	sodium-reduced soy sauce	75 mL
½ to 1 tsp	sesame oil	2 to 5 mL
⅛ tsp	black pepper	0.5 mL

1. In a small bowl, whisk eggs until well blended. Pour into a large nonstick skillet; cook, undisturbed, over low heat for 4 to 5 minutes or until bottom is lightly browned and mixture is almost set. Flip eggs over and cook for 1 to 2 minutes. Remove from pan; cool slightly. Cut into ¼-inch (5 mm) strips. Set aside.

2. In the same skillet, heat oil over medium-high heat. Add mushrooms; cook for 4 to 5 minutes or until lightly browned. Add garlic and ginger; cook for 1 minute. Stir in rice, peas and onions until combined. Stir in soy sauce, sesame oil and pepper; add cooked egg strips. Cook for 2 minutes or until piping hot.

PER SERVING	
Calories: 284	
Dietary Fiber: 2 g	Carbohydrate: 39 g
Fat: 8 g	Protein: 12 g

SERVES 4

P

Bev Callaghan, Dietitian

Enjoy this as a meal or snack — it's a great way to use up frozen leftover rice. You can easily divide the ingredients in half to serve 2.

TIP

Using a small amount of highly flavored sesame oil adds great taste without adding too much fat.

DIETITIAN'S MESSAGE

This is a great meal for a busy weeknight. Serve with a green salad or an extra vegetable such as broccoli, if desired. Add frozen yogurt and fresh berries for dessert.

....

Daryle Ryo Nagata, Chef
Jane Thornthwaite,
Dietitian

This vegetarian version of the well-loved hamburger gets its flavor from the variety of ingredients — a combination of lentils, grains, beans and vegetables. For a spicier version, add finely chopped hot pepper, such as jalapeño or banana pepper, along with the bell peppers.

TIP

Be sure to use extra-firm tofu in this recipe as other textures are not firm enough to be shredded.

DIETITIAN'S MESSAGE

Tofu, lentils, walnuts and grains provide a great meat substitute in these delicious burgers. The combination provides plenty of taste along with fiber. Serve this as the focal point of a casual meal along with veggie sticks.

Garden Path Burger

Preheat oven to 375°F (190°C)
Baking sheet

¼ cup	dried lentils	50 mL
¼ cup	quinoa	50 mL
3 cups	fine dry bread crumbs	750 mL
¼ cup	quick-cooking rolled oats	50 mL
¼ cup	chopped walnuts	50 mL
1 cup	coarsely chopped canned chickpeas, drained and rinsed	250 mL
⅔ cup	each finely chopped carrot, celery and Spanish onion	150 mL
½ cup	each finely chopped red and green bell pepper	125 mL
½ cup	shredded extra-firm tofu	125 mL
¼ cup	sliced green onions	50 mL
¼ cup	toasted pumpkin seeds	50 mL
1 tbsp	coarsely cracked black pepper	15 mL
12	onion *or* vegetable kaiser buns, split and toasted	12

Toppings

Light mayonnaise, bean sprouts, sliced tomato, chopped fresh cilantro, shredded lettuce

1. In a medium saucepan, combine lentils, quinoa and 1½ cups (375 mL) water; bring to a boil. Reduce heat and simmer for 10 minutes; drain.

2. In a large bowl, mix together lentil mixture, bread crumbs, rolled oats, walnuts, chickpeas, carrot, celery, onion, red and green peppers, tofu, green onions, pumpkin seeds and black pepper. Using 1 cup (250 mL) for each, form into ½-inch (1 cm) thick patties about 3 inches (8 cm) in diameter.

3. Bake on baking sheet in preheated oven for about 20 minutes or until hot and golden brown. Serve on buns with favorite toppings.

PER SERVING	
Calories: 408	
Dietary Fiber: 4 g	Carbohydrate: 71 g
Fat: 7 g	Protein: 15 g

Falafel

SERVES 8
....

Margaret Howard, Dietitian

1	can (19 oz/540 mL) chickpeas, drained (reserve liquid)	1
2	large cloves garlic	2
1	small onion, chopped	1
½ cup	packed parsley leaves	125 mL
⅓ cup	tahini (sesame seed paste)	75 mL
2 tbsp	lemon juice	25 mL
1 tbsp	ground cumin	15 mL
1 tsp	ground coriander	5 mL
1 tsp	ground turmeric	5 mL
½ tsp	salt	2 mL
¼ tsp	black pepper	1 mL
¼ cup	dry bread crumbs	50 mL
1 tbsp	vegetable oil	15 mL
4	whole-wheat pita breads	4
	Shredded lettuce, chopped tomatoes, diced cucumber, alfalfa sprouts, plain yogurt	

Residents of Middle Eastern countries enjoy falafels in much the same way as North Americans enjoy hamburgers. Traditionally, falafels are made from cooked chickpeas, ground and seasoned, then shaped into balls and deep-fried. Several balls are then placed in pita bread and topped with tahini yogurt salad. The following adaptation shapes the chickpea mixture into patties and uses much less oil. Seasonings may be increased to suit your taste, and extra bread crumbs will give a drier patty.

1. In a food processor or blender, process chickpeas, 2 tbsp (25 mL) of the reserved liquid, garlic, onion, parsley, tahini, lemon juice and seasonings; process until almost smooth. Stir in bread crumbs; shape into 8 patties.

2. In a large nonstick skillet over medium-high heat, heat oil. Add patties; cook for 2 to 3 minutes per side or until lightly browned. Cut pita breads in half; serve each patty in pocket of half a pita bread; garnish as desired.

TIP

Tahini is available in health food stores and the specialty foods section of many supermarkets.

DIETITIAN'S MESSAGE

Legumes are an economical source of protein and B vitamins. Serve the falafels in whole-wheat pita pockets, topped with fresh vegetables and Tabbouleh (see recipe, page 169) for a vegetarian meal that provides complete protein and is rich in fiber.

PER SERVING	
Calories: 253	
Dietary Fiber: 3 g	Carbohydrate: 38 g
Fat: 8 g	Protein: 9 g

TAHINI YOGURT SALAD
Combine plain yogurt with chopped tomato and cucumber, minced garlic and parsley; add some tahini paste and freshly ground pepper to taste.

SERVES 6
....
Marilynn Small, Dietitian

Vegetarian chili is a great meal planner today as most people are trying to reduce their intake of fat and increase dietary fiber. If desired, garnish with chopped green or red onion and a dollop of light sour cream.

TIPS

Substitute 1 cup (250 mL) dried beans, soaked, cooked and drained, for the canned beans, if desired.

If you have a slow cooker, use it to prepare dried beans for use in this recipe. Soak the beans, either overnight or using the quick-soak method (see technique, page 118). In a slow cooker, combine 1 cup (250 mL) soaked beans, drained, and 3 cups (750 mL) water. Cover and cook on Low setting for 8 to 10 hours. For convenience, cook the beans overnight, drain and refrigerate until ready to use.

DIETITIAN'S MESSAGE

Although a rich source of vegetable protein, beans do not contain the full range of essential amino acids to be classified as a "complete" protein. Strict vegetarians must ensure they eat adequate amounts of grains and cereals, seeds and nuts and, if appropriate, dairy products and eggs, in addition to legumes.

Crowd-Pleasing Vegetarian Chili

1 tbsp	vegetable oil	15 mL
1	onion, chopped	1
1	red bell pepper, chopped	1
2	cloves garlic, minced	2
1	stalk celery, chopped	1
1 to 2 tbsp	chili powder	15 to 25 mL
2 tsp	ground cumin	10 mL
1	can (28 oz/796 mL) tomatoes	1
1	can (14 oz/398 mL) black *or* red kidney beans, drained and rinsed	1
1	can (12 oz/355 mL) corn kernels, drained	1
1 cup	bran cereal	250 mL
3 cups	cooked rice	750 mL
½ cup	shredded Cheddar cheese	125 mL

1. In a large saucepan, heat oil over medium-high heat. Add onion, red pepper, garlic and celery; cook until vegetables are tender. Stir in chili powder and cumin; cook for 1 minute.

2. Add tomatoes, breaking up with spoon. Stir in beans, corn and cereal; bring to a boil. Reduce heat, cover and simmer for 5 minutes. Serve over rice, sprinkled with cheese.

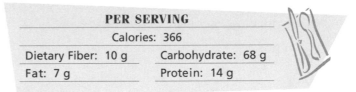

PER SERVING	
Calories: 366	
Dietary Fiber: 10 g	Carbohydrate: 68 g
Fat: 7 g	Protein: 14 g

Vegetarian Chili

²/₃ cup	bulgur (4 oz/125 g)	150 mL
1 tbsp	vegetable oil	15 mL
1	medium onion, diced	1
2	cloves garlic, minced	2
½ cup	each diced celery and carrots	125 mL
¼ cup	diced green bell pepper	50 mL
1	can (28 oz/796 mL) tomatoes	1
1	can (5½ oz/156 mL) tomato paste	1
2 to 3 tbsp	chili powder	25 to 45 mL
1	can (19 oz/540 mL) kidney beans, drained and rinsed	1
2 tsp	Worcestershire sauce	10 mL
	Hot pepper sauce	

1. Cover bulgur with hot water; let stand.

2. Meanwhile, in a large saucepan, heat oil over medium heat; cook onion, garlic, celery, carrots and green pepper, stirring, for 3 to 5 minutes or until softened. Stir in tomatoes, breaking up with spoon; stir in tomato paste, chili powder, beans and Worcestershire sauce. Cook for 10 to 15 minutes, stirring occasionally, until heated through. Stir in bulgur. Season with hot pepper sauce to taste.

PER SERVING	
Calories: 350	
Dietary Fiber: 20 g	Carbohydrate: 66 g
Fat: 6 g	Protein: 16 g

SERVES 4

Martin Wilkinson, Chef
Marianna Fiocco, Dietitian

Here's a new take on an old favorite — replacing meat with bulgur in a traditional kidney bean chili. The bulgur, which is made from cracked wheat that has been parboiled and roasted, adds a pleasant texture to this chili.

TIP

To turn up the heat a notch, try adding finely chopped banana or jalapeño pepper to taste along with the bell pepper.

DIETITIAN'S MESSAGE

This meatless version of chili is a great way to introduce friends and family to vegetarian meals. The recipe can be doubled to feed a larger crowd. Serve with hot cheese bread and an assortment of raw vegetables with dip.

Here's a chili you can have ready in about half an hour, made from ingredients you're likely to have on hand.

TIP

Transform leftovers into a Chili Baked Potato. Scrub a medium potato and pierce with a fork. Microwave on High for 3 to 4 minutes. Let stand for 2 minutes. Cut an X in the top of potato and squeeze open. Top with hot chili and shredded cheese.

DIETITIAN'S MESSAGE

This chili provides an incredible 18 g of fiber per serving — more than most people eat in a day.

Fast Chili

1 lb	lean ground beef	500 g
1	can (19 oz/540 mL) stewed tomatoes	1
2	cans (each 14 oz/398 mL) beans in tomato sauce	2
2	cans (each 19 oz/540 mL) kidney beans, drained and rinsed	2
1 cup	sliced white *or* red onions	250 mL
2 cups	diced green bell peppers	500 mL
1 tbsp	chili powder	15 mL

1. In a large saucepan or Dutch oven over medium-high heat, brown meat until no longer pink inside. Drain fat.

2. Add tomatoes, beans, onions, green peppers and chili powder. Reduce heat and simmer, covered and stirring occasionally, for 20 to 30 minutes.

PER SERVING	
Calories: 338	
Dietary Fiber: 18 g	Carbohydrate: 50 g
Fat: 6 g	Protein: 24 g

There are many variations on the theme of Chickpeas in Tomato Sauce, most of which can be found in Mediterranean or Indian cooking.

TIP

If you prefer a zippier version of this dish, add 1 tbsp (15 mL) minced ginger root along with the garlic. If you don't have fresh parsley in the fridge, garnish with finely chopped red or green onion instead.

Chickpeas in Tomato Sauce

1	large onion, cut into thin wedges	1
2	cloves garlic, minced	2
1 tbsp	olive oil	15 mL
1	can (28 oz/796 mL) chickpeas, drained and rinsed	1
1½ cups	canned crushed tomatoes	375 mL
½ tsp	salt	2 mL
½ tsp	black pepper	2 mL
½ tsp	dried thyme	2 mL
¼ tsp	cayenne pepper	1 mL
1	bay leaf	1
	Chopped fresh parsley	

1. In a large saucepan over medium-high heat, cook onion and garlic in oil for about 5 minutes or until tender. Add chickpeas; cook for 3 to 4 minutes. Add tomatoes and seasonings except parsley; cook over low heat for about 25 minutes. Remove bay leaf before serving; garnish with chopped parsley.

PER SERVING	
Calories: 306	
Dietary Fiber: 9 g	Carbohydrate: 54 g
Fat: 6 g	Protein: 11 g

Chickpea Hot Pot

2 tsp	olive oil	10 mL
½ cup	chopped onions	125 mL
1 tbsp	curry paste	15 mL
2	cans (each 28 oz/796 mL) diced plum tomatoes, with juice	2
1	can (19 oz/540 mL) chickpeas, drained and rinsed	1
1 cup	diced sweet potatoes	250 mL
1 tbsp	granulated sugar	15 mL
1 tsp	minced garlic	5 mL
1 cup	cubed firm tofu	250 mL
2 cups	bok choy, cut into strips	500 mL
2 cups	broccoli florets	500 mL
½ tsp	black pepper	2 mL

1. In a saucepan, heat oil over medium-high heat. Add onions and cook until softened. Stir in curry paste. Add tomatoes, chickpeas, sweet potatoes, sugar and garlic; bring to a boil. Reduce heat and simmer, covered, until sweet potatoes are tender.

2. Stir in tofu, bok choy, broccoli and pepper. Cook, uncovered, for 2 minutes or until broccoli is tender-crisp. Adjust seasoning to taste.

PER SERVING	
Calories: 229	
Dietary Fiber: 6 g	Carbohydrate: 37 g
Fat: 6 g	Protein: 11 g

SERVES 6

Shannon Crocker, Dietitian

This is a quick, easy and nutritious vegetarian dish

TIPS
Curry paste is available in Asian markets or the specialty section of some supermarkets.

You can substitute black beans or red kidney beans for the chickpeas. Add more curry paste if you like spice.

SERVES 6

Lisa Hamilton

These enchiladas will be softer if cooked in the microwave and crisper if cooked in a conventional oven. Add salsa to suit your taste, or a finely chopped jalapeño pepper along with the seasonings. Garnish with chopped red or green onion and a dollop of light sour cream, if desired.

TIP

For a spicier version, add ¼ to ½ tsp (1 to 2 mL) cayenne pepper along with the seasonings.

DIETITIAN'S MESSAGE

Legumes are a great source of vegetable protein and fiber. The combination of legumes and cereal protein in this recipe ensures a complete protein intake. Serve with veggie sticks and finish with frozen yogurt and fresh fruit.

Spicy Vegetable Enchiladas

Preheat oven to 350°F (180°C)
Baking sheet

1	can (14 oz/398 mL) kidney beans, drained and rinsed	1
1	can (14 oz/398 mL) crushed tomatoes	1
1 cup	firm tofu, cubed	250 mL
½ cup	finely chopped peanuts	125 mL
2 tbsp	salsa	25 mL
½ tsp	chili powder	2 mL
½ tsp	salt	2 mL
6	large soft corn *or* flour tortillas	6
1 cup	shredded Monterey Jack *or* Cheddar cheese	250 mL

1. In a saucepan, combine kidney beans, tomatoes, tofu, peanuts, salsa and seasonings; heat until hot and bubbling, stirring constantly to prevent sticking.

2. Spread filling evenly over tortillas; roll tortillas around filling. Place seam side down on a baking sheet; sprinkle with cheese. Bake in preheated oven for about 5 minutes, or microwave on High for about 3 minutes, or until cheese melts.

PER SERVING	
Calories: 377	
Dietary Fiber: 6 g	Carbohydrate: 38 g
Fat: 17 g	Protein: 21 g

Mixed Winter Beans

2 cups	assorted dried beans (romano, white, kidney, pinto)	500 mL
1	can (28 oz/796 mL) tomatoes	1
1	can (19 oz/540 mL) chickpeas, drained and rinsed	1
2	medium carrots, sliced	2
1	medium onion, chopped	1
1	clove garlic, minced	1
1 cup	shredded cabbage	250 mL
½ cup	diced peeled turnip	125 mL
1 tbsp	chili powder	15 mL
1 tsp	Worcestershire sauce	5 mL
½ tsp	salt	2 mL
¼ tsp	black pepper	1 mL
	Chopped fresh parsley	

1. Cover beans with water and soak overnight; drain and rinse. In a 4-quart (4 L) saucepan, cover beans with fresh water; bring to a boil. Reduce heat and simmer, covered, for 40 to 50 minutes or until tender. Drain and rinse; return to saucepan.

2. Add tomatoes, chickpeas, carrots, onion, garlic, cabbage, turnip, chili powder, Worcestershire sauce, salt and pepper. Add water to cover; bring to a boil. Reduce heat and simmer, uncovered, for 30 to 40 minutes or until vegetables are tender. Garnish with parsley.

PER SERVING	
Calories: 356	
Dietary Fiber: 18 g	Carbohydrate: 66 g
Fat: 3 g	Protein: 21 g

SERVES 6
....
Janice Mitchell, Chef
Jane Henderson, Dietitian

You need only 1 pot to prepare this economical meatless dish. It uses an assortment of dried beans with lots of winter produce, to produce a tasty pot of old-fashioned baked beans.

TIP
Keep single servings on hand in the freezer for quick microwave meals.

DIETITIAN'S MESSAGE
This meatless, lower-fat dish is chock-full of protein, fiber, vitamins and antioxidants. Complete the meal with a tossed green salad and Steamed Brown Bread (see recipe, page 42). Serve fresh or canned fruit for dessert.

Main Meals

To kick-start your nutritional health, this chapter includes an array of tasty meals featuring a variety of lean proteins and colorful combinations of vegetables rich in vitamins and antioxidants. Most are easy to prepare, to meet your needs for busy weeknights. We have also included a few dishes that are more involved, which you may want to save for entertaining. The recipes in this chapter include beef, pork, lamb, chicken, fish and seafood, as well as delicious vegetarian dishes. Whether it is a simple stir-fry, an easy one-pot dinner or a more elaborate presentation, these recipes will appeal to a wide variety of tastes and help you to establish a pattern of healthy eating.

mealtimes and well-being

In recent years, there has been a growing recognition that enjoyment of food affects psychological and emotional as well as physical well-being. Although meal times are one of the best times for socializing and communicating with families and friends, many of us say we don't have enough time to prepare healthy meals. Common sense tells us we need to change our mind-set. Delicious, nutritious food is a key component of a healthy lifestyle based on pleasure, a zest for all that life has to offer and a pervading sense of well-being.

the importance of protein

Meat, poultry, fish and meat alternatives (legumes, eggs, nuts and seeds) supply such essential nutrients as iron, zinc and B vitamins (thiamin, riboflavin, niacin, vitamin B12). They are also our main source of high-quality protein. Aim for two to three servings a day from the Meat and Alternatives food group.

boost your zinc intake!

Limiting food choices can make getting enough zinc a challenge. Lean cuts of meat, fish and poultry provide zinc. If you are a vegetarian, you may have difficulty getting enough of this valuable mineral in your diet. Be sure to eat the following foods often:

- tofu, tempeh, texturized vegetable protein;
- legumes such as lentils, chickpeas, kidney beans, black beans and lima beans;
- grains such as oatmeal, millet, wheat germ and fortified cereals;
- nuts such as cashews, peanuts and pecans.

make lower-fat choices more often

A diet high in fat, saturated fat and excess calories will contribute to high blood cholesterol, high triglycerides and obesity. Control the fat in your diet by emphasizing lean sources of protein and foods rich in carbohydrates and fiber (whole-grain breads and cereals, vegetables, fruit, and legumes). Use preparation methods that minimize fat, such as broiling, roasting or steaming, and enhance flavors with herbs and spices. These choices can help you to control cholesterol and body fat levels, reducing your risk of heart disease, obesity, cancer and diabetes.

watch the heat

Foods cooked at high temperatures present a risk for cancer. Barbecuing, frying, broiling and roasting are OK once in a while but not every day. Serve cured or smoked meat only occasionally.

meet your iron needs and increase your endurance

Everyone needs iron, in varying degrees. An adequate intake of iron keeps you feeling energetic and healthy. Not having enough can lead to iron-deficiency anemia, which can cause you to look pale and feel tired or run down.

Getting enough iron can be a real challenge for children, women, pregnant women, female athletes and vegetarians. The best sources of this valuable mineral include clams, oysters, meat, eggs and fish. If you are a vegetarian, eat plenty of legumes, tofu, pumpkin and sesame seeds, nuts, dark leafy green vegetables, dried fruits, whole grains, iron-enriched breads, pasta and cereals.

Iron comes in two forms. Plant sources of iron are called non-heme iron. This type is not absorbed as well as the heme type of iron found in animal foods. To improve iron absorption, consume foods rich in vitamin C with any iron-rich food. For example, combine beans with tomatoes and accompany cereal with a glass of orange juice. And drink coffee or tea between (not with) meals since these beverages can interfere with iron absorption.

bump up protein while reducing fat

- Choose leaner meat cuts — round steak, lean ground beef, flank steak and pork tenderloin — as well as chicken and turkey.
- Trim any visible fat from meat, and choose skinless poultry or remove the skin after cooking.
- Watch serving sizes, bearing in mind that one serving is about 3 oz (90 g) of meat, approximately the size of a deck of cards.
- Use meat, poultry and fish as complements to the grains, vegetables, fruit and beans in your meals. For example, the meat portion might account for only one-quarter of your meal.
- Use lower-fat cooking methods. Instead of frying, try baking, roasting, poaching, broiling, grilling or microwaving. Stir-fry in a nonstick pan using only a small amount of oil or vegetable spray.
- Enhance the natural flavor of meats and fish with herbs and spices, marinades and natural juices, rather than rich gravies and sauces.
- Experiment with the taste of meat alternatives, such as legumes.

explore new foods and new flavors

In today's multicultural society, a multitude of cuisines and culinary influences is reflected in our grocery stores and restaurants. If your mealtimes have become predictable and lackluster, practise adding variety to your menu as a way of adding zest to your life. Experiment with new foods or ethnic dishes. Spice up your life by using vegetables to add bursts of flavor and texture to traditional recipes — for instance, Skillet Pork Chops with Sweet Potatoes and Couscous, or Broiled Ham Steak with Pineapple Mango Salsa, found in this chapter.

Try one of these marinades to add flavor to the meat of your choice.

TIPS

To prepare, combine ingredients for the chosen marinade. Set aside 2 tbsp (25 mL) for basting. Place meat in plastic bag or shallow pan; pour marinade over meat. Refrigerate for 8 hours or overnight, turning meat once or twice. Just before cooking, drain meat.

Each of these recipes makes sufficient marinade for up to 3 lb (1.5 kg) meat.

Sauce that is used to marinade raw meat, poultry or seafood should not be used on cooked food. Boil leftover marinade or prepare extra for basting cooked food.

DIETITIAN'S MESSAGE

These marinades are lower in fat than many commercial marinades.

Marinades for Meat

Apple Rosemary Marinade

For lamb or pork
Makes about 1 1/2 cups (375 mL)

3/4 cup	unsweetened frozen concentrated apple juice, thawed	175 mL
1/2 cup	cider vinegar	125 mL
1/4 cup	liquid honey	50 mL
1 tbsp	soy sauce	15 mL
1 tsp	dried rosemary	5 mL

Ginger Yogurt Marinade

For poultry or pork
Makes about 1 cup (250 mL)

1 cup	lower-fat plain yogurt	250 mL
1 tbsp	minced ginger root	15 mL
2 tsp	ground coriander	10 mL
1 tsp	grated orange zest	5 mL
1/4 tsp	hot pepper sauce	1 mL

Lemon Pesto Marinade

For chicken, fish, veal or lamb
Makes about 3/4 cup (175 mL)

1/2 cup	chicken broth	125 mL
2 tbsp	Lemon Pesto Sauce (see recipe, page 75)	25 mL
2 tbsp	white wine vinegar	25 mL

Beer Carbonara Marinade

For lamb, beef or pork
Makes about 1 cup (250 mL)

1 cup	beer	250 mL
1/2 cup	chopped onions	125 mL
2 tbsp	vegetable oil	25 mL
2 tsp	each brown sugar and Dijon mustard	10 mL
	Freshly ground black pepper to taste	

Main Meals

Slow-Cooked Beef Stew

Electric slow cooker

1 lb	lean stewing beef, cut into 1-inch (2.5 cm) cubes and patted dry	500 g
1 tbsp	all-purpose flour	15 mL
2 tsp	vegetable oil	10 mL
2 cups	cubed turnips	500 mL
2 cups	cubed carrots	500 mL
1 cup	sliced onions	250 mL
1½ cups	boiling water	375 mL
2	beef bouillon cubes *or* sachets	2
3 tbsp	red wine vinegar	45 mL
3 tbsp	ketchup	45 mL
4 tsp	prepared mustard	20 mL
1 tsp	Worcestershire sauce	5 mL
2 tbsp	all-purpose flour	25 mL
3 tbsp	cold water	45 mL

1. In a large bowl, toss beef cubes with flour; set aside. In a large nonstick skillet, heat oil over medium-high heat; add beef and cook for 4 to 5 minutes or until browned on all sides. Place in slow cooker. Add turnips, carrots and onions.

2. In a medium bowl, blend together water, bouillon, vinegar, ketchup, mustard and Worcestershire sauce. Add to slow cooker; stir gently. Cook, covered, on Low heat setting for 9 hours.

3. In a measuring cup, whisk together flour and water. Add flour mixture to stew; stir gently to blend. Increase heat setting to High; cook, covered, for 15 minutes or until thickened.

PER SERVING	
Calories: 308	
Dietary Fiber: 4 g	Carbohydrate: 24 g
Fat: 11 g	Protein: 28 g

SERVES 4
....
Bonnie Conrad, Dietitian

In the winter, there's nothing more comforting than a plate of hearty beef stew served over mashed potatoes.

TIPS

If desired, substitute 1 can (10 oz/284 mL) condensed beef broth (undiluted) for the water and bouillon cubes.

Freeze in airtight containers or resealable plastic bags for up to 3 months.

DIETITIAN'S MESSAGE

This comforting stew provides 1 meat, and 2 vegetable servings. Adding rice or noodles and ending the meal with Orange Crème Caramel (see recipe, page 423) ensures that all the food groups are represented.

*This easy-to-make curry
is perfect for an everyday
meal or for a buffet
casserole at a party. To
turn up the heat, add
a finely chopped chili
pepper or a pinch (or
two!) of cayenne pepper
along with the seasonings.*

TIP

This dish freezes well, so
double the quantity and
freeze the extra in units
that are suitable for your
family's needs.

DIETITIAN'S MESSAGE

Serve this curry with rice
and Raita Cucumber Salad
(see recipe, page 155)
or Cool Cucumber Salad
(see recipe, page 154)
for a meal that is rich
in protein, iron and
B vitamins. Boost the
fiber content by using
brown rice.

Easy Beef Curry

1 lb	stewing beef, cubed	500 g
1	medium Spanish onion, sliced	1
1 tbsp	butter *or* margarine	15 mL
1	can (19 oz/540 mL) tomatoes	1
3 tbsp	flaked coconut	45 mL
	or	
⅓ cup	raisins	75 mL
1 tbsp	lemon juice	15 mL
1 tsp	granulated sugar	5 mL
1 tsp	chili powder	5 mL
1 tsp	ground turmeric	5 mL
½ tsp	curry powder	2 mL
½ tsp	salt	2 mL
¼ tsp	ground cinnamon	1 mL
Pinch	ground cloves	Pinch

1. In a large Dutch oven or stockpot over medium-high heat,
   brown beef and onion in butter for about 10 minutes. Add
   tomatoes, coconut, lemon juice, sugar and seasonings.

2. Cook, covered, over low heat for about 2 hours or until
   meat is tender. Taste and add extra curry powder if
   required. Serve over cooked rice or noodles.

With Coconut

PER SERVING	
Calories: 208	
Dietary Fiber: 3 g	Carbohydrate: 12 g
Fat: 9 g	Protein: 20 g

With Raisins

PER SERVING	
Calories: 222	
Dietary Fiber: 2 g	Carbohydrate: 18 g
Fat: 8 g	Protein: 20 g

Ginger Vegetable Beef Medley

1½ cups	brown rice	375 mL
4 cups	boiling water	1 L
¼ cup	safflower oil, divided	50 mL
2	small onions, cut into wedges	2
1	clove garlic, minced	1
½ lb	green beans, diagonally sliced	250 g
1 lb	mushrooms, sliced	500 g
1 cup	sliced water chestnuts	250 mL
2 tsp	chopped ginger root	10 mL
½ tsp	black pepper	2 mL
1½ lb	sirloin or top round steak, cut into thin strips	750 g
3 tbsp	cornstarch	45 mL
2 tsp	ground ginger	10 mL
½ cup	water	125 mL
⅓ cup	chili sauce	75 mL
¼ cup	soy sauce	50 mL

1. In a saucepan, add rice to boiling water. Cover and cook for 45 minutes or until tender and water is absorbed.

2. In a wok or nonstick skillet, heat 2 tbsp (25 mL) of the oil over high heat. Add onions and garlic; stir-fry for 1 minute. Add green beans, mushrooms and water chestnuts. Cover and steam for 4 minutes. Stir in ginger root and pepper. Remove mixture and keep warm.

3. Coat beef strips in cornstarch and ground ginger. In wok, stir-fry beef over high heat in remaining oil until brown. Stir in water, chili sauce and soy sauce.

4. Arrange rice on platter; top with vegetable mixture and beef strips.

PER SERVING
Calories: 552	
Dietary Fiber: 5 g	Carbohydrate: 63 g
Fat: 20 g	Protein: 31 g

SERVES 6

Maisie S. Vanriel, Dietitian

Vegetables can be varied in this beef stir-fry — red or white onions, sliced carrots, snow peas, chopped broccoli or cauliflower. Remember that brown rice is not only more flavorful than white, it is also more nutritious.

TIP

Be sure to use a tomato-based chili sauce in this recipe rather than one made from chili peppers; otherwise the result will be overwhelmingly spicy.

DIETITIAN'S MESSAGE

This hearty dish is almost a meal in itself. It is loaded with high-quality protein, B vitamins, iron and fiber. Complete the meal with Lemon Pudding (see recipe, page 425).

M. Kathy Dyck

This classic stir-fry marries Asian flavors with beef and vegetables. All you need to add is cooked rice.

TIP

When preparing food for stir-frying, cut into small pieces of approximately equal size so that they will cook through rapidly and in the same period of time. Have sauce and ingredients prepared and easily accessible before starting to cook.

DIETITIAN'S MESSAGE

This Asian-style meal is perfect for a busy weeknight. For a quick and easy dessert that continues the Asian theme, serve sliced melon, such as cantaloupe, sprinkled with gingered sugar (granulated sugar mixed with ground ginger to taste).

Beef with Broccoli

1 lb	sirloin steak, cut into thin strips	500 g
¼ cup	soy sauce	50 mL
2 tbsp	cornstarch, divided	25 mL
1	clove garlic, minced	1
1	thin slice ginger root, minced	1
2 tbsp	safflower oil, divided	25 mL
2	medium onions, cut into wedges	2
3	large carrots, sliced into coins	3
1	head broccoli, cut into florets	1
1¼ cups	water, divided	300 mL
1 tbsp	oyster sauce	15 mL
1 tsp	granulated sugar	5 mL

1. Place steak in a medium bowl. In a separate bowl, combine soy sauce, 1 tbsp (15 mL) of the cornstarch, garlic and ginger root; pour over steak.

2. In a wok or nonstick skillet, heat 1 tbsp (15 mL) of the oil over high heat. Add beef and stir-fry until browned. Set aside.

3. In wok, heat remaining oil over high heat. Add onions and stir-fry for 1 minute. Add carrots, broccoli and 1 cup (250 mL) of the water; cover and steam for 4 minutes.

4. Combine remaining water, oyster sauce, remaining cornstarch and sugar. Stir sauce into wok; cook until smooth and thickened. Return meat to wok. Reheat to serving temperature.

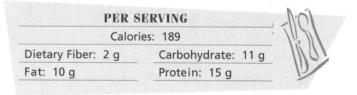

PER SERVING	
Calories: 189	
Dietary Fiber: 2 g	Carbohydrate: 11 g
Fat: 10 g	Protein: 15 g

Hoisin Beef and Broccoli Stir-Fry

2 tsp	vegetable oil	10 mL
12 oz	sirloin *or* inside round steak, cut into 3- by ½-inch (7.5 by 1 cm) strips	375 g
1 tbsp	chopped ginger root	15 mL
1 tsp	minced garlic	5 mL
3 cups	small broccoli florets	750 mL
⅓ cup	sliced water chestnuts	75 mL
½ tsp	cornstarch	2 mL
⅓ cup	orange juice *or* beef stock	75 mL
2 tbsp	hoisin sauce	25 mL
½ tsp	sesame oil (optional)	2 mL
	Black pepper	
1 tbsp	toasted sesame seeds (optional)	15 mL

1. In a large nonstick skillet, heat oil over medium-high heat; add beef strips and stir-fry for 1 to 2 minutes or until browned. Add ginger, garlic, broccoli and water chestnuts; stir-fry for another 2 to 3 minutes or until broccoli is tender-crisp.

2. In a small bowl or glass measuring cup, whisk together cornstarch, orange juice, hoisin sauce and, if using, sesame oil. Add to skillet; cook, stirring, for 1 to 2 minutes or until thickened and heated through. Season with pepper to taste. If desired, sprinkle with sesame seeds.

PER SERVING
Calories: 178

Dietary Fiber: 2 g	Carbohydrate: 11 g
Fat: 6 g	Protein: 20 g

SERVES 4
....
Bev Callaghan, Dietitian

There are endless variations on the theme of stir-fried beef and broccoli. This one highlights flavorful hoisin sauce, a spicy-sweet condiment made from fermented soybeans. Serve over cooked rice.

TIP

Hoisin sauce also makes a great glaze for fish fillets or chicken breasts. Look for it in the Asian food section of most supermarkets. Refrigerate after opening.

DIETITIAN'S MESSAGE

Using a nonstick skillet helps you cook with very small amounts of oil — and makes cleanup a breeze. Adding a tiny amount of flavored oil, such as sesame oil, provides taste without adding too much fat. End the meal with Fruit Plate with Creamy Dip (see recipe, page 386).

Beef and Rice Noodles

Marinade

1 tbsp	vegetable oil	15 mL
2 tsp	tamari *or* soy sauce	10 mL
1 tsp	cornstarch	5 mL
1 tsp	dry sherry	5 mL
Pinch	granulated sugar	Pinch

Beef and Noodles

½ lb	lean boneless beef (round, sirloin *or* flank)	250 g
¼ lb	rice vermicelli	125 g
2	slices ginger root	2
3 tsp	vegetable oil, divided	15 mL
1	clove garlic, chopped	1
1 tbsp	tamari *or* soy sauce	15 mL
2	green onions, cut into 1-inch (2.5 cm) pieces	2
2	stalks celery, cut into julienne strips	2
1	medium carrot, cut into julienne strips	1
1	medium green bell pepper, cut into julienne strips	1

1. *Marinade:* In a bowl, whisk together ingredients.

2. *Beef and Noodles:* Cut beef across the grain into strips; toss with marinade. Let marinate for 15 minutes. Meanwhile, cover rice vermicelli with boiling water; let stand for 15 minutes. Drain well.

3. In a wok or skillet over high heat, stir-fry ginger root in 1 tsp (5 mL) of the oil until lightly browned; discard ginger. Add garlic and beef; stir-fry until beef is desired degree of doneness. Remove from wok and keep warm.

4. Add remaining oil; stir-fry rice vermicelli for 1 minute. Stir in tamari sauce. Remove from wok and keep warm. Add onions, celery, carrot and green pepper to wok; stir-fry until tender-crisp. Return beef and noodles to wok; stir-fry for 1 minute. Makes 2 main-course servings or 4 servings for a multi-course meal.

PER SERVING (4-SERVING SIZE)	
Calories: 273	
Dietary Fiber: 2 g	Carbohydrate: 29 g
Fat: 10 g	Protein: 16 g

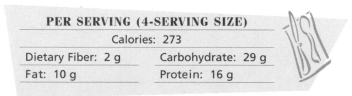

Main Meals

Spiced Veal Stir-Fry

1 tsp	ground ginger	5 mL
½ tsp	garlic powder	2 mL
¼ tsp	red pepper flakes	1 mL
Pinch	ground cinnamon	Pinch
Pinch	each allspice and ground cloves	Pinch
1¼ lb	veal scaloppine, cut into thin strips	625 g
1 cup	chicken broth	250 mL
¼ cup	dry white wine (optional)	50 mL
3 tbsp	soy sauce	45 mL
2 tbsp	cornstarch	25 mL
2 tbsp	vegetable oil, divided	25 mL
1	medium onion, chopped	1
2 cups	mushrooms, quartered	500 mL
3	medium carrots, sliced	3
3	stalks celery, diagonally sliced	3
1	medium green bell pepper, chopped	1

1. Combine ginger, garlic powder, red pepper flakes, cinnamon, allspice and cloves. Transfer one-third of the spice mixture to bowl; add veal and toss to coat. Chill for 1 to 2 hours.

2. Combine remaining spice mixture, chicken broth, wine, if using, soy sauce and cornstarch; set sauce aside.

3. In a large skillet, heat 1 tbsp (15 mL) of the oil over medium-high heat; sauté onion, mushrooms, carrots, celery and green pepper for 5 minutes or until tender. Remove from pan. Add remaining oil to skillet; brown veal for about 2 minutes. Add sauce and bring to a boil; cook, stirring, until thickened. Return vegetables to skillet and heat through.

PER SERVING	
Calories: 200	
Dietary Fiber: 2 g	Carbohydrate: 12 g
Fat: 7 g	Protein: 23 g

SERVES 6

Tyrone Miller, Chef
Karen Jackson, Dietitian

This delicious stir-fry recipe uses veal seasoned with ginger, garlic, red pepper flakes — and cinnamon! Serve over rice.

TIPS

Stir-frying and sautéing are basically the same method of cooking: food is cooked quickly in a pan with sloping sides.

If desired, replace the white wine in this recipe with additional chicken stock.

DIETITIAN'S MESSAGE

It is unusual to find veal in a stir-fry. Make this a special meal by serving with Chilled Melon Soup with Mango (see recipe, page 96). Serve Lemon Pudding (see recipe, page 425) for dessert.

SERVES 6

·····················

Lynn Homer, Dietitian

This recipe is a delicious way to cook a less tender cut of beef. Be sure to have plenty of mashed potatoes to enjoy with the savory gravy.

TIPS

To tenderize steaks, place meat between 2 pieces of plastic wrap and pound with a flat wooden or rubber mallet until flattened slightly. This process helps to break down the tough fibers in the meat.

If desired, replace the red wine in this recipe with beef stock.

For best results when making mashed potatoes, use potatoes with a high starch component, such as Yukon Gold. For a garlicky twist, cook peeled garlic with the potatoes (1 clove garlic per medium potato). When the potatoes are cooked, mash with the garlic and 1 tbsp (15 mL) milk or buttermilk per potato. Season to taste.

DIETITIAN'S MESSAGE

Serve this delicious and comforting dish with steamed green beans and garlic mashed potatoes. Finish with Orange Crème Caramel (see recipe, page 423).

Salisbury Steak in Wine Sauce

Preheat oven to 350°F (180°C)
11- by 7-inch (2 L) baking dish, greased

2 tbsp	vegetable oil, divided	25 mL
6	4-oz (125 g) tenderized round steaks (see Tip, at left), pounded to ½-inch (1 cm) thickness and patted dry	6
1 cup	sliced onions	250 mL
2 cups	sliced mushrooms	500 mL
3 tbsp	all-purpose flour	45 mL
1	beef bouillon cube	1
1½ cups	hot water	375 mL
½ cup	dry red wine	125 mL
2 tsp	Worcestershire sauce	10 mL
½ tsp	each garlic powder and paprika	2 mL
1	bay leaf	1
⅛ tsp	black pepper	0.5 mL
1 tbsp	chopped fresh parsley (optional)	15 mL

1. In a nonstick skillet, heat 1 tsp (5 mL) of the oil over medium-high heat; cook steaks in 2 batches, turning once, until brown on both sides. Transfer to prepared dish.

2. Heat another 1 tsp (5 mL) of the oil in skillet. Add onions and mushrooms; cook until softened. Transfer to baking dish, placing vegetables on top of steaks. Remove skillet from heat and add remaining oil; blend in flour.

3. In a small bowl, dissolve bouillon cube in hot water. Slowly add bouillon to flour mixture, whisking constantly until well combined. Return skillet to medium heat; stir in wine, Worcestershire sauce, garlic powder, paprika, bay leaf and pepper. Whisk constantly until sauce is thickened and smooth. Pour sauce over steaks.

4. Cook, covered, in preheated oven for 45 to 50 minutes or until meat is fork-tender. Remove bay leaf before serving. Sprinkle with parsley, if desired.

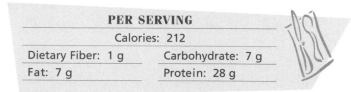

PER SERVING	
Calories: 212	
Dietary Fiber: 1 g	Carbohydrate: 7 g
Fat: 7 g	Protein: 28 g

Simple Steak Dinner

Spinach Salad

2 tbsp	lower-fat plain yogurt	25 mL
2 tbsp	light mayonnaise	25 mL
2 tsp	cider vinegar	10 mL
1 tsp	liquid honey	5 mL
	Salt and black pepper	
½	bunch spinach	½
5	small white turnips, peeled (*or* red-skinned potatoes)	5

Steak

8 oz	striploin steak	250 g
	Black pepper	
1	small onion, sliced	1
1 cup	quartered mushrooms	250 mL
¼ cup	water, red wine *or* beef broth	50 mL

1. *Spinach Salad:* Combine yogurt, mayonnaise, vinegar and honey; season with salt and pepper to taste. Break spinach into bite-size pieces. Set aside.

2. In a saucepan of boiling water or in the microwave, cook or steam turnips until tender. Slice into wedges.

3. *Steak:* Meanwhile, trim all visible fat from steak; cut into 2 pieces. Season with pepper to taste. In a nonstick skillet sprayed with vegetable oil cooking spray, brown steak over high heat on both sides. Reduce heat to medium. Add onion and mushrooms; cook, stirring, until steak is done as desired, 3 to 5 minutes for medium. Remove steak from pan. Stir water into vegetables; cook over high heat until 2 tbsp (25 mL) liquid remains.

4. To serve, toss spinach with dressing. Place on dinner plates along with steak and turnips. Top with vegetable sauce.

PER SERVING

Calories: 358	
Dietary Fiber: 9 g	Carbohydrate: 33 g
Fat: 12 g	Protein: 32 g

SERVES 2

Chris Klugman, Chef
Susie Langley, Dietitian

Sometimes it's not just coming up with a recipe that's a challenge, it's deciding what to serve with it. This recipe offers a total mealtime solution.

TIP
If using unpackaged spinach, be sure to wash it thoroughly as it can be gritty. Submerge the leaves in a large container of tepid water and swish to loosen any grit. Rinse thoroughly and drain in a colander.

DIETITIAN'S MESSAGE

This dinner can be made in less than 30 minutes. Pan-broiling without fat makes this lean red meat and seasonal fresh vegetable combo a treat. The spinach salad with honey yogurt dressing completes the meal.

Yannick Vincent, Chef
Debra Reid, Dietitian

This variation of a classic pot-au-feu is sophisticated enough for even the most elegant dinner.

TIP

Use this recipe as the basis for a superb beef fondue. Cut the beef into ¾-inch (2 cm) cubes. Bring the consommé and soup can of water to a boil, then pour all but 1 cup (250 mL) of the liquid into fondue pot and maintain at a simmer. Proceed with Step 2, using reserved liquid (beef will not have been cooked in it) and serve sauce as a dipping sauce. (Or skip this step and serve cooked beef with Dijon mustard, horseradish or other dipping sauce of your choice.) Spear beef pieces with a fondue fork and cook until desired doneness (about 3 minutes).

DIETITIAN'S MESSAGE

Although beef tenderloin, a lean meat option, is more likely to be grilled than poached, poaching produces a moist, flavorful result. Balance this meal with abundant vegetables and tasty grain products.

Poached Beef Tenderloin

1	can (10 oz/284 mL) beef consommé	1
1½ lb	beef tenderloin	750 g
1	can (5½ oz/156 mL) tomato paste	1
1 tbsp	butter, melted	15 mL
1 tbsp	all-purpose flour	15 mL
2 tbsp	Madeira	25 mL
¼ tsp	black pepper	1 mL
	Watercress	

1. In a covered skillet, bring consommé and 1 soup can of water to a boil. Add beef; cover and simmer for 25 to 30 minutes or until desired doneness. Remove beef and keep warm.

2. Reserve 1 cup (250 mL) of the cooking liquid in skillet; stir in tomato paste. Combine butter and flour; stir into skillet and cook, stirring, until thickened and bubbly. Add Madeira and pepper; heat through.

3. To serve, slice beef. Serve sauce on the side. Garnish with watercress.

PER SERVING	
Calories: 158	
Dietary Fiber: 1 g	Carbohydrate: 6 g
Fat: 7 g	Protein: 18 g

Flank Steak Stir-Fry

1 lb	flank steak	500 g
¼ cup	soy sauce	50 mL
1 tbsp	water	15 mL
2 tsp	cornstarch	10 mL
1 tsp	dry sherry	5 mL
1	clove garlic, minced	1
1 tbsp	vegetable oil	15 mL
2½ cups	cubed green bell pepper	625 mL
2	large tomatoes, cut into wedges	2
¼ tsp	black pepper	1 mL

1. Trim steak and thinly slice across the grain; cut into bite-size pieces. In a medium bowl, combine soy sauce, water, cornstarch, sherry and garlic. Stir in steak and let stand for 10 minutes.

2. In a nonstick skillet, heat oil over medium heat; cook green peppers, stirring, until almost tender. Add beef; cook to desired doneness, about 2 minutes. Stir in tomatoes and pepper; cook just until heated through.

PER SERVING	
Calories: 174	
Dietary Fiber: 2 g	Carbohydrate: 7 g
Fat: 8 g	Protein: 18 g

SERVES 6

**William King, Chef
Rosemary Duffenais,
Dietitian**

Finding recipes the whole family will like and that can be made in less than 20 minutes is a challenge. This tasty stir-fry, made with green peppers and tomatoes, fits the bill on both counts! Serve with rice.

TIP

For variety, replace the green pepper in this recipe with shredded cabbage, chopped napa cabbage or broccoli florets.

DIETITIAN'S MESSAGE

Serve this tasty stir-fry with rice and a yellow or orange vegetable, such as Honey-Glazed Carrots (see recipe, page 360) or Roasted Red Pepper Salad (see recipe, page 149), to complement the color of the green peppers and add vitamin A.

James Kennedy, Chef
Pat Scarlett, Dietitian

This classic stroganoff uses sauce made from scratch as a lower-fat alternative to those made with roux. Serve with egg noodles and garnish with chopped fresh parsley.

TIPS

This recipe makes about 2 cups (500 mL) of brown sauce, twice the quantity of sauce required. Freeze the remainder for future use.

To save time, use a prepackaged brown sauce in this recipe. Add red wine and fresh thyme leaves for extra flavor.

DIETITIAN'S MESSAGE

This recipe offers a lower-fat alternative to traditional beef stroganoff recipes, which are usually finished with sour cream. Make the sauce ahead and serve with egg noodles and a green vegetable for a great winter meal. Finish with Fluffy Pumpkin Cheesecake (see recipe, page 409).

Beef Stroganoff

Brown Sauce

¼ cup	each diced onion, leek and celery	50 mL
2 tbsp	diced carrot	25 mL
2 tbsp	tomato paste	25 mL
½ cup	red wine	125 mL
4 cups	strong beef broth	1 L
1	clove garlic, chopped	1
1 tsp	dried thyme	5 mL
1	bay leaf	1
3 tbsp	cornstarch, dissolved in 2 tbsp (25 mL) water	45 mL

Beef

2 cups	sliced mushrooms	500 mL
¾ cup	diced onion	175 mL
1 cup	Brown Sauce	250 mL
⅓ cup	lower-fat plain yogurt	75 mL
1½ tsp	Dijon mustard	7 mL
1 lb	boneless trimmed sirloin steak, cut into thin strips	500 g
¼ cup	diced seeded tomato	50 mL

1. *Brown Sauce:* In a skillet sprayed with nonstick cooking spray, cook vegetables over medium-high heat, stirring, until well browned. Mix in tomato paste. Add half of the wine; cook, stirring, until evaporated. Repeat with remaining wine.

2. Add beef broth, garlic, thyme and bay leaf; bring to a boil. Reduce heat and simmer until reduced by half. Strain, discard vegetables and return liquid to skillet. Add dissolved cornstarch and cook, stirring, until thickened.

3. *Beef:* Spray a medium skillet with nonstick cooking spray; heat over medium heat. Cook mushrooms and onion, stirring, for 2 to 3 minutes or until onion is softened. Whisk together Brown Sauce, yogurt and mustard; mix into mushroom mixture and heat over low heat. Set aside.

4. Spray a large skillet with nonstick cooking spray; heat over high heat. Add beef; cook, stirring, until browned. Stir in sauce and tomato; heat through.

PER SERVING	
Calories: 208	
Dietary Fiber: 1 g	Carbohydrate: 10 g
Fat: 5 g	Protein: 28 g

Sesame Steak

¼ cup	light soy sauce	50 mL
1	clove garlic, minced	1
1	small onion, finely chopped	1
1 tbsp	liquid honey	15 mL
1 tbsp	sesame seeds	15 mL
1 tsp	grated ginger root	5 mL
1 tsp	black pepper	5 mL
1 lb	flank steak	500 g

1. In a shallow nonaluminum pan, mix together soy sauce, garlic, onion, honey, sesame seeds, ginger and pepper. Add steak, turning to coat. Cover and marinate in refrigerator for at least 4 to 6 hours or preferably overnight.

2. Preheat barbecue or broiler; place steak on greased grill or under broiler; cook for 4 to 5 minutes per side for medium-rare. Slice across the grain to serve.

PER SERVING	
Calories: 200	
Dietary Fiber: Trace	Carbohydrate: 2 g
Fat: 9 g	Protein: 26 g

SERVES 4

**Janice Mitchell, Chef
Jane Henderson, Dietitian**

Flank steak is a popular cut of beef because it is versatile and extremely flavorful. In this recipe, the steak is marinated in a soy, garlic, ginger and honey sauce. The result is both tender and packed with flavor. Serve with stir-fried vegetables or salad and garlic bread.

TIP

Marinating meat adds flavor while it tenderizes. For convenience, marinate meat in a resealable plastic freezer bag.

DIETITIAN'S MESSAGE

Flank steak is a lean cut of meat that can be quite elegant when grilled and cut across the grain. Serve this delicious steak with rice and stir-fried vegetables or Sautéed Spinach with Pine Nuts (see recipe, page 355). Finish the meal with Peach Cobbler (see recipe, page 403).

Serve these satays as a main meal with rice and stir-fried vegetables. They're also great as an appetizer or snack anytime. If the weather isn't suitable for barbecuing, the satays can be broiled instead.

TIP

Remember to use a clean plate to transfer cooked satays from the barbecue. Raw meat juices can contaminate cooked foods.

MAKE AHEAD

Start marinating the beef strips the night before and the satays will only take a few minutes to prepare the next day. Soak wooden skewers for about 30 minutes to prevent them from burning on the barbecue. Be careful with skewers when young children are around.

DIETITIAN'S MESSAGE

Serve as an appetizer with raw vegetables and Cottage Cheese Herb Dip (see recipe, page 78), or as a meal with rice and a tossed green salad. Complete the meal with Peachy Upside-Down Cake (see recipe, page 407).

Barbecued Beef Satays

8 bamboo skewers, soaked (see Make Ahead)

1¼ lb	sirloin *or* round steak, cut into 3- by ½-inch (7.5 by 1 cm) strips	625 g
¼ cup	sodium-reduced soy sauce	50 mL
1 tbsp	lemon juice	15 mL
1 tbsp	brown sugar	15 mL
½ tsp	minced garlic	2 mL
½ tsp	ground coriander	2 mL
¼ tsp	ground cumin	1 mL
¼ tsp	ground ginger	1 mL
	Prepared peanut sauce	

1. Place beef strips in a large freezer bag. Set aside.

2. In a small bowl, blend together soy sauce, lemon juice, brown sugar, garlic, coriander, cumin and ginger. Pour over beef strips; seal bag. Marinate in refrigerator for at least 4 hours or overnight.

3. Preheat barbecue or broiler. Remove meat from marinade; thread onto small wooden skewers. Discard marinade.

4. Barbecue or broil over medium-high heat, turning once, for 4 to 5 minutes or until browned and cooked to desired doneness. Serve with your favorite peanut dipping sauce.

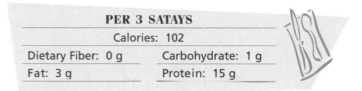

PER 3 SATAYS	
Calories: 102	
Dietary Fiber: 0 g	Carbohydrate: 1 g
Fat: 3 g	Protein: 15 g

Meat Loaf "Muffins" with Barbecue Sauce

Preheat oven to 375°F (190°C)
12-cup muffin tin, greased

Meat Loaf "Muffins"

1½ lb	lean ground beef	750 g
¾ cup	oatmeal *or* dry bread crumbs *or* cracker crumbs	175 mL
¼ cup	wheat bran	50 mL
1	can (5.4 oz/160 mL) 2% evaporated milk	1
1	egg	1
1 tsp	chili powder	5 mL
½ tsp	garlic powder	2 mL
¼ tsp	salt	1 mL
¼ tsp	black pepper	1 mL

Barbecue Sauce

1 cup	ketchup	250 mL
¼ cup	finely chopped onion	50 mL
2 tbsp	brown sugar	25 mL
½ tsp	hot pepper sauce (optional)	2 mL

1. *Meat Loaf "Muffins":* In a large bowl, combine ground beef, oatmeal, bran, milk, egg, chili powder, garlic powder, salt and pepper. Divide mixture evenly among muffin cups, pressing down lightly.

2. *Barbecue Sauce:* In another bowl, combine ketchup, onion, sugar and, if using, hot pepper sauce. Spoon about 1 tbsp (15 mL) sauce over each muffin.

3. Bake in preheated oven for 25 to 30 minutes or until meat is no longer pink in center.

PER SERVING	
Calories: 396	
Dietary Fiber: 3 g	Carbohydrate: 29 g
Fat: 19 g	Protein: 27 g

SERVES 6

Diana Callaghan

These meaty "muffins" are a favorite of kids and adults. Instead of making the sauce, substitute 1 cup (250 mL) of your favorite prepared barbecue sauce.

TIP

If your kids don't like onion pieces in the sauce, substitute ¼ tsp (1 mL) onion or garlic powder. Limit use of onion and garlic salt, as they add unnecessary sodium.

DIETITIAN'S MESSAGE

Adding wheat bran is a great way to boost the fiber content of meat loaf, meatballs and hamburgers. Use about ¼ cup (50 mL) per 1½ lb (750 g) ground meat. Adding canned evaporated milk or skim-milk powder helps to increase calcium.

**Larry DeVries, Chef
Jackie Kopilas and
Rachel Barkley, Dietitians**

*Although it is costly, beef
tenderloin is both lean
and tender, and there is
no waste as there is with
some less expensive cuts
of meat. This elegant
recipe picks up on the
higher-fat approach of
serving steak with
Roquefort butter.*

TIPS

If fresh thyme is available,
use 1 tsp (5 mL) leaves in
the sauce instead of the
dried thyme.

There are many different
types of blue cheese,
ranging in flavor from
very mild to very strong.
You may want to sample
some at the cheese
counter before deciding
which is for you.

DIETITIAN'S MESSAGE

In this recipe, the strong
tastes of the blue cheese
and the garlic complement
the lower-fat preparation.
Complete this rich-
tasting meal with simple
and light accompaniments
such as parsleyed
potatoes and a steamed
green vegetable. For a
special meal, finish with
Fruit Meringues with
Cinnamon Crème Fraîche
(see recipe, page 382).

Beef Tenderloin with Blue Cheese Herb Crust

Preheat oven to 350°F (180°C)
Baking sheet

Sauce

1 cup	beef broth	250 mL
1 tbsp	cornstarch	15 mL
¼ tsp	crushed dried thyme	1 mL

Beef

⅓ cup	crumbled blue cheese	75 mL
¼ cup	fresh white bread crumbs	50 mL
2 tbsp	chopped fresh parsley	25 mL
2 tbsp	chopped fresh chives *or* green onions	25 mL
1	clove garlic	1
4	beef tenderloin medallions (3 oz/90 g each)	4

1. *Sauce:* In a small saucepan, bring broth, cornstarch and thyme to a boil, stirring; simmer for 1 minute. Keep warm.

2. *Beef:* In a food processor, process cheese, crumbs, parsley, chives and garlic until in fine crumbs.

3. In a nonstick skillet, brown medallions quickly on each side. Remove from skillet and place on baking sheet. Pack cheese mixture evenly on top of each. Bake in preheated oven for about 20 minutes for medium doneness or as desired. Spoon sauce onto plates and top with beef.

PER 3 SATAYS	
Calories: 171	
Dietary Fiber: Trace	Carbohydrate: 4 g
Fat: 8 g	Protein: 19 g

Beef Fajitas

Preheat oven to 350°F (180°C)
13- by 9-inch (3 L) baking dish, greased

1 tbsp	vegetable oil	15 mL
1	each medium green and red bell pepper, cut into thin strips	1
2	medium onions, thinly sliced	2
1 lb	beef steak (round, flank *or* sirloin), trimmed and thinly sliced across the grain	500 g
2	medium tomatoes, diced	2
2	cloves garlic, minced	2
2 tsp	chili powder	10 mL
1 tsp	hot pepper sauce	5 mL
½ tsp	each black pepper, dry mustard and ground ginger	2 mL
10	8-inch (20 cm) soft flour tortillas	10
⅔ cup	shredded light Cheddar-style cheese	150 mL

1. In a large nonstick skillet, heat oil over medium-high heat; cook green and red peppers and onions, stirring, for 4 to 5 minutes. Remove from pan.

2. Add beef to pan; brown for 2 minutes. Stir in tomatoes, garlic, chili powder, hot pepper sauce, pepper, mustard and ginger; heat through. Return vegetables to skillet; heat through.

3. Divide mixture among tortillas; sprinkle mixture with 1 tbsp (15 mL) cheese and roll up. Place in greased 13- by 9-inch (3 L) baking dish. Bake in preheated oven for about 10 minutes to heat through.

PER SERVING	
Calories: 256	
Dietary Fiber: 2 g	Carbohydrate: 30 g
Fat: 8 g	Protein: 17 g

SERVES 5

**Robert Neil, Chef
Denise Hargrove, Dietitian**

Fajitas have become popular, in part because they are fun to put together as well as to eat. This version is assembled, then baked.

TIP

For convenience, you can assemble these fajitas early in the day and bake just before serving.

DIETITIAN'S MESSAGE

All the food groups are represented in this combination of lean beef with lots of vegetables and a bit of cheese, wrapped in a tortilla. Serve with fresh salad greens or veggie sticks for a complete finger food meal. For a Mexican-themed party, double the recipe and start the festivities with Black Bean Salsa (see recipe, page 80) or Fiery Verde Dip (see recipe, page 80).

••••••••••••••••••••
Ronald Davis, Chef
Debra McNair, Dietitian

*This marvelously moist
dish (which you can
make the day before) is
excellent served as part
of a cold buffet with
salads and bread.*

TIP

If making this dish ahead
of time, refrigerate
the veal in a clean
container within 2 hours
of cooking.

DIETITIAN'S MESSAGE

Using vegetables, herbs
and lemon to flavor the
meat in this recipe
increases the taste
without increasing the
fat content. Serve with
Orange Broccoli (see
recipe, page 351) and,
for a treat, Simple Risotto
(see recipe, page 213).
For a special meal,
finish with Baked Alaska
Volcano (see recipe,
page 390).

Braised Roasted Veal

Preheat oven to 475°F (240°C)
Roasting pan

2 lb	veal leg (top portion)	1 kg
½ tsp	each crumbled dried rosemary and thyme	2 mL
Pinch	dried tarragon	Pinch
1	stalk celery, chopped	1
1	medium onion, chopped	1
1	medium carrot, diced	1
⅓ cup	water	75 mL
¼ cup	vinegar	50 mL
¼ cup	white wine	50 mL
1 tsp	grated lemon zest	5 mL
1 tbsp	lemon juice	15 mL

1. Place veal in roasting pan; sprinkle with rosemary, thyme and tarragon. Place celery, onion and carrot around veal. Roast in preheated oven for 10 minutes.

2. Reduce temperature to 375°F (190°C). Add water, vinegar, wine, lemon zest and juice. Cover and roast for 1 hour. Remove from pan and cool. Chill. Slice to serve.

PER SERVING	
Calories: 144	
Dietary Fiber: 0 g	Carbohydrate: 0 g
Fat: 4 g	Protein: 25 g

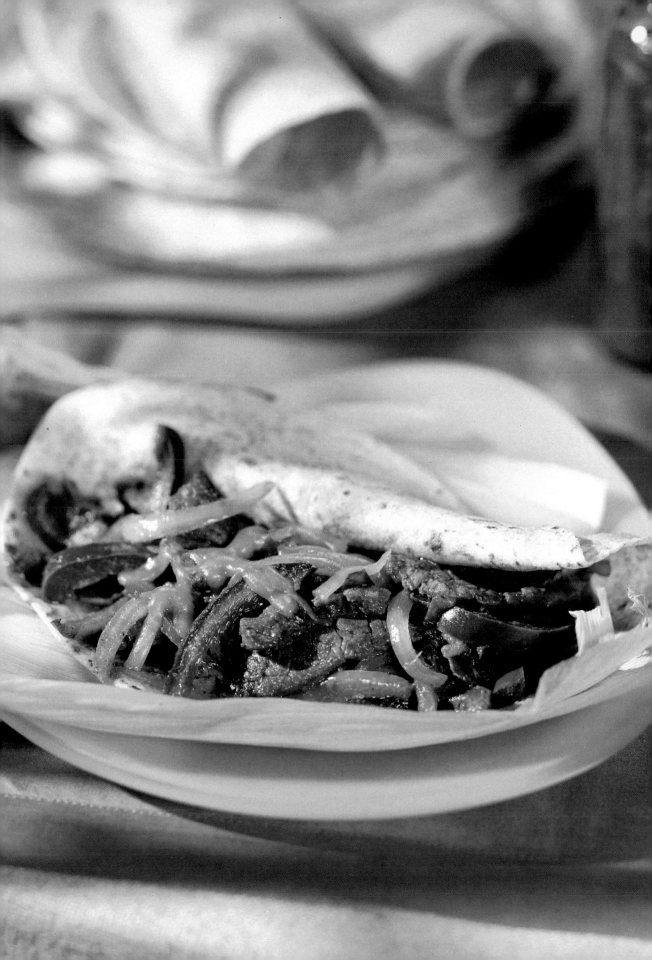

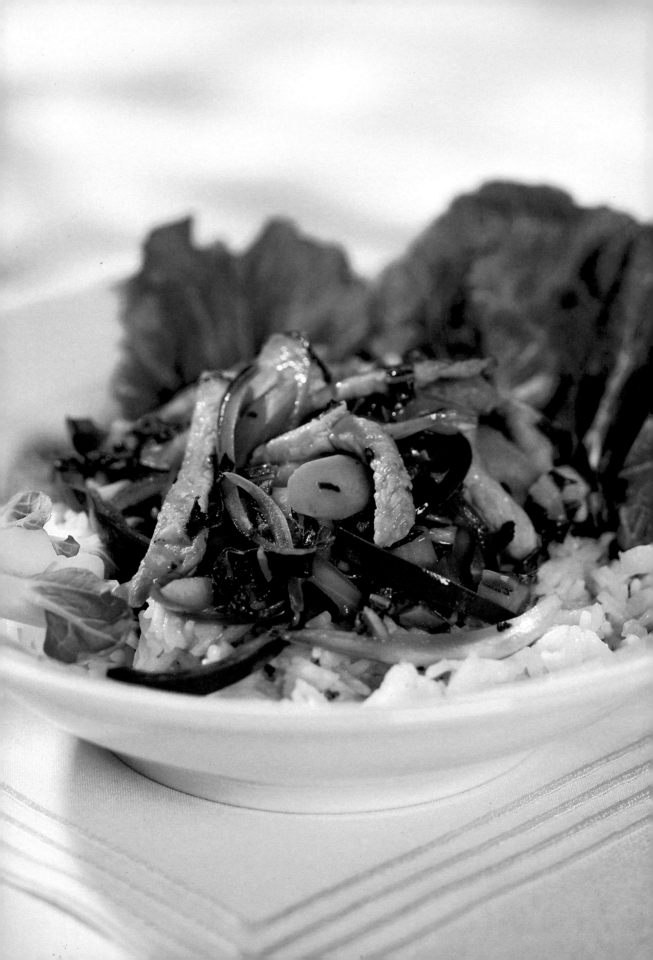

Orange Ginger Pork and Vegetables

SERVES 4
....

**David Powell, Chef
Rosanne E. Maluk,
Dietitian**

2 tbsp	vegetable oil	25 mL
1	medium onion, sliced	1
2	medium carrots, sliced	2
1	each medium green and red bell pepper, cut into thin strips	1
1 cup	sliced celery	250 mL
1 lb	well-trimmed boneless pork loin, cut into thin strips	500 g
1	clove garlic, minced	1
2 tsp	grated ginger root	10 mL
1/4 tsp	red pepper flakes	1 mL
2 cups	shredded bok choy	500 mL
1/2 cup	orange juice	125 mL
	Salt	

1. In a large skillet, heat 1 tbsp (15 mL) of the oil over medium-high heat; sauté onion, carrots, green and red peppers and celery for about 5 minutes or until tender. Remove from pan.

2. Add remaining oil to skillet. Brown pork with garlic, ginger root and red pepper flakes until pork is no longer pink. Return vegetables to skillet; add bok choy. Add orange juice; heat through, 2 to 3 minutes. Season with salt to taste.

b pts

PER SERVING	
Calories: 291	
Dietary Fiber: 4 g	Carbohydrate: 16 g
Fat: 14 g	Protein: 26 g

In Chinese cooking, ginger root is valued as much for its healthful properties — it is believed to have stimulating and cleansing benefits — as its zesty flavor. Here, it brings out the best of both the pork and vegetables in this easy stir-fry.

TIPS

Adjust the quantity of red pepper flakes to suit your taste. Or, for a more Asian version of this dish, omit the red pepper flakes and substitute an Asian chili paste instead. Sambal oelek, a bottled chili paste, easily identified by its bright red color, is readily available in Asian markets. Try adding 1/2 tsp (2 mL) of this zesty mix to the pan after the pork is browned.

Bok choy is a Chinese green frequently used in stir-fries. Use both stalks and leaves.

DIETITIAN'S MESSAGE

The peppers, orange juice and red pepper flakes add flavor to this dish. Serve with brown rice for additional fiber.

Not only is pork tenderloin one of the leanest cuts of pork, it is also extremely tender and succulent. Here, its delicate flavor is enhanced with a yogurt, honey and lemon sauce, and the unique taste of unripened green peppercorns, which are available packed in brine in most supermarkets.

TIP

When using leeks, wash them carefully as they are grown in sandy soil and can be gritty. Slice them lengthwise without cutting through the bottom layers, then soak them in lots of tepid water. Rinse thoroughly in tepid water to remove any remaining grit.

DIETITIAN'S MESSAGE

Use leeks to add variety to your vegetable choices. Serve with steamed green beans or Stuffed Tomatoes (see recipe, page 348). Finish with Strawberries in Phyllo Cups (see recipe, page 380) for a grand dessert.

Pork with Leeks and Noodles

¾ lb	pork tenderloin	375 g
	Black pepper	
	Strips of zest from 1 lemon	
2 tbsp	vegetable oil, divided	25 mL
3	leeks (white part only), cut into julienne strips	3
½ cup	dry white wine	125 mL
⅔ cup	lower-fat plain yogurt	150 mL
2 tbsp	liquid honey	25 mL
1 tsp	lemon juice	5 mL
¼ tsp	salt	1 mL
1 tsp	cornstarch	5 mL
1 tbsp	cold water	15 mL
1 tsp	green peppercorns, packed in brine, drained	5 mL
Noodles		
3 cups	egg noodles	750 mL
1 tbsp	butter	15 mL
Pinch	each salt and ground nutmeg	Pinch

1. Slice pork diagonally into 8 pieces. Place between plastic wrap and pound with meat mallet to ¼-inch (5 mm) thickness. Sprinkle with pepper to taste. Cover lemon zest with boiling water; drain and set aside for garnish.

2. In a large skillet, heat 1 tbsp (15 mL) of the oil over medium-high heat; brown pork on both sides until no longer pink. Remove from pan and keep warm.

3. Add remaining oil to skillet; cook leeks, stirring, for 5 minutes. Add wine; simmer until reduced by half. Over low heat, stir in yogurt, honey, lemon juice and salt. Dissolve cornstarch in water; add to skillet and stir until thickened. Stir in peppercorns.

4. *Noodles:* Meanwhile, cook noodles according to package directions; drain and add butter, salt and nutmeg. Divide noodles among 4 plates. Top each with 2 pork escallops; spoon sauce over top. Garnish with lemon zest.

PER SERVING	
Calories: 389	
Dietary Fiber: 3 g	Carbohydrate: 40 g
Fat: 14 g	Protein: 25 g

Pork Teriyaki

1 lb	pork tenderloin, cut into thin strips	500 g
¼ cup	teriyaki sauce	50 mL
1 cup	water	250 mL
½ cup	dried apricots, halved	125 mL
2½ cups	pineapple *or* orange juice	625 mL
1¼ cups	white rice	300 mL
1 tbsp	vegetable oil	15 mL
1	medium onion, chopped	1
1	medium red bell pepper, chopped	1
1	small yellow bell pepper, chopped	1
¼ cup	slivered almonds	50 mL

1. Marinate pork in teriyaki sauce for several hours in refrigerator.

2. Bring water and apricots to a boil in a small saucepan. Cook for about 20 minutes or until tender. Remove apricots, reserving liquid. Add pineapple juice to saucepan; return to boil. Add rice and cook for about 15 minutes or until rice is tender and liquid is absorbed.

3. In a large skillet over medium-high heat, stir-fry pork in hot oil for about 5 minutes or until browned. Add onion and peppers; stir-fry for 5 minutes. Stir in apricots and almonds. Serve over rice.

PER SERVING	
Calories: 471	
Dietary Fiber: 4 g	Carbohydrate: 69 g
Fat: 10 g	Protein: 27 g

SERVES 5

Marilyn Grisé

Teriyaki is a Japanese soy-based sauce that is usually used to glaze fish or meat that is grilled or stir-fried. Here, it is used as a marinade and combines with fruit, vegetables and almonds to create a uniquely flavored dish.

TIP
Vary the vegetables in this stir-fry — add sliced red or white onions, sliced carrots, snow peas, broccoli or cauliflower florets or chopped green or red pepper, as desired. Cut pieces about the same size to ensure even cooking.

DIETITIAN'S MESSAGE
Stir-fried vegetables retain their crunchy texture and bright colors. They also retain more nutrients because of the fast cooking time. This dish, which delivers a healthy dose of iron, contains foods from all the food groups, except for Milk Products. Complete the meal with a dairy-rich dessert such as a baked custard.

These colorful kebabs are perfect for casual entertaining or for a special family meal.

TIPS

Soak wooden skewers for 30 minutes to prevent them from burning on the barbecue.

To prevent bacterial contamination, use a clean platter to transfer kebabs back from the barbecue.

Fresh pineapple works best in this recipe; it has a firmer texture and, unlike canned pineapple, can be cut into larger chunks.

DIETITIAN'S MESSAGE

This recipe provides a meat serving as well as 2 servings from the Vegetables and Fruit group. Serve these kebabs on a bed of couscous with a green salad. For dessert, serve Country Apple Berry Crisp (see recipe, page 404).

Polynesian Pork Kebabs

Eight 8-inch (20 cm) wooden skewers

¼ cup	sodium-reduced soy sauce	50 mL
2 tbsp	lemon juice	25 mL
2 tbsp	liquid honey *or* brown sugar	25 mL
1 tsp	vegetable oil	5 mL
1 tsp	ground ginger (*or* ½ tsp/2 mL minced ginger root)	5 mL
1 lb	lean pork loin *or* tenderloin, cubed	500 g
1½ cups	cubed fresh pineapple	375 mL
1	red bell pepper, cut into chunks	1
1	green bell pepper, cut into chunks	1

1. In a medium bowl, combine soy sauce, lemon juice, honey, oil and ginger; add pork cubes, tossing to coat. Cover and marinate for at least 30 minutes or overnight in refrigerator.

2. Thread skewers alternately with pieces of pork, pineapple, red pepper and green pepper. Brush kebabs with marinade; discard any left over.

3. Preheat barbecue or broiler. Barbecue kebabs over medium-high heat, turning once, for 10 to 12 minutes or until pork is just slightly pink in the center. Alternatively, grill under broiler, turning once, for 8 to 10 minutes or until cooked through.

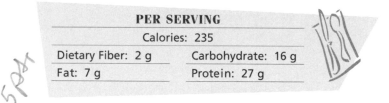

PER SERVING	
Calories: 235	
Dietary Fiber: 2 g	Carbohydrate: 16 g
Fat: 7 g	Protein: 27 g

QUICK COUSCOUS

Place 1 cup (250 mL) couscous in a medium ovenproof bowl with a dash of olive oil. Pour 1 cup (250 mL) boiling water on top of couscous; stir. Cover and let stand for 5 minutes. Fluff with a fork. Makes 3 cups (750 mL). One half cup (125 mL) couscous provides 1 Grain Products serving.

Pork Chops with Peaches and Kiwi

¾ cup	chicken stock	175 mL
½ cup	orange juice	125 mL
4 tsp	cornstarch	20 mL
2 tsp	granulated sugar	10 mL
1 tsp	minced garlic	5 mL
1 tsp	minced ginger root (or ¼ tsp/ 1 mL ground ginger)	5 mL
½ tsp	grated lemon zest (optional)	2 mL
1 tsp	olive oil	5 mL
4	lean boneless or bone-in pork chops	4
1½ cups	sliced peaches	375 mL
½ cup	sliced (cut lengthwise) peeled kiwi fruit	125 mL
	Salt and black pepper	

1. In a medium bowl, combine stock, orange juice, cornstarch, sugar, garlic, ginger and, if using, lemon zest. Set aside.

2. In a large nonstick skillet, heat oil over medium-high heat. Add pork chops and sear for 1 to 2 minutes per side or until golden. Add stock mixture; bring to a boil. Reduce heat to medium-low and simmer for 5 to 6 minutes or until pork is cooked and just slightly pink at the center. Stir in peaches and kiwi. Season with salt and pepper to taste. Simmer for 1 to 2 minutes or until heated through.

PER SERVING	
Calories: 234	
Dietary Fiber: 2 g	Carbohydrate: 19 g
Fat: 7 g	Protein: 23 g

SERVES 4

Johanne Thériault, Dietitian

Pork and fruit are a delicious combination usually reserved for special occasions. Here's an easy-to-make recipe that allows you to experience these great taste sensations on weeknights.

TIPS

Use 1 can (14 oz/398 mL) drained sliced peaches instead of fresh peaches for a year-round recipe. Or use fresh nectarines or mangoes.

Young children often prefer fruit "straight up" — that is, without sauce. In this case, prepare extra fruit and serve it alone as a side dish.

FOOD FAST

If you are serving this dish with rice, start cooking it while you prepare the rest of the meal.

DIETITIAN'S MESSAGE

Experiment with new ways to include more fruit in your main meals. Dark orange fruits such as peaches, mangoes and nectarines provide vitamins A and C, as well as some fiber.

This "meal in a skillet" is the perfect solution for a busy weeknight supper.

TIP

If desired, substitute 1 cup (250 mL) chicken stock for the bouillon cube and water. If you are concerned about salt intake, choose a low-sodium alternative.

DIETITIAN'S MESSAGE

Start your meal planning around the couscous and the vegetables in this recipe. Focusing meal planning on grains and vegetables helps to keep fat intake under control. Whenever possible, choose nutrient-rich vegetables that are dark orange, red or green.

All the food groups except Milk Products are represented in this one-dish meal.

Skillet Pork Chops with Sweet Potatoes and Couscous

2 tsp	vegetable oil	10 mL
4	boneless pork loin chops, trimmed and patted dry (about 1 lb/500 g)	4
½ cup	chopped onions	125 mL
½ cup	chopped celery *or* fennel	125 mL
2 cups	diced sweet potatoes	500 mL
1	chicken bouillon cube dissolved in 1 cup (250 mL) water	1
½ to 1 tsp	crumbled dried rosemary	2 to 5 mL
¾ cup	orange juice *or* apple juice	175 mL
1 cup	quick-cooking couscous	250 mL
	Black pepper	

1. In a large nonstick skillet, heat 1 tsp (5 mL) of the oil over medium-high heat. Add pork chops and cook, turning once, for 7 to 8 minutes or until slightly pink at center and juices run clear when pierced with a fork. Transfer pork to a plate and keep warm.

2. Add remaining oil to skillet. Add onions and celery; cook for 3 minutes. Add sweet potatoes, bouillon mixture and rosemary; bring to a boil. Reduce heat and simmer, covered, for 7 to 8 minutes or until potatoes are barely tender.

3. Stir in orange juice and couscous. Return pork to skillet and simmer, covered, for 2 minutes. Remove pan from heat and let stand for 3 minutes. Fluff couscous with fork. Season with pepper to taste.

PER SERVING	
Calories: 462	
Dietary Fiber: 4 g	Carbohydrate: 59 g
Fat: 9 g	Protein: 33 g

Pork Tenderloin with Roasted Potatoes

Preheat oven to 375°F (190°C)
11- by 7-inch (2 L) baking dish, greased

1	12-oz (375 g) pork tenderloin	1
2 tsp	orange marmalade	10 mL
2 tsp	Dijon mustard	10 mL
1 tsp	vegetable oil	5 mL
2 cups	potatoes, cut into 1-inch (2.5 cm) pieces	500 mL
1 tbsp	lemon juice	15 mL
1 tsp	crumbled dried rosemary	5 mL

1. Pat pork tenderloin dry; place in center of baking dish.

2. In a small bowl, combine marmalade, mustard and ½ tsp (2 mL) of the oil; brush over pork.

3. In a medium bowl, toss potatoes with remaining oil; arrange around pork in baking dish. Sprinkle potatoes with lemon juice. Sprinkle pork and potatoes with rosemary. Bake in preheated oven for 40 to 45 minutes or until pork is just slightly pink at center and potatoes are tender. Cut pork into ½-inch (1 cm) slices before serving.

PER SERVING	
Calories: 236	
Dietary Fiber: 2 g	Carbohydrate: 17 g
Fat: 5 g	Protein: 29 g

SERVES 3
....
Bev Callaghan, Dietitian

This dish takes only 10 minutes to prepare. And because it cooks in 1 baking dish, cleanup is a snap!

TIP

If you need to feed more than 3 people, just buy another pork tenderloin and double the remaining ingredients. If you have leftovers, add slices of tenderloin to Egg and Mushroom Fried Rice (see recipe, page 225) or use in sandwiches.

DIETITIAN'S MESSAGE

Serve with green beans, applesauce, whole-grain rolls and a glass of cold milk. To boost your vitamin A intake, replace 1 cup (250 mL) white potatoes with sweet potatoes.

The Pineapple Mango Salsa in this recipe is also great with grilled salmon or swordfish. For lunch, try it stuffed in a pita with chicken salad or rolled up in a tortilla with light cream cheese and some thinly sliced ham or smoked turkey.

TIPS

Fresh pineapple tastes best in this recipe, but you can use canned pineapple instead.

Choose a ripe mango that is red or orange-yellow and soft to the touch.

MAKE AHEAD

The salsa can be made ahead and kept in the refrigerator for several days.

DIETITIAN'S MESSAGE

Ham, bacon and many processed deli meats are often high in salt. If you are concerned about excess sodium, you may want to limit your consumption of these foods.

Broiled Ham Steak with Pineapple Mango Salsa

Preheat broiler
Shallow baking dish, greased

2	6-oz (175 g) packaged ham steaks	2
2 tsp	Dijon *or* other mustard	10 mL
2 tsp	brown sugar	10 mL
1 tbsp	orange juice *or* pineapple juice	15 mL
Pineapple Mango Salsa		
1 cup	diced fresh mango	250 mL
1 cup	diced fresh pineapple	250 mL
½ cup	chopped red onion	125 mL
¼ cup	finely chopped fresh cilantro	50 mL
2 tbsp	lime juice	25 mL

1. Place ham steaks in baking dish and spread with mustard. Sprinkle with brown sugar, then orange juice. Broil for 2 to 3 minutes or until golden and bubbling.

2. *Pineapple Mango Salsa:* In a bowl, stir together mango, pineapple, onion, cilantro and lime juice. Chill until ready to use. Warm to room temperature before serving with ham steak.

PER SERVING	
Calories: 175	
Dietary Fiber: 2 g	Carbohydrate: 17 g
Fat: 4 g	Protein: 18 g

Grilled Lamb and Vegetables with Roasted Garlic

Preheat oven to 400°F (200°C)

2	stalks celery, cut into 1-inch (2.5 cm) thick slices	2
1	medium red bell pepper, cut into strips	1
1	medium zucchini, sliced	1
1	medium eggplant, cut into ¼-inch (5 mm) thick slices	1
1 tsp	crushed dried thyme	5 mL
2	heads garlic	2
¼ cup	olive oil, divided	50 mL
2 tbsp	white wine vinegar	25 mL
¼ tsp	each salt and black pepper	1 mL
1	pkg (400 g) frozen boneless lamb loins, thawed	1
	Fresh thyme (optional)	

1. In a bowl, combine celery, red pepper, zucchini, eggplant and thyme; let stand for 1 hour.

2. Cut top off garlic heads; place in a small baking dish or custard cups. Set aside 1 tbsp (15 mL) of the oil. Cover garlic with remaining oil. Bake in preheated oven for 30 to 35 minutes or until cloves come out of their skins. (Do not burn.) Remove garlic from skins and mash with fork. Stir in vinegar, salt and pepper. Keep warm (or reheat in microwave for 15 seconds).

3. Preheat broiler. Brush lamb and vegetables with reserved oil. Grill lamb loins and vegetables for 2 to 3 minutes per side. (Or heat reserved oil in large skillet; brown lamb for about 5 minutes. Remove; keep warm. Add vegetables to skillet and sauté for about 5 minutes or until tender.)

4. To serve, pour 1 tbsp (15 mL) garlic sauce onto 1 side of each of 4 plates. Slice lamb and place on top. Place vegetables beside lamb. Garnish with fresh thyme, if desired.

PER SERVING	
Calories: 268	
Dietary Fiber: 4 g	Carbohydrate: 16 g
Fat: 13 g	Protein: 23 g

The subtle flavor of roasted garlic blends perfectly with the warm vegetables and thinly sliced lamb in this delicious recipe. Although it will impress guests, it is easy enough to serve for a family weeknight dinner if you are feeling a bit celebratory.

TIPS

Roasted garlic has a milder taste than fresh garlic and is also easier on the digestive system.

Use 1 tbsp (15 mL) fresh thyme instead of dried, and fresh rather than frozen lamb, if available.

If desired, cook this dish on the barbecue, bearing in mind that because foods cooked at high temperatures may present a risk for cancer, they should be served less often.

DIETITIAN'S MESSAGE

Feature all food groups by serving this dish with pita bread and Quick Roasted Red Pepper Dip (see recipe, page 81).

*Lamb, cumin, couscous
and chickpeas are used
often in Middle Eastern
cuisine. Served with
vegetables lightly cooked
in olive oil, this dish does
justice to that region's
rich culinary heritage.*

TIP

Soak wooden skewers
for 30 minutes to prevent
them from burning.

DIETITIAN'S MESSAGE

Serve this as a special
meal and expect even the
most discriminating guest
to be impressed. Begin
with an antipasto platter
or Eggplant Tapas (see
recipe, page 83). Complete
the meal with a Spicy
Fruit Compote (see
recipe, page 383).

Lamb with Couscous and Mixed Vegetables

Six 8-inch (20 cm) wooden skewers

6	lamb loins (3 oz/90 g each), cut into 1-inch (2.5 cm) cubes	6
1	medium Spanish onion, cut into 1-inch (2.5 cm) cubes	1
1 cup	dry red wine	250 mL
¼ cup	finely chopped onion	50 mL
2 tbsp	olive oil	25 mL
1	bay leaf	1
8	black peppercorns	8
¼ tsp	ground cumin	1 mL
½ cup	beef broth	125 mL
1 tbsp	cornstarch, dissolved in 2 tbsp (25 mL) cold water	15 mL

Couscous

1 cup	couscous	250 mL
1½ cups	boiling water	375 mL
1 tsp	olive oil	5 mL
½ tsp	salt	2 mL
¼ tsp	black pepper	1 mL

Vegetables

1 tbsp	olive oil	15 mL
2	stalks celery, diced	2
1	each small green and red bell pepper, diced	1
1	small zucchini, chopped	1
½ cup	drained canned chickpeas	125 mL
¼ cup	chopped onion	50 mL

1. Alternately thread lamb and onion cubes onto skewers. In a glass dish, combine wine, onion, oil, bay leaf, peppercorns and cumin; add skewers, coat with marinade and refrigerate for 6 to 12 hours, basting occasionally.

2. Remove brochettes. Strain marinade into saucepan and bring to a boil; cook until reduced by half. Add beef broth; bring to a boil. Add dissolved cornstarch and stir until thickened. Keep warm. Preheat barbecue or broiler.

3. *Couscous:* Pour boiling water over couscous; cover and let stand for 10 minutes. Stir in oil, salt and pepper.

4. Broil or grill lamb to desired doneness.

5. *Vegetables:* Meanwhile, in a skillet, heat oil over medium heat; cook vegetables until tender, about 5 minutes. To serve, place brochette on couscous on each plate. Arrange vegetables to one side and sauce on the side.

PER SERVING

Calories: 315

Dietary Fiber: 3 g	Carbohydrate: 36 g
Fat: 11 g	Protein: 15 g

Barbecued Butterflied Leg of Lamb

1	2-lb (1 kg) butterflied leg of lamb, trimmed	1
1 tsp	minced garlic	5 mL
2 tbsp	lemon juice	25 mL
2 tbsp	chopped fresh oregano (*or* 2 tsp/10 mL dried)	25 mL
2 tbsp	chopped fresh mint (*or* 2 tsp/10 mL dried)	25 mL
1 tbsp	olive oil	15 mL
	Black pepper	

1. Place lamb in a large shallow dish, fat side down. Spread with garlic. Sprinkle with lemon juice, oregano, mint and olive oil. Season with pepper to taste.

2. Cover and marinate in refrigerator, turning once or twice, for 2 hours or overnight. Remove from refrigerator 30 minutes before grilling.

3. Preheat barbecue or broiler. For medium-rare, barbecue on greased grill for 10 to 12 minutes per side, depending on thickness of lamb or, if using a meat thermometer, until the internal temperature of lamb registers 140° to 150°F (60° to 65°C).

PER SERVING

Calories: 177

Dietary Fiber: 0 g	Carbohydrate: 1 g
Fat: 7 g	Protein: 26 g

SERVES 6

Bev Callaghan, Dietitian

This simple Greek-style marinade is the perfect companion to grilled lamb, which is best served medium-rare.

TIP
Ask your butcher to prepare a butterflied leg of lamb for you. You may need to order it a day or two in advance.

DIETITIAN'S MESSAGE

To conform to healthy eating guidelines, a serving size of meat should be about 2 to 3 oz (60 to 90 g), about the size of the palm of your hand. To make this dish part of a special meal, begin with Apple Watercress Vichyssoise (see recipe, page 99) and accompany the lamb with minted green peas and parsleyed potatoes. Complete this elegant dinner with Creamy Fruit Crêpes (see recipe, page 401).

*Here's a dish that may
seem exotic, but it's easy
to make from ingredients
that are readily available.
It demonstrates how the
use of fruit, herbs and
spices can add zest to
the simplest recipes.
Here, oranges, kiwi fruit,
currants, curry powder
and ginger root are used
to give lamb chops an
Eastern aura.*

TIP

For a richer-tasting sauce,
use white wine or beef
broth instead of the
water in this recipe.

DIETITIAN'S MESSAGE

Lamb provides high-
quality protein and is a
good source of iron.

Serve with rice and
Cool Cucumber Salad
(see recipe, page 154)
and end the meal with a
slice of Lazy Daisy Cake
(see recipe, page 411).

Curried Lamb Chops

6	loin lamb chops, 1½ inches (4 cm) thick	6
2 tbsp	white wine vinegar	25 mL
1 tsp	salt	5 mL
¼ tsp	black pepper	1 mL
2 tsp	vegetable oil	10 mL
1 tsp	curry powder	5 mL
1 tsp	finely chopped ginger root	5 mL
1	clove garlic, minced	1
¼ tsp	ground cloves	1 mL
¼ tsp	ground cinnamon	1 mL
¾ cup	water, divided	175 mL
1	medium onion, chopped	1
2 tbsp	all-purpose flour	25 mL
2 tbsp	currants	25 mL
1	kiwi fruit, peeled and sliced	1
1	orange, peeled and sliced	1

1. Place lamb chops in shallow pan. Combine vinegar, salt and pepper; spoon over chops. Set aside for 5 minutes.

2. In a heavy skillet, cook oil, curry, ginger root, garlic and seasonings until mixture bubbles. Add ½ cup (125 mL) water and onion. Cook over medium heat for about 5 minutes.

3. Sprinkle flour over lamb chops; add chops to onion in skillet. Cook for about 4 minutes per side or until chops lose pink color. Stir in remaining water and currants. Cook, covered, over low heat for about 30 minutes or until chops are tender. Add kiwi fruit and oranges and cook for about 3 minutes.

PER SERVING	
Calories: 217	
Dietary Fiber: 1 g	Carbohydrate: 11 g
Fat: 8 g	Protein: 25 g

Grilled Lamb Chops with Sautéed Peppers and Zucchini

Preheat broiler or barbecue

¼ cup	balsamic *or* red wine vinegar	50 mL
2 tbsp	olive oil, divided	25 mL
1 tbsp	Dijon mustard	15 mL
1 tsp	dried thyme leaves	5 mL
1 tsp	minced garlic	5 mL
⅛ tsp	black pepper	0.5 mL
8 to 12	bone-in, center-cut loin lamb chops, trimmed of fat (about 1½ lb/750 g in total)	8 to 12
1½ cups	sliced zucchini	375 mL
1½ cups	julienned red bell peppers	375 mL
1 cup	sliced sweet onion	250 mL

1. In a large bowl, blend together vinegar, 1 tbsp (15 mL) of the oil, mustard, thyme, garlic and pepper. Transfer 2 to 3 tbsp (25 to 45 mL) of the mixture to a small bowl; set aside.

2. Place chops on broiling pan or grill; spoon reserved vinaigrette on top. Cook, turning once, for 8 to 10 minutes or until cooked to desired doneness.

3. Meanwhile, in a large nonstick skillet, heat remaining 1 tbsp (15 mL) oil over medium-high heat. Add zucchini, peppers and onion; stir-fry for 6 to 8 minutes or until tender-crisp. Add remaining vinaigrette to pan; cook, stirring, for 1 to 2 minutes or until heated through.

PER SERVING	
Calories: 233	
Dietary Fiber: 2 g	Carbohydrate: 12 g
Fat: 12 g	Protein: 19 g

SERVES 4

··························

Bev Callaghan, Dietitian

Try this impressive dish for your next dinner party. Your guests need never know how easy it is to make!

TIPS

For extra-easy cleanup, line the broiler pan with foil.

If weather permits, grill chops on the barbecue; you'll improve their flavor — and enjoy some time outdoors!

To cook the vegetables on the grill, place vegetables and sauce in a heavy-duty foil packet and barbecue for about 10 minutes, turning once.

DIETITIAN'S MESSAGE

This easy but delicious meal, which provides 2 servings of vegetables in addition to the meat, can be rounded out with couscous or rice. Serve Hot Water Gingerbread (see recipe, page 410) with applesauce for dessert.

· ·

**John Cordeaux, Chef
Kim Arrey, Dietitian**

*Here's a recipe that's
ideal for a special
occasion when you need
to pull out all the stops
and impress your guests.*

TIP

The Apple Mango Relish
can be made ahead and
refrigerated until ready
to use.

DIETITIAN'S MESSAGE

For an elegant meal,
begin with an antipasto
platter using a selection
of recipes from the
Appetizers and Dips
chapter of this book,
such as Hummus with
Tahini, Eggplant and Olive
Antipasto or Lemon Pesto
Spread. Complete the
meal with green beans
or a simple green salad
and Pear Gingerbread
Upside-Down Cake
(see recipe, page 426).

Party-Style Lamb

Preheat oven to 450°F (230°C)
Piping bag

1	boneless lamb loin (1 lb/500 g)	1
	Fresh thyme for garnish	

Sweet Potato Purée

1	large sweet potato, peeled and cut into 1-inch (2.5 cm) pieces	1
1	clove garlic, minced	1
2 tbsp	butter *or* margarine	25 mL
¼ tsp	salt	1 mL

Carrot Thyme Sauce

1 tbsp	vegetable oil	15 mL
2	shallots, chopped	2
1½ cups	chicken broth	375 mL
½ cup	dry red wine	125 mL
¼ tsp	crushed dried thyme	1 mL
3	medium carrots, diced	3

Apple Mango Relish

1	small apple, peeled and diced	1
½ cup	diced peeled mango	125 mL
2 tbsp	lemon juice	25 mL
1 tbsp	liquid honey	15 mL
½ tsp	chopped fresh mint	2 mL

1. *Sweet Potato Purée:* Cook potato, covered, until tender; drain. Purée; blend in seasonings. Keep warm.

2. *Carrot Thyme Sauce:* In a saucepan, heat oil over medium heat; cook shallots until softened. Stir in remaining ingredients; bring to a boil. Reduce heat and simmer, uncovered, for 30 minutes. Purée until smooth.

3. *Apple Mango Relish:* Combine ingredients; cover and chill.

4. Coat lamb generously with pepper. Cook in preheated oven for 8 to 10 minutes. Slice; arrange 2 loins into rings on each plate. Using piping bag, pipe purée into rosette in center. Spoon sauce on lamb; add relish. Garnish with thyme.

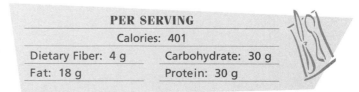

PER SERVING	
Calories: 401	
Dietary Fiber: 4 g	Carbohydrate: 30 g
Fat: 18 g	Protein: 30 g

Grilled Chicken with Stir-Fried Vegetables

Preheat barbecue or broiler

4	boneless skinless chicken breasts (3 oz/90 g each)	4
1	lime	1
1 tsp	soy sauce	5 mL
4	stalks celery	4
1	each medium red and green bell pepper	1
1	large onion	1
1	medium carrot	1
1½ tsp	each ground cumin and chili powder	7 mL
1 tsp	lemon pepper	5 mL
½ cup	chicken broth	125 mL

1. Using meat mallet, pound chicken between plastic wrap to ⅜-inch (9 mm) thickness. Place chicken in glass dish; squeeze lime juice over all. Coat with soy sauce. Set aside.

2. Cut celery on angle ⅛ inch (3 mm) thick and 2 inches (5 cm) long. Cut red and green peppers and onion into long thin strips. Using peeler, peel carrot into long thin strips. Combine vegetables with cumin, chili powder and lemon pepper. Set aside.

3. Broil or barbecue chicken until no longer pink, 4 to 5 minutes per side.

4. Meanwhile, in a large nonstick skillet sprayed with nonstick cooking spray, cook vegetables, stirring, until hot. Stir in chicken broth; cook until vegetables are tender, about 8 minutes. Serve over chicken.

PER SERVING

Calories: 152	
Dietary Fiber: 3 g	Carbohydrate: 13 g
Fat: 2 g	Protein: 22 g

SERVES 4

P

**Donald Pattie, Chef
Joan Rew, Dietitian**

Quick, easy and light, this recipe combines grilled chicken and stir-fried vegetables and uses both Asian and Tex-Mex spices to create a tasty "fusion" dish.

TIP

To prevent food from sticking when stir-frying, heat the pan before adding the oil. Tip the pan to distribute the oil evenly across the bottom and around the sides. Return the pan to the element. When the oil is just smoking, begin to fry, using large spatulas to stir the vegetables.

DIETITIAN'S MESSAGE

When a small amount of oil is used, stir-frying can help to reduce fat intake. Because the food is cooked so quickly, it maintains many of the nutrients that are often lost in prolonged cooking.

Say "salsa" and you probably think of tomatoes, onions and peppers. But this salsa uses dried fruit — raisins, apricots and pears — for a delicious change with a Mediterranean flair.

TIPS

For variety, try poaching the chicken instead of grilling. It can also be served cold.

Like most salsas, this one can be prepared ahead of time. Leftovers make a great accompaniment to grilled meats.

DIETITIAN'S MESSAGE

Salsas are a great way to include vegetables and fruit in your diet.

Grilled Chicken Breast with Dried Fruit Salsa

Dried Fruit Salsa

1	medium red bell pepper, diced	1
⅓ cup	raisins *or* diced pitted prunes	75 mL
⅓ cup	each diced dried apricots and pears	75 mL
¼ cup	diced red onion	50 mL
¼ cup	coarsely chopped fresh cilantro	50 mL
⅓ cup	lime juice	75 mL
1 tbsp	olive oil	15 mL
¼ tsp	each salt and black pepper	1 mL

Chicken

6	boneless skinless chicken breasts (3 oz/90 g each)	6

1. *Dried Fruit Salsa:* In a glass bowl, combine red pepper, raisins, apricot, pears, onion, cilantro, lime juice, oil, salt and pepper. Cover and chill for at least 1 hour.

2. Preheat barbecue or grill. Grill or broil chicken for 4 to 5 minutes per side or until no longer pink inside. Serve topped with salsa.

PER SERVING	
Calories: 195	
Dietary Fiber: 3 g	Carbohydrate: 22 g
Fat: 4 g	Protein: 20 g

Chicken in Pita

Tabbouleh

¾ cup	bulgur	175 mL
3	medium tomatoes, seeded and diced	3
2 cups	chopped fresh parsley	500 mL
¼ cup	lemon juice	50 mL
2 tbsp	chopped fresh mint	25 mL
½ tsp	salt	2 mL
¼ tsp	black pepper	1 mL

Hummus

1	clove garlic, minced	1
1	can (19 oz/540 mL) chickpeas, drained	1
3 tbsp	sesame oil	45 mL
2 tbsp	lemon juice	25 mL
½ tsp	salt	2 mL
¼ tsp	black pepper	1 mL

Chicken and Vegetables

6	boneless skinless chicken breasts	6
1 tbsp	olive oil	15 mL
	Salt and black pepper	
½	English cucumber, diced	½
2	medium tomatoes, seeded and diced	2
½	box (145 g) alfalfa sprouts	½
6	whole-wheat pitas, halved and warmed	6

1. *Tabbouleh:* Cover bulgur with 1½ cups (375 mL) boiling water; soak for 30 minutes. Drain. Stir in remaining ingredients.

2. Preheat barbecue or grill.

3. *Hummus:* In a food processor, purée garlic and chickpeas. Add remaining ingredients; process until blended.

4. Brush chicken with oil; grill or broil until no longer pink inside. Season to taste. Slice into thin strips.

5. *Chicken and Vegetables:* Place chicken, cucumber, tomatoes, sprouts, hummus and tabbouleh in separate bowls. Use to fill pitas.

PER SERVING

Calories: 554	
Dietary Fiber: 12 g	Carbohydrate: 69 g
Fat: 13 g	Protein: 41 g

SERVES 6
....

**James McLean, Chef
Jane Curry, Dietitian**

Here's a perfect recipe for a family lunch or dinner, as everyone can put his or her own pita together.

TIP

The hummus in this recipe is easy to make. If you have any leftover Hummus with Tahini or Italian-Style Hummus (see recipes, page 72), use it up in this recipe.

DIETITIAN'S MESSAGE

Although sprouts are nutritious, recently they have been linked with outbreaks of salmonella and E. coli, likely because bacteria can lodge in the tiny cracks in the seeds and multiply when the seeds are germinating. Exercise caution when using sprouts. A thorough cleaning will ensure their safety.

*Here is an easy "fusion"
recipe that combines a
variety of toothsome
flavors from around
the world.*

TIP

Sauce used to marinate
raw meat, poultry or
seafood should not be
used on cooked foods as
it may contain harmful
bacteria. Boil leftover
marinade or prepare extra
for basting cooked food.
Wash and sanitize your
brush or use separate
brushes when marinating
raw and cooked foods.

DIETITIAN'S MESSAGE

For an Eastern flair,
complete this meal with
Cool Cucumber Salad
(see recipe, page 154),
jasmine rice and fresh
berries. A slice of
Geraldine's Almond Cake
(see recipe, page 408)
would be an ideal finish
to this meal.

Grilled Chicken with Curry Sauce

Chicken

4	boneless skinless chicken breasts (about 1 lb/500 g)	4
2 tsp	grated lemon *or* lime zest	10 mL
1/3 cup	lemon *or* lime juice	75 mL
2 tbsp	chopped fresh basil (*or* 2 tsp/10 mL dried)	25 mL
4 tsp	Dijon mustard	20 mL
2 tsp	chopped fresh thyme (*or* 1/4 tsp/1 mL dried)	5 mL
	Black pepper	

Curry Sauce

1/4 cup	light mayonnaise	50 mL
1/4 cup	lower-fat plain yogurt	50 mL
1 tsp	grated lime zest	5 mL
1 tbsp	lime juice	15 mL
1/2 tsp	curry powder	2 mL

1. *Chicken:* Place chicken in single layer in glass dish. Combine lemon zest and juice, basil, mustard, thyme, and pepper to taste; pour over chicken. Cover and refrigerate for 3 to 12 hours, turning chicken occasionally.

2. Preheat barbecue or grill. Remove chicken from marinade. Grill for 6 to 8 minutes per side or until no longer pink inside.

3. *Curry Sauce:* In a bowl, combine mayonnaise, yogurt, lime zest and juice, and curry powder. Serve with chicken.

PER SERVING WITH CURRY SAUCE	
Calories: 186	
Dietary Fiber: Trace	Carbohydrate: 3 g
Fat: 6 g	Protein: 28 g

Spiced Chicken with Peach Chutney

SERVES 4
....

Chris Klugman, Chef
Susie Langley, Dietitian

Peach Chutney

1 lb	peaches, peeled and thinly sliced (4 medium)	500 g
½ cup	packed brown sugar	125 mL
½ cup	finely chopped red onion	125 mL
⅓ cup	cider vinegar	75 mL
¼ cup	lemon juice	50 mL
1	clove garlic, minced	1
1 tsp	chopped ginger root	5 mL
1 tsp	chopped green chilies	5 mL

Spiced Chicken

4 tsp	dried oregano	20 mL
1 tbsp	minced garlic	15 mL
1 tbsp	vegetable oil	15 mL
¾ tsp	fennel seeds	4 mL
¾ tsp	ground cinnamon	4 mL
¾ tsp	chopped green chilies	4 mL
4	chicken breasts (about 6 oz/175 g each)	4

1. *Peach Chutney:* In a saucepan, bring ingredients to a boil. Reduce heat and simmer for 5 minutes. With slotted spoon, remove peaches and set aside. Simmer liquid until reduced to thick syrup. Return peaches to saucepan and return to boil. Remove from heat. Cool.

2. *Spiced Chicken:* Preheat barbecue or oven. In a small food processor, combine ingredients for spice mixture; process until smooth. Lift up skin from chicken but do not remove. Spread spices on chicken and replace skin. Let stand for 30 minutes.

3. Barbecue on greased grill for about 35 minutes or until no longer pink inside. Or bake on greased baking sheet in 400°F (200°C) oven. Remove skin before serving with Peach Chutney.

PER SERVING	
Calories: 341	
Dietary Fiber: 2 g	Carbohydrate: 42 g
Fat: 8 g	Protein: 26 g

Adding a spice rub both on and under the skin before barbecuing ensures moist and tasty chicken. If you are watching your fat intake, remove the skin before serving.

TIPS

You can make the Peach Chutney ahead and refrigerate until ready to serve.

Use ¼ cup (50 mL) chopped fresh oregano instead of dried, if desired.

DIETITIAN'S MESSAGE

Improper handling of poultry can spread bacteria throughout the kitchen. To reduce the possibility of cross-contamination, keep poultry — and all raw meats — away from other foods during storage and preparation. Use separate cutting boards for meats and vegetables. Clean and sanitize countertops, cutting boards and utensils with a mild bleach solution (1 tsp/5 mL bleach per 3 cups/750 mL water) before and after preparing food.

*Stuffed chicken breasts
are easier to make than
you may think. They add
a touch of elegance and
surprise at serving time.*

TIP

Prepared pesto sauce can
be found in supermarkets
near fresh pasta or in
the deli.

DIETITIAN'S MESSAGE

Lean and tender,
boneless chicken breasts
are a great convenience
food and a valuable asset
in a program of healthy
eating. Evaporated milk is
an excellent substitute for
cream in this rich-tasting,
velvety sauce. Add a
serving of Spinach Fancy
(see recipe, page 354),
along with jasmine or
basmati rice, and you have
a special-occasion meal.

Brie-Stuffed Breast of Chicken

Preheat oven to 350°F (180°C)
4-cup (1 L) covered casserole

4	boneless skinless chicken breasts (4 oz/125 g each)	4
4 tsp	pesto sauce	20 mL
2 oz	Brie cheese, rind removed and diced (½ cup/125 mL)	60 g
¾ cup	chicken broth	175 mL
¼ cup	white wine	50 mL
2 tbsp	lemon juice	25 mL
½ cup	2% evaporated milk	125 mL

1. With meat mallet, pound chicken between plastic wrap to ¼-inch (5 mm) thickness. Spread 1 tsp (5 mL) pesto over each breast; place Brie cheese in middle. Fold up sides and ends, overlapping to cover cheese completely; secure with toothpick if necessary. Place seam side down in 4-cup (1 L) covered casserole.

2. In a saucepan, bring chicken broth, wine and lemon juice just to a boil; pour over chicken. Cover and bake in preheated oven for 15 to 20 minutes or until no longer pink.

3. Reduce temperature to 200°F (100°C). Drain liquid from breasts into rinsed saucepan; return covered breasts to oven to keep warm. Boil liquid until reduced by half. Stir in evaporated milk; simmer until hot.

4. Slice chicken breasts and fan on warmed plates; drizzle with sauce.

PER SERVING	
Calories: 234	
Dietary Fiber: Trace	Carbohydrate: 5 g
Fat: 8 g	Protein: 33 g

Yogurt-Marinated Chicken

Preheat oven to 350°F (180°C)
Baking pan

1¼ cups	lower-fat plain yogurt	300 mL
3	cloves garlic, minced	3
1 tbsp	minced ginger root (*or* 2 tsp/10 mL ground ginger)	15 mL
1 tbsp	lemon juice	15 mL
1 tbsp	vegetable oil	15 mL
2 tsp	paprika	10 mL
1 tsp	chili powder	5 mL
1 tsp	crumbled dried rosemary	5 mL
1 tsp	black pepper	5 mL
½ tsp	turmeric	2 mL
8	boneless skinless chicken breasts (about 1½ lb/750 g)	8

1. In a large bowl, combine yogurt, garlic, ginger root, lemon juice, oil, paprika, chili powder, rosemary, pepper and turmeric; whisk until smooth. Add chicken, turning to coat all over. Cover and refrigerate for 24 hours.

2. Place chicken in single layer in baking pan, reserving marinade. Bake in preheated oven for 20 to 25 minutes or until no longer pink inside, spooning additional marinade over chicken halfway through baking.

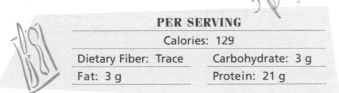

PER SERVING	
Calories: 129	
Dietary Fiber: Trace	Carbohydrate: 3 g
Fat: 3 g	Protein: 21 g

SERVES 8
··············
Nanak Chand Vig, Chef
Fabiola Masri, Dietitian

Here's an interesting variation on Chicken Tandoori, a grilled chicken that is an Indian specialty.

TIP

Instead of using chicken breasts only, you can substitute one 3-lb (1.5 kg) chicken, cut into 8 pieces; bake for 45 to 60 minutes.

DIETITIAN'S MESSAGE

Most marinated recipes call for vinegar, lemon juice or wine. This Indian-style recipe uses yogurt, which enhances the taste and tenderizes the texture. Serve with Rice Pilaf (see recipe, page 212) and a green salad.

Tyrone Miller, Chef
Karen Jackson, Dietitian

Here's a traditional chicken pot pie, but with a twist: the yummy filling is baked, "popover" style, in a flavorful cottage cheese pastry. Like its antecedent, chicken pot pie, this is infinitely comforting food.

TIP

Cottage cheese makes a pastry that's thicker and firmer than traditional flaky pastry, which makes it easier to work with.

DIETITIAN'S MESSAGE

Use this lower-fat pastry option with similar dishes. Its lighter ingredients make it a great choice for all kinds of fillings that are baked in pastry. Serve with Hot and Spicy Fruit Slaw (see recipe, page 158).

Chicken in Light Pastry

Preheat oven to 375°F (190°C)
Baking sheet

2 tbsp	vegetable oil, divided	25 mL
1	medium onion, chopped	1
1	clove garlic, minced	1
1 cup	sliced carrots	250 mL
½ cup	diced celery	125 mL
1 lb	boneless skinless chicken breasts, cut into thin strips	500 g
3 tbsp	all-purpose flour	45 mL
1 cup	chicken broth	250 mL
½ tsp	crushed dried thyme	2 mL
¼ tsp	crushed dried rosemary	1 mL
¼ tsp	each salt and black pepper	1 mL
1	medium potato, peeled, cooked and diced	1

Cottage Cheese Pastry

⅔ cup	lower-fat creamed cottage cheese	150 mL
3 tbsp	vegetable oil	45 mL
2	egg whites	2
2¾ cups	all-purpose flour	675 mL
2 tsp	baking powder	10 mL
½ tsp	salt	2 mL
1	egg, lightly beaten	1

1. In a large skillet, heat 1 tbsp (15 mL) of the oil over medium heat; cook onion, garlic, carrots and celery for 5 minutes. Remove from pan.

2. Add remaining oil to skillet; brown chicken until no longer pink inside. Stir in flour. Add chicken broth, thyme, rosemary, salt and pepper; bring to a boil. Add cooked vegetables and potato; heat through. Cool slightly.

3. *Cottage Cheese Pastry:* In a blender or food processor, process cottage cheese until smooth; blend in oil and egg whites. In a bowl, combine flour, baking powder and salt; stir in cheese mixture until dough forms, adding a little cold water, if necessary. Form into a ball; wrap in plastic wrap. Refrigerate for at least 1 hour.

4. On a floured board, form dough into 8-inch (20 cm) oblong tube and cut into 8 pieces. Roll each piece into 7-inch (18 cm) circle; top with about ½ cup (125 mL) chicken mixture. Brush edges with egg; fold pastry over filling to form half-moon shape. Crimp edges. Brush with egg and cut slits to vent. Bake on baking sheet in preheated oven for 15 to 20 minutes or until lightly browned.

PER SERVING	
Calories: 371	
Dietary Fiber: 2 g	Carbohydrate: 43 g
Fat: 11 g	Protein: 23 g

Honey Dijon Chicken

Preheat oven to 350°F (180°C)
Baking sheet, greased

2 tbsp	all-purpose flour	25 mL
¼ tsp	each salt and black pepper	1 mL
4	boneless skinless chicken breasts (3 oz/90 g each)	4
2 tbsp	liquid honey	25 mL
2 tbsp	Dijon mustard	25 mL
1 tbsp	olive oil	15 mL

1. On a piece of waxed paper, combine flour, salt and pepper; coat chicken with mixture. In a small dish, combine honey and mustard; set aside.

2. In a skillet, heat oil over medium-high heat; quickly brown chicken on both sides. Place on greased baking sheet; spread with honey mixture. Bake in preheated oven for 10 to 15 minutes or until chicken is no longer pink inside.

PER SERVING	
Calories: 177	
Dietary Fiber: Trace	Carbohydrate: 12 g
Fat: 5 g	Protein: 21 g

SERVES 4 P

Alastair Gray, Chef
Mary Margaret Laing,
Dietitian

You'd never guess by the taste just how quick and easy this recipe is to make!

TIP
When sautéing, make sure your pan is large enough to hold the ingredients comfortably. If not, cook ingredients in batches. If food is jammed together, it will steam, which causes it to lose flavor.

DIETITIAN'S MESSAGE
To add flavor without adding fat, honey and mustard are a superb combination. For a quickly prepared dinner, this chicken dish has it all: it's easy, nutritious and has a great, zippy taste.

*Tofu, cilantro, ginger and
lime give this tasty
chicken an Asian flair.
The unusual Yogurt Lime
Sauce, which is flavored
with Dijon mustard, adds
a "fusion" element to the
dish.*

TIP

When mincing ginger
root, peel off the skin
and chop finely, or use a
fine grater. If you have
leftover chopped ginger
root, cover it with sherry
and refrigerate in a
sealed jar. Use the
drained ginger to flavor
oil before sautéing meat.

DIETITIAN'S MESSAGE

Poaching, rather than
frying, the chicken and
using a lower-fat yogurt
for the sauce make this
tangy entrée lower in
calories and fat. Serve
with Orange Broccoli
(see recipe, page 351)
and rice.

Shrimp-Stuffed Chicken

Preheat oven to 350°F (180°C)
9-inch (2.5 L) square baking pan
Roasting pan

25	medium raw shrimp, peeled and deveined	25
½ cup	firm tofu	125 mL
¼ cup	chopped onion	50 mL
2	cloves garlic, minced	2
1 tbsp	grated ginger root	15 mL
1 tbsp	lime juice	15 mL
1 tbsp	chopped fresh cilantro	15 mL
2 tsp	soy sauce	10 mL
¼ tsp	each salt and white pepper	1 mL
6	boneless skinless chicken breasts (about 1½ lb/750 g)	6
1	egg white, lightly beaten	1
	Grated lime zest	

Yogurt Lime Sauce

1 cup	strong chicken broth	250 mL
1 tbsp	chopped shallots	15 mL
2 tbsp	cornstarch	25 mL
2 tbsp	lime juice	25 mL
1 tbsp	Dijon mustard	15 mL
¼ cup	lower-fat plain yogurt	50 mL

1. In a food processor, chop shrimp very finely. Add tofu, onion, garlic, ginger root, lime juice, cilantro, soy sauce, salt and pepper; process to form paste.

2. With meat mallet, pound chicken between plastic wrap to flatten. Divide shrimp mixture among breasts. Brush edges with egg white; fold chicken around filling to seal. Wrap individually in plastic wrap; place in 9-inch (2.5 L) square baking pan. Place in roasting pan (or broiler pan). Add boiling water to come three-quarters of the way up sides of square pan. Cover and bake in preheated oven for 25 to 30 minutes or until firm and moist.

3. *Yogurt Lime Sauce:* In a saucepan, bring broth and shallots to a boil. Combine cornstarch, lime juice and mustard; stir into broth until boiling and thickened. Over low heat, add yogurt and heat through. Serve with chicken. Garnish with lime zest.

PER SERVING WITH SAUCE	
Calories: 210	
Dietary Fiber: 1 g	Carbohydrate: 7 g
Fat: 4 g	Protein: 35 g

Creamy Mustard Chicken

Preheat oven to 350°F (180°C)
Lightly greased baking dish

2 lb	chicken pieces, skinned	1 kg
½ cup	lower-fat plain yogurt	125 mL
⅓ cup	light mayonnaise	75 mL
¼ cup	sliced green onions	50 mL
1 tbsp	Dijon mustard	15 mL
1 tbsp	Worcestershire sauce	15 mL
½ tsp	dried thyme	2 mL
½ tsp	salt	2 mL
¼ tsp	white pepper	1 mL
2 tbsp	grated Parmesan cheese	25 mL
	Chopped fresh parsley	

1. Place chicken in single layer in lightly greased ovenproof casserole. Combine yogurt, mayonnaise, onions, mustard and seasonings. Spoon sauce over each chicken piece. Bake in preheated oven for about 45 minutes or until chicken is no longer pink inside. Sprinkle with Parmesan cheese and brown under the broiler. Serve garnished with chopped parsley.

PER SERVING	
Calories: 217	
Dietary Fiber: Trace	Carbohydrate: 3 g
Fat: 11 g	Protein: 25 g

SERVES 6

Diane Felker

In this recipe, yogurt, light mayonnaise, Dijon mustard and Worcestershire sauce combine to create this toothsome sauce, which is flavorful and light.

TIP
Worcestershire sauce, a pungent mix of onions, garlic, tamarind and anchovies, among other ingredients, is a handy tool for enhancing the flavor of many sauces.

DIETITIAN'S MESSAGE
The rich, tangy sauce makes this dish a family favorite. Balance the meal with steamed carrots and a tossed green salad. Serve with rice — brown rice for extra fiber. Finish with Lemon Sherbet (see recipe, page 399).

Making pizza at home is a fun-filled family activity and a celebratory way to end a busy week. If you have difficulty coming up with topping combinations, here's a recipe that will get you started.

TIPS

Keep pizza dough rounds in the freezer to make this recipe quickly, or make your own homemade dough or Whole-Wheat Pizza Dough (see recipe, page 49).

Try baking the pizza on a preheated baking stone. Heat the stone for about 45 minutes before adding the pizza.

DIETITIAN'S MESSAGE

This pizza has something from every food group. If desired, add a tossed green salad.

Chicken Pizza

Preheat oven to 350°F (180°C)
Large baking sheet

1	12-inch (30 cm) pizza dough round, prepared *or* homemade	1
⅓ cup	tomato paste	75 mL
⅓ cup	water	75 mL
1 tbsp	vegetable oil	15 mL
½ tsp	dried oregano	2 mL
¼ tsp	celery seed	1 mL
Dash	hot pepper sauce	Dash
Pinch	black pepper	Pinch
1 cup	sliced mushrooms	250 mL
1 cup	diced cooked chicken	250 mL
½ cup	diced canned pineapple	125 mL
¼ cup	minced ham (optional)	50 mL
¼ cup	diced green bell pepper	50 mL
1½ cups	shredded part-skim mozzarella cheese	375 mL
2 tbsp	grated Parmesan cheese	25 mL
	Dried oregano and celery seed	

1. Place pizza dough round on large baking sheet. Combine tomato paste, water, oil and seasonings. Spread over dough. Arrange mushrooms, chicken, pineapple, ham, if using, and green pepper on top. Top with mozzarella and Parmesan cheese. Sprinkle with oregano and celery seed. Bake in preheated oven for 12 to 15 minutes. Cut into wedges to serve.

PER SERVING	
Calories: 245	
Dietary Fiber: 2 g	Carbohydrate: 21 g
Fat: 10 g	Protein: 17 g

Chicken and Broccoli Bake

Preheat oven to 350°F (180°C)
Oblong baking dish, lightly greased

6	chicken breast halves, skinned and boned	6
1	green onion, finely chopped	1
3 tbsp	butter *or* margarine	45 mL
2 tsp	lemon juice	10 mL
3 tbsp	all-purpose flour	45 mL
2 cups	2% milk	500 mL
1 tbsp	chopped fresh parsley	15 mL
½ tsp	salt	2 mL
¼ tsp	dried basil	1 mL
Pinch	black pepper	Pinch
1 cup	shredded Cheddar cheese, divided	250 mL
1 cup	egg noodles	250 mL
2	medium tomatoes, sliced	2
2 cups	chopped broccoli, blanched	500 mL

1. In a large skillet over medium-high heat, cook chicken and onion in butter on 1 side until golden brown. Turn chicken to brown other side; sprinkle with lemon juice. Remove chicken. Whisk flour into pan juices; cook, stirring, for 2 minutes. Gradually whisk in milk, stirring constantly until smooth and thickened. Stir in seasonings and half of the cheese.

2. In a large pot of boiling water, cook noodles according to package directions or until tender but firm; drain well. Place cooked noodles in lightly greased oblong baking dish. Top with half of the sauce. Arrange tomato slices, broccoli and chicken on top of noodles. Cover with remaining sauce. Sprinkle with remaining cheese. Bake, uncovered, in preheated oven for about 30 minutes or until bubbling hot.

PER SERVING

Calories: 384	
Dietary Fiber: 2 g	Carbohydrate: 20 g
Fat: 17 g	Protein: 38 g

SERVES 6
....
Patrick Mullin

This tasty combination of noodles, cheese, chicken and vegetables in a creamy sauce is comfort food. Make this casserole the day before you intend to serve it and reheat for even better flavor.

TIP

Substitute Swiss cheese for the Cheddar if you prefer.

DIETITIAN'S MESSAGE

All the food groups are represented in this one-dish meal. Complete the meal with a tossed salad with Lemon Pesto Dressing (see recipe, page 132) and Autumn Crumble (see recipe, page 402) for dessert.

Kay Dallimore

Apricot jam or orange marmalade and Asian flavors add flair to this easy-to-make dish.

TIP

Mustard is a versatile condiment and has many uses in cooking. Dry mustard, used here, is hot and pungent. It adds flavor without fat.

DIETITIAN'S MESSAGE

Serve this tasty dish with Rice Pilaf (see recipe, page 212) and steamed green beans or Sweet Baked Tomatoes (see recipe, page 350). End the meal with sherbet sprinkled with fresh berries.

Tangy Glazed Chicken

Preheat oven to 350°F (180°C) • Baking pan, lightly greased

1 lb	chicken breasts, skinned and boned	500 g
2 tbsp	sugar-reduced apricot jam *or* orange marmalade	25 mL
2 tbsp	unsweetened orange juice	25 mL
1	small clove garlic, minced	1
2 tsp	soy sauce	10 mL
½ tsp	ground ginger	2 mL
¼ tsp	dry mustard	1 mL

1. Place chicken in pan. Combine remaining ingredients and spoon over chicken. Bake in preheated oven until chicken is glazed and no longer pink inside, about 45 minutes.

PER SERVING	
Calories: 151	
Dietary Fiber: 0 g	Carbohydrate: 3 g
Fat: 3 g	Protein: 26 g

Shelagh Rowney

Fast and easy, these wings are perfect for a bunch of hungry teens.

TIP

Remove tips of wings and split into 2 pieces at joint before baking.

DIETITIAN'S MESSAGE

Serve with rice and Mandarin Orange Salad with Almonds (see recipe, page 143). For a snack, serve with raw vegetables and Honey Mustard Dip (see recipe, page 81) and whole-grain rolls.

Sticky Chicken Wings

Preheat oven to 425°F (220°C) • 13- by 9-inch (3 L) nonstick pan

3 lb	chicken wings (see Tip, at left)	1.5 kg
⅓ cup	liquid honey	75 mL
¼ cup	packed brown sugar	50 mL
3 tbsp	soy sauce	45 mL
2 tbsp	lemon juice *or* vinegar	25 mL
1 tsp	garlic powder	5 mL
½ tsp	ground ginger (optional)	2 mL

1. Bake wings in a single layer in preheated oven for 20 minutes; drain. Blend remaining ingredients; pour over wings. Reduce temperature to 400°F (200°C); bake, turning twice, until browned.

PER SERVING (4 WINGS)	
Calories: 307	
Dietary Fiber: 0 g	Carbohydrate: 26 g
Fat: 14 g	Protein: 20 g

Pepper-Stuffed Chicken with Cantaloupe Sauce

Preheat broiler
Baking sheet

½	each large red and green bell pepper, seeded	½
4	boneless skinless chicken breasts (4 oz/125 g each)	4
	Salt and black pepper	
2 cups	water	500 mL
1	stalk celery, cut into ½-inch (1 cm) pieces	1
1	small onion, sliced	1
1	bay leaf	1
¼	large cantaloupe, peeled	¼
2 tsp	lemon juice	10 mL
	Chopped fresh parsley	

1. Roast peppers (see instructions, page 127). Cut each into 4 long strips.

2. Place chicken between plastic wrap; flatten with mallet. Sprinkle with salt and pepper to taste. Place 1 green and 1 red pepper strip on each chicken breast; roll up tightly and secure with toothpick.

3. In a skillet, bring water, celery, onion, bay leaf and ¼ tsp (1 mL) each salt and pepper to a boil; add chicken rolls. Cover and simmer for 10 to 15 minutes or until chicken is no longer pink inside. Remove from liquid; drain.

4. In a food processor or blender, purée cantaloupe with lemon juice. Heat gently in small saucepan. Divide among 4 plates. Slice each chicken breast into 3 diagonal pieces. Place on cantaloupe purée. Sprinkle with parsley.

PER SERVING
Calories: 169	
Dietary Fiber: 1 g	Carbohydrate: 10 g
Fat: 2 g	Protein: 28 g

SERVES 4

**Vern Dean, Chef
Jane Thornthwaite, Dietitian**

Roasted peppers add flavor and color to this unusual dish.

TIP
Remove bay leaf before serving as it might cause someone to choke if eaten.

DIETITIAN'S MESSAGE

The red pepper and cantaloupe boost the vitamin A and C content of this dish. Team it up with a spinach salad for a meal with eye appeal. With this lighter meal, you can splurge on Cranberry Surprise (see recipe, page 393) for dessert.

Chinese Almond Chicken with Noodles

SERVES 4
••••••••••••••••••••••
**Stephanie Buckle,
Dietitian**

*This is a great dish for
busy weekday dinners.*

TIPS

To toast almonds: In a
nonstick skillet over
medium heat, toast
almonds, stirring
constantly, for 3 to
4 minutes or until golden
brown. Alternatively,
microwave on High for
3 to 5 minutes, stirring
at 1-minute intervals, or
bake on baking sheet in
350°F (180°C) oven
for 3 to 5 minutes or
until fragrant.

For a change of pace,
replace the carrots with
snow peas, broccoli,
cauliflower or green or
red bell peppers. Or, to
really save time, try using
3 cups (750 mL) frozen
oriental mixed vegetables
as a substitute for the
onions, carrots, celery
and bamboo shoots,
reducing stock in Step 1
by ¼ cup (50 mL).

DIETITIAN'S MESSAGE

If you have leftover
chicken, use it to make
this recipe. Start the meal
with a bowl of Oriental
Mushroom Soup (see
recipe, page 111).

Sauce

1½ cups	chicken stock	375 mL
¼ cup	sodium-reduced soy sauce	50 mL
1 tbsp	cornstarch	15 mL
1 tsp	minced garlic	5 mL
1 tsp	granulated sugar	5 mL

Stir-Fry

1 tsp	vegetable oil	5 mL
12 oz	boneless skinless chicken breasts, cubed	375 g
1 cup	sliced onion	250 mL
1 cup	thinly sliced carrots	250 mL
½ cup	chopped celery	125 mL
1	can (6 oz/175 g) bamboo shoots, drained (optional)	1
½ cup	toasted sliced almonds (see Tip, at left)	125 mL
8 oz	thin egg noodles	250 g

1. *Sauce:* In a medium bowl, combine 1 cup (250 mL) of the stock, soy sauce, cornstarch, garlic and sugar. Set aside.

2. *Stir-Fry:* In a large nonstick skillet, heat oil over medium-high heat. Add chicken and stir-fry for 6 to 8 minutes or until no longer pink inside. Set aside.

3. Add onion to skillet along with carrots, celery and remaining chicken stock; cook for 4 to 5 minutes. Add bamboo shoots, if using. Add sauce, cooked chicken and almonds; bring to a boil. Reduce heat and simmer for 2 minutes or until thickened.

4. Meanwhile, in a large pot of boiling water, cook noodles until tender but firm; drain. Serve chicken mixture over noodles.

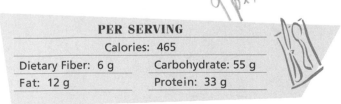

PER SERVING	
Calories: 465	
Dietary Fiber: 6 g	Carbohydrate: 55 g
Fat: 12 g	Protein: 33 g

Chicken with Sun-Dried Tomatoes

4	boneless skinless chicken breasts (4 oz/125 g each)	4
4	large basil leaves (*or* 1 tsp/5 mL dried)	4
4	sun-dried tomatoes, softened (see Tip, at right)	4
2 oz	fontina *or* mozzarella cheese, cut in 4 long strips	60 g
1 cup	chicken broth	250 mL
Sauce		
8	sun-dried tomatoes, softened	8
1 tbsp	chopped fresh basil (*or* 1 tsp/5 mL dried)	15 mL

1. Cut slit in underside of thickest part of chicken breast. Insert 1 basil leaf (or sprinkle with dried basil), 1 sun-dried tomato and 1 strip of cheese into each breast; seal with toothpick.

2. In a skillet, bring chicken broth to a boil; add chicken and return to boil. Cover and reduce heat to simmer for 10 to 15 minutes or until chicken is no longer pink inside. Remove chicken from pan and keep warm.

3. *Sauce:* Add sun-dried tomatoes and dried basil, if using, to stock in skillet; bring to a boil and cook until reduced to ½ cup (125 mL). In a food processor or blender, purée until smooth. Add fresh basil, if using. Serve over chicken.

PER SERVING	
Calories: 206	
Dietary Fiber: 1 g	Carbohydrate: 4 g
Fat: 6 g	Protein: 32 g

4 pts.

Takashi Ito and Scott Brown, Chefs
Mary Sue Waisman, Dietitian

Here's a yummy Italian-inspired recipe for chicken breasts stuffed with cheese, basil and flavor-packed sun-dried tomatoes.

TIPS

Sun-dried tomatoes are available in packages in many produce shops and Italian delis. To keep the fat content down, choose tomatoes that are not packed in oil.

To soften sun-dried tomatoes, cover with boiling water and let stand for 10 minutes; drain.

DIETITIAN'S MESSAGE

This recipe has a definite Italian flair. Serve it with Heart to Heart Salad (see recipe, page 155) and whole-wheat pasta to increase your fiber intake. If you are feeling festive, finish with Light Tiramisu (see recipe, page 422).

SERVES 4
....

Anton Koch, Chef
Kim Arrey, Dietitian

You can make this quick curry in minutes. The fruit adds a soothing note to the spices as well as great color and texture. Just be careful not to boil or the yogurt is likely to curdle.

TIP

To toast almonds, bake on a baking sheet in 350°F (180°C) oven for 3 to 5 minutes or until fragrant.

DIETITIAN'S MESSAGE

The plain yogurt makes a creamy sauce with lower fat. Serve with jasmine rice, Raita Cucumber Salad (see recipe, page 155) and naan, a type of Indian bread often available at supermarkets. End the meal with a light fruit dessert.

Quick Chicken Curry

¾ cup	long-grain rice	175 mL
1 tbsp	olive oil	15 mL
¾ lb	boneless skinless chicken breasts, cut into thin strips	375 g
2	medium oranges, peeled and cubed	2
1	medium (unpeeled) apple, cubed	1
¾ cup	red seedless grapes	175 mL
1	can (8 oz/227 mL) pineapple chunks, drained	1
1 tbsp	curry powder	15 mL
1 tsp	ground cumin	5 mL
½ tsp	salt	2 mL
¼ tsp	black pepper	1 mL
1 cup	lower-fat plain yogurt	250 mL
2 tbsp	sliced almonds, toasted (see Tip, at left))	25 mL

1. Cook rice according to package directions.
2. Meanwhile, in a large skillet, heat oil over medium-high heat; brown chicken on all sides until no longer pink inside, about 3 minutes. Reduce heat; stir in oranges, apple, grapes and pineapple and heat gently for 3 minutes. Sprinkle with curry powder, cumin, salt and pepper; mix well. Stir in yogurt and heat through.
3. Divide rice among 4 plates. Top with chicken curry; sprinkle with almonds.

PER SERVING	
Calories: 414	
Dietary Fiber: 4 g	Carbohydrate: 59 g
Fat: 8 g	Protein: 27 g

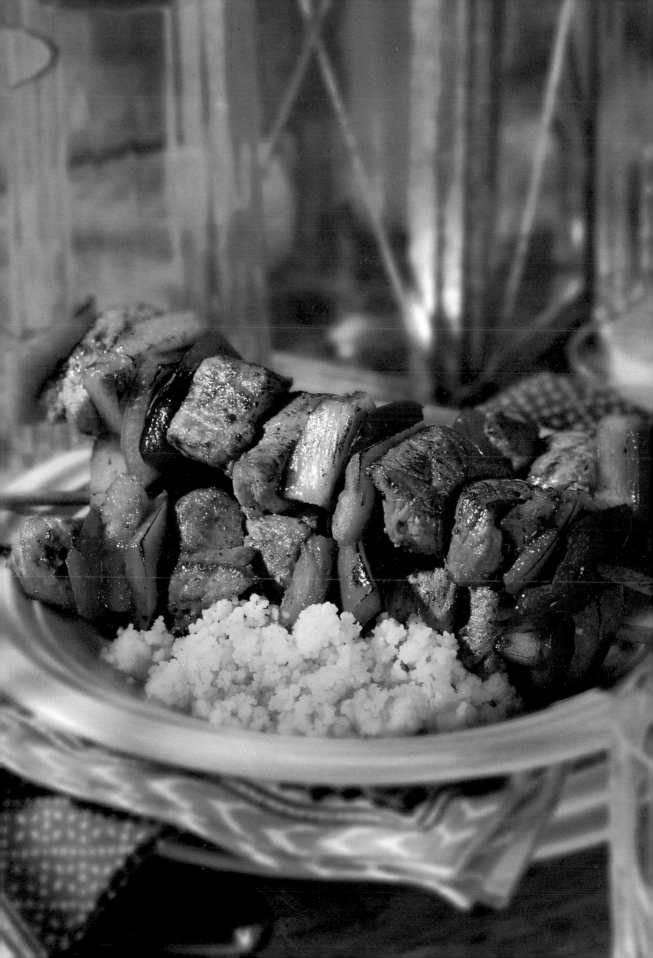

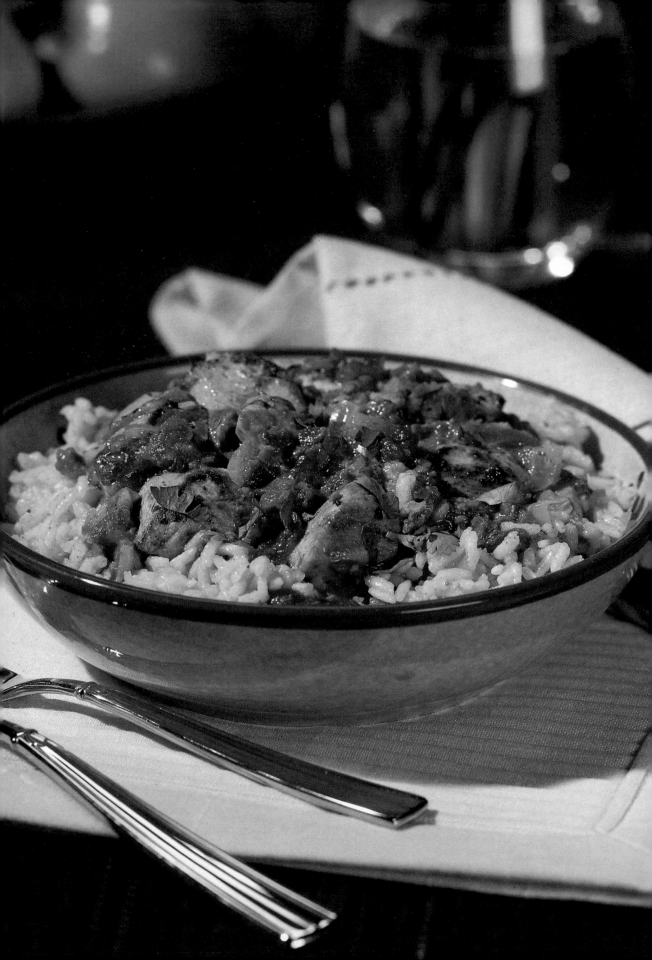

Curried Chicken with Apples and Bananas

SERVES 6   **P**

Ronald Smedmor

Here's a great chicken dish from the Kashmir region of India that you can make using ingredients you're likely to have on hand.

2 tbsp	vegetable oil	25 mL
1	3-lb (1.5 kg) chicken, skin removed and cut into 6 to 8 pieces	1
1 cup	chopped onion	250 mL
1 tbsp	minced garlic	15 mL
2 tbsp	mild *or* medium curry powder	25 mL
2 tsp	ground turmeric	10 mL
½ tsp	ground cumin	2 mL
½ tsp	ground coriander	2 mL
1 cup	diced peeled tart apples	250 mL
1½ cups	diced bananas	375 mL
1½ cups	diced tomatoes	375 mL
1 cup	chicken stock	250 mL
1 cup	lower-fat plain yogurt	250 mL
	Salt	

TIP

This recipe can be made ahead without adding the yogurt. When ready to serve, reheat on medium until mixture is simmering, then stir in the yogurt.

DIETITIAN'S MESSAGE

The sweetness of the fruit, combined with the spiciness of the sauce, makes this a perfect meal for a cold winter evening. The recipe provides a serving each of fruit and meat. Serve with brown rice to complete the meal.

1. In a large saucepan or Dutch oven, heat 1 tbsp (15 mL) of the oil over medium-high heat. Add half of the chicken pieces and cook, turning once, until brown. Repeat with remaining oil and chicken. Transfer chicken to a plate and set aside.

2. Reduce heat to medium. Add onion and garlic; cook for 5 minutes or until soft. Stir in curry powder, turmeric, cumin and coriander; sauté for 1 minute.

3. Add apples, bananas, tomatoes and chicken stock; bring to a boil. Reduce heat and simmer, uncovered and stirring frequently, for 5 minutes or until liquid is reduced by half. Return chicken to pan; simmer, covered, for 30 minutes or until juices run clear when chicken is pierced with a fork.

4. Stir in yogurt; simmer for 15 minutes, stirring occasionally and watching for curdling. Season to taste with salt.

PER SERVING	
Calories: 273	
Dietary Fiber: 2 g	Carbohydrate: 20 g
Fat: 9 g	Protein: 28 g

≺ Exotic Ginger Cumin Chicken (Page 292)

Main Meals

P

Curried Red Pepper Chicken

DIETITIAN'S MESSAGE

Transform this into an exotic meal by serving the chicken over Coconut Rice: prepare rice using lower-fat unsweetened coconut milk in place of water. Serve Raita Cucumber Salad (see recipe, page 155) on the side and finish with Poached Pears with Tea Ice Cream (see recipe, page 396).

2 tsp	vegetable oil	10 mL
1¼ lb	boneless skinless chicken breasts, cut into strips	625 g
1 cup	thinly sliced carrots	250 mL
2 cups	julienned red bell peppers	500 mL
3 tbsp	curry paste	45 mL
1 cup	chicken stock	250 mL
1 tsp	minced garlic	5 mL
¼ tsp	black pepper	1 mL
¼ cup	water	50 mL
1 tbsp	cornstarch	15 mL

1. In a large nonstick skillet, heat 1 tsp (5 mL) of the oil over medium-high heat. Add chicken strips and cook for 4 to 5 minutes or until browned on all sides. Remove chicken and set aside.

2. In same skillet, heat remaining oil over medium-high heat. Add carrots and peppers; cook for 3 minutes. Add curry paste and cook, stirring, for 1 minute or until thoroughly combined.

3. Return chicken to skillet. Stir in stock, garlic and pepper; bring to a boil. Reduce heat and simmer for 5 to 6 minutes or until chicken is cooked through and vegetables are tender-crisp.

4. In a small bowl, whisk together water and cornstarch; add to skillet. Cook over medium heat for 1 to 2 minutes or until thickened.

PER SERVING	
Calories: 188	
Dietary Fiber: 1 g	Carbohydrate: 6 g
Fat: 7 g	Protein: 23 g

Skillet Chicken and Shrimp Paella

SERVES 6 **P**
....

Kelly Husband, Dietitian

1 tbsp	olive oil	15 mL
12 oz	boneless skinless chicken breasts, cut into strips	375 g
½ cup	chopped onion	125 mL
2 tsp	minced garlic	10 mL
1	can (10 oz/284 mL) chicken broth	1
1¼ cups	water	300 mL
1	can (19 oz/540 mL) stewed tomatoes, with juice	1
1¼ cups	uncooked long-grain rice	300 mL
1 tsp	dried oregano	5 mL
½ tsp	paprika	2 mL
¼ tsp	salt	1 mL
¼ tsp	black pepper	1 mL
¼ tsp	ground turmeric *or* crumbled saffron	1 mL
1 cup	julienned red bell peppers	250 mL
1 cup	snow peas, trimmed and cut into bite-size pieces *or* frozen peas	250 mL
8 oz	cooked large shrimp (about 15)	250 g

1. In a large nonstick skillet, heat 2 tsp (10 mL) of the oil over medium-high heat. Add chicken and cook until browned and no longer pink inside. Remove from pan and set aside.

2. In same skillet, heat remaining oil over medium-high heat. Add onion; reduce heat to medium and cook for 3 to 4 minutes or until softened but not brown. Add garlic, broth, water, tomatoes, rice, oregano, paprika, salt, pepper and turmeric; bring to a boil. Reduce heat and simmer, covered, for 15 minutes.

3. Add red peppers and simmer, covered, for 4 to 5 minutes or until rice is tender. Stir in snow peas, cooked chicken and shrimp; simmer, uncovered, for 2 to 3 minutes or until heated through.

Don't be daunted by the long ingredient list. This one-pot meal is a snap to prepare — the perfect dish for casual entertaining.

VARIATION

For a change, replace the shrimp with 8 oz (250 g) cooked Italian sausage (hot or mild), cut into slices; add to recipe in Step 3 when chicken is returned to skillet. Keep in mind, though, that using sausage will increase the fat content. For an all-chicken dish, substitute an equal amount of additional chicken for the shrimp. Or try a combination of chicken, shrimp and sausage.

DIETITIAN'S MESSAGE

Three food groups are represented in this one-pot meal. It is easily balanced by adding a serving from the Milk Products group, such as yogurt.

PER SERVING	
Calories: 317	
Dietary Fiber: 2 g	Carbohydrate: 40 g
Fat: 5 g	Protein: 28 g

P

Here's another curry-style chicken dish you can make using ingredients you're likely to have on hand.

TIP

Try using canola oil in this and other recipes calling for vegetable oil. Canola oil is high in monounsaturated fat. It is inexpensive and widely available. And because of its neutral flavor, it is an excellent all-purpose oil for baking, cooking and salad dressings.

DIETITIAN'S MESSAGE

Serve this flavorful chicken dish over basmati rice, a long-grain rice grown in India that is aged before it is husked. Accompany with a cool, creamy Raita Cucumber Salad (see recipe, page 155) and Indian bread such as pappadums or naan, if available. Finish with a serving of fruit, if desired.

Exotic Ginger Cumin Chicken
4 p^{ts}

1 tbsp	vegetable oil, divided	15 mL
2 lb	boneless skinless chicken breasts, cut into bite-size pieces	1 kg
2 tsp	minced garlic	10 mL
½ cup	chopped onion	125 mL
1 tbsp	finely chopped ginger root (*or* ½ tsp/2 mL ground ginger)	15 mL
¼ to ½ tsp	cayenne pepper	1 to 2 mL
1 tsp	each ground coriander and cumin	5 mL
1 tsp	ground turmeric	5 mL
½ cup	chicken stock	125 mL
1	can (19 oz/540 mL) stewed tomatoes	1
2 tbsp	tomato paste	25 mL
2 tsp	granulated sugar	10 mL
½ tsp	salt	2 mL
¾ cup	lower-fat plain yogurt	175 mL
2 tbsp	chopped fresh cilantro (optional)	25 mL

1. In a large saucepan or Dutch oven, heat 2 tsp (10 mL) of the oil over medium high heat. Add half of the chicken and cook for 2 to 3 minutes or until brown. Remove from pan and set aside. Repeat with remaining chicken.

2. Add remaining oil to pan; add garlic, onion and ginger. Reduce heat to medium and cook, stirring constantly, for 4 to 5 minutes or until softened but not brown. Stir in cayenne, coriander, cumin and turmeric; sauté for 1 minute or until fragrant.

3. Stir in stock, tomatoes, tomato paste, sugar and salt; return chicken to pan. Bring to a boil; reduce heat and simmer for 5 minutes or until chicken is no longer pink inside.

4. Stir in yogurt and cilantro, if using; simmer over very low heat for 1 to 2 minutes.

PER SERVING	
Calories: 193	
Dietary Fiber: 1 g	Carbohydrate: 10 g
Fat: 4 g	Protein: 28 g

Tarragon Chicken Stew

4	chicken breasts (about 7 oz/200 g each)	4
1 tbsp	butter	15 mL
¼ cup	all-purpose flour	50 mL
2 cups	chicken broth	500 mL
1 cup	dry white wine	250 mL
2 tsp	crushed dried tarragon	10 mL
1 tsp	grated lemon zest	5 mL
½ tsp	granulated sugar	2 mL
¼ tsp	each salt and black pepper	1 mL
4	medium carrots, cut into 1-inch (2.5 cm) pieces	4
2	large potatoes, peeled and cut into 1-inch (2.5 cm) pieces	2
2	cloves garlic	2
½ lb	mushrooms, sliced	250 g
½ cup	frozen peas	125 mL

1. Remove skin from chicken and trim any fat. In a large skillet, melt butter over medium-high heat; brown chicken for 3 minutes per side. Remove from pan.

2. Dissolve flour in chicken broth; add to skillet along with wine, tarragon, lemon zest, sugar, salt and pepper. Cook, stirring, until boiling. Return chicken to pan along with carrots, potatoes and garlic; cover and simmer for 25 to 30 minutes or until vegetables are tender and chicken is no longer pink inside.

3. Remove chicken from skillet; debone and cut into bite-size pieces. Remove garlic and mash with fork. Add mushrooms and increase heat until sauce boils gently. Return chicken and garlic to pan; add peas and heat through.

PER SERVING
Calories: 374

Dietary Fiber: 6 g	Carbohydrate: 40 g
Fat: 6 g	Protein: 38 g

SERVES 4
....

William King, Chef
Rosemary Duffenais, Dietitian

This quick version of chicken stew has its roots in classic French cooking. It is flavored with tarragon and lemon and skips the heavy cream that is usually used to thicken the sauce.

TIP

If you have fresh tarragon on hand, use 2 whole sprigs instead of the dried and garnish with finely chopped leaves, to taste.

DIETITIAN'S MESSAGE

Enjoy this delicious stew with a slice of pumpernickel bread and a glass of milk.

This is perfect for a family meal or a brunch with a green salad. You can make this casserole ahead, refrigerate and bake before serving, allowing a slightly longer baking time.

TIPS
To reduce the fat in the dish, omit the almonds and increase the cornflakes crumbs by half.

You can use a garlic press to mince garlic, if desired.

DIETITIAN'S MESSAGE
This make-ahead casserole is a great family meal. All of the food groups, with the exception of the Milk Products group, are represented. Add a glass of milk or finish with yogurt to complete the meal.

Almond Chicken Dinner

Preheat oven to 350°F (180°C)
12-cup (3 L) shallow baking dish, greased

1 tsp	vegetable oil	5 mL
1	large onion, chopped	1
1	medium carrot, grated	1
1½ cups	sliced mushrooms	375 mL
1 cup	chopped celery	250 mL
½ cup	chopped red *or* green bell pepper	125 mL
2 tbsp	all-purpose flour	25 mL
1½ cups	1% milk	375 mL
2	cloves garlic, minced	2
½ tsp	each crushed dried thyme and basil	2 mL
¼ tsp	each crushed dried rosemary and salt	1 mL
½ cup	light sour cream	125 mL
2 tbsp	lemon juice	25 mL
1 tsp	Worcestershire sauce	5 mL
3 cups	cubed cooked chicken	750 mL
2 cups	cooked rice	500 mL
1	can (10 oz/284 mL) sliced water chestnuts, drained	1

Topping

1 cup	cornflakes, coarsely crushed	250 mL
½ cup	slivered almonds	125 mL

1. In a skillet, heat oil over medium-high heat; cook onion, carrot, mushrooms, celery and green pepper, stirring, for 5 minutes. Dissolve flour in milk; stir into skillet along with garlic, thyme, basil, rosemary and salt. Cook, stirring, until thickened and bubbling. Remove from heat.

2. Stir in sour cream, lemon juice and Worcestershire sauce. Add remaining ingredients; mix well. Pour into prepared dish.

3. *Topping:* Combine ingredients and sprinkle over casserole. Bake in preheated oven for 35 to 40 minutes or until hot.

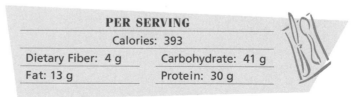

PER SERVING	
Calories: 393	
Dietary Fiber: 4 g	Carbohydrate: 41 g
Fat: 13 g	Protein: 30 g

Baked Chicken and Potato Dinner

Preheat oven to 400°F (200°C)
13- by 9-inch (3 L) baking dish

4	bone-in skinless chicken breasts	4
2	medium unpeeled russet potatoes, cut into 1-inch (2.5 cm) cubes	2
1 cup	green *and/or* red bell peppers, cut into 1-inch (2.5 cm) cubes	250 mL
1	medium onion, cut into 8 pieces	1
2 tbsp	olive oil	25 mL
1 tsp	garlic powder	5 mL
1 tsp	Hungarian paprika	5 mL
¼ cup	grated Parmesan cheese	50 mL

1. Pat chicken breasts dry with paper towel; place 1 breast in each corner of baking dish. Put potatoes, peppers and onion in center of dish. Drizzle olive oil over chicken and vegetables; sprinkle with garlic powder, paprika and cheese.

2. Bake in preheated oven, stirring vegetables once halfway through cooking time, for 40 to 50 minutes or until juices run clear when chicken is pierced with a fork and vegetables are tender.

PER SERVING	
Calories: 387	
Dietary Fiber: 3 g	Carbohydrate: 33 g
Fat: 11 g	Protein: 38 g

SERVES 4   P
....
Gabriella Barna-Adorjan

In this recipe, Gabriella uses Hungarian paprika from the city of Szeged, which is available from Hungarian and fine food delicatessens. If you can't find it, regular paprika will do.

TIPS

Paprika is the mildest member of the pepper family. There are 2 main varieties, Hungarian and Spanish paprika, and both are available in sweet or hot versions.

If you need to feed a crowd, just double this recipe and use 2 baking dishes. For color contrast, use a mixture of red and green bell peppers.

DIETITIAN'S MESSAGE

This recipe has 2 generous servings of vegetables. Serve with Honey-Glazed Carrots (see recipe, page 360) and whole-grain rolls.

P

Here's another kid-friendly dinner that can be made using ingredients you're likely to have on hand. Serve over rice or pasta for a complete meal.

TIP

After preparing uncooked meat and poultry, be sure to clean cutting boards and utensils in hot soapy water and sanitize by rinsing in hot water that has a capful of bleach added to it. Having 2 cutting boards — 1 for raw meat and the other for everything else — helps reduce chances of bacterial contamination.

DIETITIAN'S MESSAGE

Using commercially prepared pasta sauce can increase salt intake, so if this is a concern, make your own (see recipes on pages 179 to 181). Serve this chicken casserole with pasta to complete the food groups.

Baked Chicken Parmesan

Preheat oven to 350°F (180°C)
11- by 7-inch (2 L) baking dish, greased

2 tsp	vegetable oil	10 mL
4	boneless skinless chicken breasts	4
1 cup	diced zucchini	250 mL
½ cup	sliced onions	125 mL
1½ cups	Piquant Tomato Sauce (see recipe, page 180) *or* commercially prepared tomato pasta sauce	375 mL
1 tsp	dried basil *or* dried Italian seasoning	5 mL
1 cup	shredded part-skim mozzarella cheese	250 mL
½ cup	grated Parmesan cheese	125 mL

1. In a large nonstick skillet, heat 1 tsp (5 mL) of the oil over medium-high heat. Add chicken breasts and sear for 1 to 2 minutes per side or until golden brown. Transfer to greased 11- by 7-inch (2 L) baking dish.

2. Heat remaining oil in skillet. Add zucchini and onions; sauté for 3 to 5 minutes or until lightly browned. Remove from pan and place on top of chicken.

3. In a small bowl, blend together Piquant Tomato Sauce and basil; pour over chicken and vegetables. Sprinkle with mozzarella and Parmesan cheese. Bake in preheated oven for 25 to 30 minutes or until juices run clear when chicken is pierced with a fork.

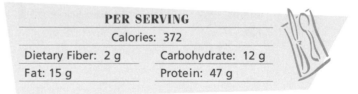

PER SERVING	
Calories: 372	
Dietary Fiber: 2 g	Carbohydrate: 12 g
Fat: 15 g	Protein: 47 g

Slow-Cooked Creole Chicken

Electric slow cooker

2 lb	boneless skinless chicken thighs	1 kg
2 cups	diced green bell peppers	500 mL
½ cup	chopped green onions *or* cooking onions	125 mL
1	can (19 oz/540 mL) stewed tomatoes	1
1	can (5.5 oz/155 g) tomato paste	1
2 tsp	minced garlic	10 mL
1 tsp	hot pepper sauce	5 mL
1	bay leaf	1
2 tsp	dried thyme leaves	10 mL
8 oz	spicy smoked Polish sausage, sliced	250 g

1. Place chicken thighs in bottom of slow cooker. Add peppers, onions, tomatoes, tomato paste, garlic, hot pepper sauce, bay leaf and dried thyme. Cook, covered, on Low heat setting for 4 to 5 hours. Increase heat setting to High; add sausage and cook for 20 to 30 minutes. Remove bay leaf.

PER SERVING	
Calories: 284	
Dietary Fiber: 2 g	Carbohydrate: 12 g
Fat: 14 g	Protein: 27 g

QUICK MICROWAVE RICE
In a large microwave-safe bowl, combine 1½ cups (375 mL) rice and 2½ cups (625 mL) hot water. Cover completely and microwave on Medium-High for 20 minutes. Let stand for 2 to 3 minutes; fluff with a fork and serve. Rice freezes well, so save any leftovers in airtight containers and use as needed.

SERVES 8
....
Enid Witt-Jaques

Children love the succulent chicken and sausage in this recipe — they'll be sure to ask for more.

TIP
If someone in your family prefers a less pronounced tomato flavor in this dish, substitute 1 can (10 oz/ 285 mL) condensed tomato soup for the tomato paste.

DIETITIAN'S MESSAGE
This recipe provides 1 serving of meat and 2 servings of vegetables. Serve with rice and enjoy milk pudding for dessert.

*This simple turkey dish
with fall slaw and
maple-herbed leeks offers
an unusual combination
of fruit and vegetables.*

TIPS

When making this dish,
double — or triple — the
quantity of slaw. The salad
will store well in the
refrigerator for a couple
of days.

To julienne vegetables,
cut them into thin
straw-like strips ⅛ inch
(5 mm) thick.

DIETITIAN'S MESSAGE

This dish offers an
unusual combination of
fruits and vegetables with
a multitude of vitamins
and minerals. Add
steamed rice and a green
vegetable. Make this into
a festive fall meal and
end with Fluffy Pumpkin
Cheesecake (see recipe,
page 409).

Turkey Skewers with Slaw and Leeks

Four 8-inch (20 cm) skewers

Slaw

1 cup	thinly sliced cabbage	250 mL
1	carrot, grated (½ cup/125 mL)	1
½ cup	finely diced red onion	125 mL
½ cup	finely chopped dried apricots	125 mL
½ cup	light sour cream	125 mL
2	small zucchini, finely chopped	2
⅓ cup	coarsely chopped cranberries	75 mL
1	red apple, seeded and diced	1
¼ cup	apple juice	50 mL
¼ tsp	dried herbes de Provence (*or* mixture of thyme, tarragon and marjoram)	2 mL

Leeks

1 cup	julienned leeks (white part only)	250 mL
1 tbsp	maple syrup	15 mL
1½ tsp	red wine *or* cider vinegar	7 mL

Turkey

4	thin turkey cutlets (2 to 3 oz/60 to 90 g each)	4
2 tbsp	all-purpose flour	25 mL
1	egg, beaten	1
⅓ cup	fine dry bread crumbs	75 mL
2 tbsp	finely chopped pecans	25 mL
2 tbsp	olive oil	25 mL
¼ cup	coarsely chopped toasted hazelnuts *or* pecans	50 mL

1. *Slaw:* In a large bowl, mix together cabbage, carrot, onion, apricots, sour cream, zucchini, cranberries, apple, apple juice and herbs; chill.

2. *Leeks:* Mix leeks with maple syrup and vinegar; set aside.

3. *Turkey:* Dip turkey cutlets in flour, then in egg, and finally in bread crumbs mixed with pecans. Weave cutlets onto 8-inch (20 cm) skewers. In a 12-inch (30 cm) nonstick skillet, heat oil over medium heat; cook turkey for 3 to 5 minutes per side or until no longer pink inside.

4. Spoon slaw onto salad plates; top with turkey skewers. Garnish with leeks and hazelnuts.

PER SERVING	
Calories: 437	
Dietary Fiber: 6 g	Carbohydrate: 45 g
Fat: 19 g	Protein: 25 g

Cajun-Style Turkey Cutlet with Citrus

SERVES 6

Dean Mitchell, Chef
Suzanne Journault-Hemstock, Dietitian

2 tbsp	paprika	25 mL
1 tbsp	dried sage	15 mL
1 tsp	black pepper	5 mL
½ tsp	each salt, garlic powder and cayenne pepper	2 mL
6	turkey cutlets (3 oz/90 g each)	6
1 tbsp	vegetable oil	15 mL
1	large orange, peeled and sectioned	1
1	medium grapefruit, peeled and sectioned	1

Turkey cutlets are available fresh and frozen in most supermarkets and are a convenient way of enjoying turkey — without the leftovers!

1. Mix together paprika, sage, pepper, salt, garlic powder and cayenne; place on waxed paper. With meat mallet, pound turkey between 2 pieces of plastic wrap to ⅜-inch (9 mm) thickness. Coat cutlets well with seasoning mixture.

2. In a large skillet, heat oil over high heat; quickly brown turkey on both sides. Reduce heat and add orange and grapefruit; cook until turkey is no longer pink inside.

DIETITIAN'S MESSAGE

In this recipe, spices reduce the need for fat. Serve this quick and easy dinner with a mixture of wild and long-grain rice, Apple-Stuffed Squash (see recipe, page 357) and broccoli florets.

PER SERVING	
Calories: 153	
Dietary Fiber: 2 g	Carbohydrate: 8 g
Fat: 4 g	Protein: 21 g

This nutritious and colorful dish brings together an unusual combination of flavors for a delicious result.

TIPS

Dried herbs are often better than fresh in casseroles and stews because they release their flavor slowly during the cooking process. To store dried herbs, keep them in airtight containers in a cool, dark place away from sunlight. They should stay fresh for up to 12 months.

If desired, substitute 2 cups (500 mL) chicken stock for the water and bouillon cubes in this recipe. Blend the stock with the cornstarch and orange juice.

DIETITIAN'S MESSAGE

Skinless turkey breast used to make cutlets is rich in protein and B vitamins and low in fat. Using orange juice and carrot in the sauce also helps to keep the fat in check in this recipe. Add fiber to the meal by serving over brown rice.

Turkey with Sunshine Sauce

6	turkey *or* chicken cutlets	6
1 cup	buttermilk	250 mL
2 cups	fine dry bread crumbs	500 mL
2 tbsp	grated Parmesan cheese	25 mL
1 tsp	paprika	5 mL
1/2 tsp	salt	2 mL
1/4 tsp	each garlic powder, turmeric and black pepper	1 mL
1/4 tsp	each dried thyme and rosemary	1 mL
2 tbsp	vegetable oil	25 mL

Sunshine Sauce

2	green onions, finely chopped	2
2 tbsp	butter *or* margarine	25 mL
2 cups	water	500 mL
2 tbsp	cornstarch	25 mL
1/4 cup	frozen concentrated orange juice, thawed	50 mL
2	chicken bouillon cubes, crumbled	2
1 cup	finely grated carrot	250 mL
1 tsp	grated orange zest	5 mL
	Salt and black pepper to taste	

1. Dip turkey pieces into buttermilk. Combine bread crumbs, cheese and seasonings. Dip turkey into bread crumb mixture, coating thoroughly on all sides.

2. In a skillet over medium-high heat, brown turkey in hot oil, about 10 minutes per side or until no longer pink inside.

3. *Sunshine Sauce:* In a medium saucepan, cook green onion in butter until tender. Blend water with cornstarch and orange juice. Stir into sauce; cook for about 5 minutes or until smooth and thickened. Add bouillon cubes, carrot and orange peel. Cook over low heat for about 5 minutes (carrot should remain crunchy). Season with salt and pepper. Spoon over cooked turkey and serve.

PER SERVING	
Calories: 444	
Dietary Fiber: 2 g	Carbohydrate: 35 g
Fat: 11 g	Protein: 47 g

Turkey Hazelnut Roll

SERVES 6
....
Denise Giguere

Preheat oven to 350°F (180°C)
Baking pan

½	turkey breast, boned and halved lengthwise	½
1	turkey thigh, boned	1
½ cup	whole hazelnuts	125 mL
½ cup	wheat germ	125 mL
1 tbsp	brandy *or* cognac	15 mL
1	egg, beaten	1
1 tsp	salt	5 mL
1 tsp	dried thyme	5 mL
½ tsp	black pepper	2 mL
	Cranberry sauce	

1. Flatten boned turkey breast pieces by pounding between 2 sheets of heavy plastic wrap. Cut one-third of turkey thigh into ½-inch (1 cm) cubes. Grind remaining two-thirds of turkey thigh to the consistency of minced meat.

2. In a bowl, combine ground turkey with turkey cubes, hazelnuts, wheat germ, brandy, egg and seasonings. Spread mixture over 1 flattened turkey breast and cover with the other to form a sandwich. Sew the edges of the sandwich closed with needle and thread. Roll up; tie with string like a roast. Wrap in aluminum foil (dull side on the outside) to form an airtight seal.

3. Place turkey roll in baking pan containing 1 inch (2.5 cm) of boiling water. Bake, uncovered, in preheated oven for 1½ hours. Slice and serve with cranberry sauce.

PER SERVING	
Calories: 208	
Dietary Fiber: 2 g	Carbohydrate: 7 g
Fat: 10 g	Protein: 23 g

Serve this tasty dish instead of a big bird for an easy-to-manage Thanksgiving or holiday meal.

TIPS

Pounding the boned turkey helps to tenderize the meat and produces a piece of breast that is even and thin enough to work in this recipe. If you don't have a wooden mallet, use a wooden rolling pin or a heavy saucepan.

To obtain firm slices of this roll, cook the night before and refrigerate. The next day, slice the chilled roll and reheat slices in the oven, or microwave at Low heat, making sure they are well covered with either aluminum foil or plastic wrap, depending upon the method used.

DIETITIAN'S MESSAGE

Make this into a festive meal by serving Hawaiian Cranberry Salad (see recipe, page 175) along with an assortment of vegetables for additional vitamins and minerals. Choose a dessert to complement the occasion, such as Fluffy Pumpkin Cheesecake (see recipe, page 409) or Spicy Fruit Compote (see recipe, page 383).

Madeleine Dunbar-Maitland

This recipe combines either ground or slivered poultry with Asian seasonings and vegetables. Add extra teriyaki sauce if a stronger flavor is desired. Serve with cooked rice.

TIPS

If using ground turkey or chicken in this recipe, ensure that the meat is cooked through and no longer pink. Ground meat is considered a high-risk food as bacteria can spread during the grinding process.

If you don't have any sesame seeds in your cupboard, stir ½ tsp (2 mL) sesame oil into the dish just before serving.

DIETITIAN'S MESSAGE

Ground turkey and chicken are lower-fat alternatives to ground beef. This recipe features all the food groups.

Turkiaki Fiesta

2 tsp	vegetable oil	10 mL
1 lb	ground *or* slivered turkey *or* chicken	500 g
2 tbsp	teriyaki sauce	25 mL
Pinch	each salt and black pepper	Pinch
1 cup	diagonally sliced celery	250 mL
¾ cup	chopped green onions	175 mL
1	large red bell pepper, cubed	1
2 cups	snow peas, trimmed	500 mL
1	can (10 oz/284 mL) water chestnuts, drained	1
1 tbsp	sesame seeds (optional)	15 mL

1. In a wok or nonstick skillet, heat oil over high heat. Add turkey and stir-fry for about 4 minutes or until lightly browned and no longer pink inside. Add teriyaki sauce, salt, pepper, celery and onion. Cover and steam for 4 minutes. Add red pepper, snow peas and water chestnuts; cover and cook for 6 minutes, stirring occasionally. Serve sprinkled with sesame seeds, if using.

PER SERVING	
Calories: 175	
Dietary Fiber: 4 g	Carbohydrate: 12 g
Fat: 4 g	Protein: 23 g

Hot 'n' Spicy Turkey Burgers

Preheat barbecue or broiler

Sauce

½ cup	ketchup	125 mL
1 tbsp	vinegar	15 mL
1 tbsp	Worcestershire sauce	15 mL
2	cloves garlic, minced	2
¼ to ½ tsp	crushed red pepper flakes	1 to 2 mL
¼ tsp	hot pepper sauce	1 mL
¼ tsp	black pepper	1 mL

Burgers

1 lb	ground turkey	500 g
⅓ cup	quick-cooking rolled oats	75 mL
4	large hamburger buns, sliced	4

1. *Sauce:* In a small bowl, combine ketchup, vinegar, Worcestershire sauce, garlic, red pepper flakes, hot pepper sauce and pepper. Set aside.

2. *Burgers:* In a large bowl, combine turkey and oats. Add half of the sauce; mix thoroughly. Form into 4 large patties.

3. Barbecue on greased grill or broil 6 inches (15 cm) from heat for 5 to 7 minutes per side. Brush with remaining sauce after burgers have been turned. Place in buns to serve.

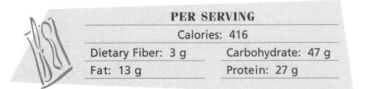

PER SERVING	
Calories: 416	
Dietary Fiber: 3 g	Carbohydrate: 47 g
Fat: 13 g	Protein: 27 g

SERVES 4

Joanne Saunders

These make a nice alternative to the usual beef burgers. When you have time, double or triple this recipe and freeze the extra patties, uncooked, for up to 3 months.

TIP

After brushing uncooked meat with sauce, be sure you don't allow the brush to contact the cooked meat; otherwise, it will become contaminated with harmful bacteria.

DIETITIAN'S MESSAGE

Serve these burgers with the usual burger fixings, including lettuce and tomatoes. Add Sweet Potato "Fries" (see recipe, page 360) to make this a fun meal for the kids. Finish with ice-cream cones, or Icy Yogurt Pops (see recipe, page 67).

P

There's nothing tastier or more comforting than a bubbling pot pie fresh from the oven. It is also an excellent way to use up leftover turkey or chicken.

TIP

If you don't have leftovers, purchase a cooked chicken at your grocery store or roast your own turkey breast. Roast 1 large bone-in turkey breast (2 lb/1 kg) in 350°F (180°C) oven for 70 to 80 minutes or until juices run clear and meat thermometer inserted in center registers 180°F (80°C); immediately transfer to the refrigerator and keep for up to 3 days.

DIETITIAN'S MESSAGE

This recipe features all the food groups and makes a complete meal on its own. Serve fruit for dessert, if desired.

Turkey Pot Pie with Biscuit Topping

Preheat oven to 400°F (200°C)
12-cup (3 L) deep baking dish, greased

3 tbsp	butter, divided	45 mL
2 cups	sliced mushrooms	500 mL
¼ cup	all-purpose flour	50 mL
1 cup	chicken stock	250 mL
2 cups	milk	500 mL
2 tbsp	sherry (optional)	25 mL
½ tsp	each dried thyme, sage and salt	2 mL
3 cups	cubed cooked turkey breast	750 mL
4 cups	frozen mixed vegetables	1 L
	Freshly ground black pepper	

Biscuit Topping

1½ cups	biscuit baking mix	375 mL
1 tsp	dried parsley	5 mL
7 tbsp	milk	105 mL

1. In a saucepan, melt 1 tbsp (15 mL) of the butter over medium heat. Add mushrooms and cook until moisture has evaporated (do not brown). Add remaining butter to pan; add flour and blend. Whisk in stock, milk and, if using, sherry. Stir in thyme, sage and salt; bring to a boil. Reduce heat to low and cook, stirring constantly, until thickened. Remove from heat.

2. Stir in turkey and frozen vegetables. Season with pepper to taste. Spoon into prepared baking dish.

3. *Biscuit Topping:* In a bowl, combine biscuit mix with parsley; stir in 6 tbsp (90 mL) of the milk. Gather dough into a ball, adding more mix as required to make dough easy to handle. On a lightly floured surface, roll out dough to fit top of dish; place over filling. Cut a small vent in center. Brush with remaining 1 tbsp (15 mL) milk.

4. Bake in preheated oven for 35 to 40 minutes or until topping is golden and casserole is bubbling hot.

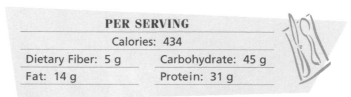

PER SERVING	
Calories: 434	
Dietary Fiber: 5 g	Carbohydrate: 45 g
Fat: 14 g	Protein: 31 g

Cedar-Baked Salmon

Soaked cedar shingles or shims
Preheat oven to 425°F (220°C)
Steamer basket

1½ lb	salmon fillets	750 g
	Grated zest and juice of 1 lime	
1½ cups	diagonally sliced asparagus	375 mL
¼ cup	julienned leek	50 mL
4	thin slices red onion	4
¼ cup	diagonally sliced celery	50 mL
½ cup	thickly sliced shiitake mushrooms	125 mL
2	medium tomatoes, seeded and cut into strips	2
8	fresh basil leaves, slivered	8
1	bag (10 oz/300 g) fresh spinach, trimmed	1
	Salt and black pepper	

1. Place soaked shingles or shims on baking sheet; lightly brush with oil. Remove skin and any bones from salmon; cut into 6 serving-size pieces and place on cedar. Sprinkle with lime zest and juice. Bake in preheated oven for 10 to 15 minutes or until fish flakes easily when tested with fork.

2. Meanwhile, in steamer basket, combine asparagus, leek, onion and celery; steam until partially cooked. Add mushrooms, tomatoes, basil and spinach; steam just until tender-crisp and spinach has wilted. Place on 6 individual plates; season with salt and pepper to taste. Top each with salmon.

PER SERVING	
Calories: 181	
Dietary Fiber: 3 g	Carbohydrate: 7 g
Fat: 7 g	Protein: 23 g

SERVES 6
....
Judson Simpson, Chef
Violaine Sauvé, Dietitian

Cedar shingles and shims, available at lumberyards, impart a unique flavor to salmon when baking. For this recipe, you'll need to soak 2 untreated cedar shingles or 1 package cedar shims in water for at least 2 hours or preferably overnight.

TIPS

Wood or wood chips, such as mesquite or grape vines, are often used in barbecuing to add flavor to foods. Soaking the wood ensures that it is damp enough to produce lots of aromatic smoke.

When soaking shingles or shims, weight them down. Otherwise they will float to the surface.

DIETITIAN'S MESSAGE

Salmon is a source of omega-3 fatty acids. Accompanied by a rice dish such as Simple Risotto (see recipe, page 213) and an array of vegetables, this recipe is a winner.

In this elegant recipe, salmon is smothered with seasoning, green onion and minced garlic, then poached in the oven on spinach leaves. Serve with a medley of fresh vegetables, if desired.

TIP

When buying spinach, look for crisp, unblemished and fresh-smelling leaves. Spinach that has passed its peak has an acrid and unpleasant taste. Spinach that hasn't been prewashed (the kind that comes in a cellophane bag) is very sandy, so wash loose spinach leaves well in a container of tepid water, then rinse thoroughly in a colander before using.

DIETITIAN'S MESSAGE

This delicious dish served with rice makes a wonderful meal. Start with a bowl of Cranberry Beet Soup (see recipe, page 108). End the meal by serving a selection of cheeses.

Smothered Salmon with Spinach

Preheat oven to 325°F (160°C)
13- by 9-inch (3 L) baking dish

12	large spinach leaves	12
2 lb	whole salmon	1 kg
1 tbsp	chopped fresh dill (*or* 1 tsp/5 mL dried dillweed)	15 mL
½ tsp	each salt and black pepper	2 mL
1 cup	cold water	250 mL
1½ tsp	margarine, melted	7 mL
1	bunch green onions, sliced (about ⅔ cup/150 mL)	1
1	clove garlic, minced	1

1. Arrange spinach leaves on bottom of 13- by 9-inch (3.5 L) baking dish. Top with salmon; sprinkle with dill, salt and pepper. Pour water and margarine over salmon. Top with green onions and garlic. Cover tightly with foil.

2. Bake in preheated oven for 25 to 30 minutes or until salmon flakes easily when tested with fork, basting twice. Arrange salmon with spinach on serving platter with pan juices.

PER SERVING	
Calories: 157	
Dietary Fiber: Trace	Carbohydrate: 1 g
Fat: 7 g	Protein: 21 g

Salmon Medallions with Two Purées

SERVES 6
....
John Cordeaux, Chef
Kim Arrey, Dietitian

Cherry Tomato Purée

10	cherry tomatoes	10
1 tbsp	sliced green onion	15 mL
1½ tsp	soy sauce	7 mL
¼ tsp	Worcestershire sauce	1 mL
¼ tsp	salt	1 mL

Beet Purée

¾ cup	chopped cooked beets	175 mL
2 tbsp	water	25 mL
1 tbsp	chopped onion	15 mL
1 tbsp	red wine vinegar	15 mL
¼ tsp	salt	1 mL
1¼ lb	salmon fillets	625 g
	Black pepper	
1 tbsp	vegetable oil	15 mL
	Chopped fresh chives	

1. *Cherry Tomato Purée:* In a food processor or blender, process tomatoes, green onion, soy sauce, Worcestershire sauce and salt until smooth. Pour into a small bowl and chill.

2. *Beet Purée:* In a food processor or blender, process beets, water, onion, vinegar and salt until smooth. Pour into a small bowl and chill.

3. Place salmon in freezer for 30 minutes to aid slicing. Slice diagonally into 6 thin medallions. Sprinkle with pepper to taste. In a skillet, heat oil over medium-high heat; quickly cook salmon, about 1 minute per side.

4. To serve, place salmon on plate; spoon purées around salmon. Garnish with chives.

PER SERVING	
Calories: 174	
Dietary Fiber: 1 g	Carbohydrate: 4 g
Fat: 8 g	Protein: 19 g

At first glance, this recipe may sound complicated but it is actually very easy. The 2 purées — cherry tomato and beet — are easily made in the food processor or blender, then chilled. The slices of salmon are quickly fried in a small amount of oil.

TIP

When puréeing a small quantity of food, such as these 2 sauces, use a hand-held blender for convenience.

DIETITIAN'S MESSAGE

Sauces do not need to be high in fat. These vegetable purées add elegance, color, flavor and nutrients to this dish, but no fat. Enjoy this salmon with rice and a side salad for a special lunch.

*Here is a stylish and
unusual dish that
couldn't be easier to
make. Prepare the tangy
vinaigrette the day
before, then warm it up
while the salmon fillets
are grilling.*

TIPS
Use ½ tsp (2 mL)
chopped fresh thyme
instead of the dried
thyme, if available.

Always preheat the
broiler when broiling
meats or fish. Lightly oil
the broiling rack and
position it 4 to 6 inches
(10 to 15 cm) from
the heat.

For best results, use
salmon fillets that
are about 1 inch
(2.5 cm) thick.

DIETITIAN'S MESSAGE

This vinaigrette adds
fabulous flavor to this
dish but it does boost
the fat content. To
maximize the vinaigrette's
value as a condiment and
keep fat under control,
serve the salmon on a
bed of greens.

Salmon with Cranberry and Caper Vinaigrette

Preheat barbecue or broiler

½ cup	red wine vinegar	125 mL
¼ cup	vegetable oil	50 mL
¼ cup	water	50 mL
¼ cup	sliced cranberries	50 mL
2 tbsp	capers	25 mL
1 tbsp	finely chopped shallots	15 mL
1 tsp	minced fresh *or* dried chives	5 mL
1 tsp	minced garlic	5 mL
½ tsp	pink peppercorns	2 mL
½	each small lemon and lime, peeled and cut into 4 wedges	½
¼ to ½ tsp	cayenne pepper	1 to 2 mL
Pinch	dried thyme	Pinch
6	salmon fillets (4 oz/125 g each), skin on	6

1. In a jar, combine vinegar, oil, water, cranberries, capers, shallots, chives, garlic, pink peppercorns, lemon and lime wedges, cayenne and thyme; shake well and let stand for 6 to 8 hours.

2. Broil or grill salmon fillets over medium-high heat for 3 to 4 minutes per side or until fish flakes easily when tested with fork.

3. Warm vinaigrette on stove or in microwave; remove lemon and lime wedges. Remove skin from salmon. Serve with vinaigrette spooned over fillets.

PER SERVING	
Calories: 237	
Dietary Fiber: Trace	Carbohydrate: 3 g
Fat: 16 g	Protein: 21 g

Barbecued Stuffed Salmon

Preheat barbecue or oven to 450°F (230°C)

1	small onion, finely chopped	1
2	cloves garlic, minced	2
1	stalk celery, finely chopped	1
1 tbsp	butter *or* margarine	15 mL
1	can (4½ oz/128 g) crabmeat, drained	1
1 cup	cooked rice	250 mL
2 tbsp	lemon juice	25 mL
1 tbsp	finely chopped parsley	15 mL
1 tsp	grated lemon zest	5 mL
½ tsp	salt	2 mL
¼ tsp	black pepper	1 mL
2	salmon fillets (1½ lb/750 g)	2
½	lemon, sliced	½

1. In a medium skillet over high heat, cook onion, garlic and celery in butter until softened. Stir in crabmeat, rice, lemon juice, parsley, lemon peel and seasonings.

2. Place stuffing over 1 fish fillet; top with second fillet. Secure with string or toothpicks. Arrange lemon slices on top. Wrap loosely in several thicknesses of aluminum foil.

3. Place on barbecue grill. Cook for about 45 minutes or until fish flakes easily with fork, or bake in preheated oven for 10 minutes per inch (2.5 cm) of thickness.

PER SERVING	
Calories: 238	
Dietary Fiber: Trace	Carbohydrate: 9 g
Fat: 9 g	Protein: 28 g

SERVES 6

Maureen Prairie

This quick and easy-to-make dish is perfect for entertaining. Your guests will be impressed, and you'll be relaxed at serving time.

TIP

To cook fish on the barbecue, put it in a fish cooker or wrap it loosely in foil left open at the top. This way the fish will remain moist yet have that great barbecue flavor.

DIETITIAN'S MESSAGE

Make this recipe the centerpiece of a summer dinner on the deck. Roast an assortment of vegetables on the grill with the salmon. Serve a cold, refreshing bowl of Babsi's Broccoli Soup (see recipe, page 109) while the main course is cooking.

SERVES 2
· ·
Lynn Roblin, Dietitian

Here's a great dish for parents who want to savor a quiet meal together after the children have been fed and put to bed. With or without the kids, it's a perfect meal for 2.

TIP

The tail end of the salmon, which contains the fewest bones, is used in this recipe. However, you can substitute two 4-oz (125 g) salmon fillets, if desired.

DIETITIAN'S MESSAGE

This recipe provides a serving of fish and 3 servings of vegetables. To complete the meal, serve with rice and finish with yogurt.

Salmon with Roasted Vegetables

Preheat oven to 425°F (220°C)
11- by 7-inch (2 L) baking dish

1 tbsp	olive oil	15 mL
2 tsp	minced garlic	10 mL
2 tsp	dried thyme, divided	10 mL
1 cup	diced peeled sweet potatoes	250 mL
1 cup	diced zucchini *or* red bell peppers	250 mL
1 cup	diced peeled parsnips *or* potatoes	250 mL
2 tbsp	lemon juice	25 mL
¼ tsp	black pepper	1 mL
1	salmon tail (8 to 12 oz/ 250 to 375 g), patted dry	1

1. In a small bowl, stir together olive oil, garlic and 1 tsp (5 mL) of the thyme. Place sweet potatoes, zucchini and parsnips in baking dish and sprinkle with oil mixture; toss to coat. Spread out vegetables in a single layer and roast in preheated oven for 15 minutes.

2. In the bowl used for oil mixture, combine remaining thyme, lemon juice and pepper. Brush mixture over salmon tail.

3. Remove vegetables from oven and stir. Place salmon skin side down on top of vegetables. Bake for 10 to 15 minutes or until fish is opaque and flakes easily with a fork. Remove skin from salmon before serving.

PER SERVING	
Calories: 415	
Dietary Fiber: 5 g	Carbohydrate: 34 g
Fat: 20 g	Protein: 25 g

Creamy Salmon Quiche

Preheat oven to 350°F (180°C)
9-inch (23 cm) pie plate, lightly greased

¼ cup	dry whole-wheat bread crumbs	50 mL
1 tbsp	100% bran cereal, crushed	15 mL
1	can (7.5 oz/213 g) salmon	1
¼ cup	chopped green onion	50 mL
¼ cup	cubed light cream cheese	50 mL
1 tbsp	chopped fresh parsley	15 mL
1¼ cups	2% milk	300 mL
3	eggs	3
½ tsp	white pepper	2 mL
	Paprika	

1. Combine bread crumbs and crushed cereal; sprinkle over bottom of prepared pie plate. Break salmon into chunks; arrange chunks over bread crumbs. Top with onion, cream cheese cubes and parsley.

2. Whisk together milk, eggs and pepper. Pour over salmon. Sprinkle lightly with paprika. Bake in preheated oven for 40 minutes or until knife inserted in center comes out clean. Let stand for 5 minutes before cutting into wedges.

PER SERVING	
Calories: 153	
Dietary Fiber: Trace	Carbohydrate: 7 g
Fat: 8 g	Protein: 14 g

Joanne E. Yaraskavitch

This crustless quiche is prepared in a pie plate and cut into wedges. For a more elegant presentation, bake it in small tart tins and serve as an appetizer.

DIETITIAN'S MESSAGE

To add a serving from the Vegetables and Fruit group, serve this nutritious quiche with Chilled Melon Soup with Mango (see recipe, page 96).

Clair Lightfoot, Dietitian

Salmon loaf is a perennial favorite for no-fuss family dinners. Grated carrot and part-skim mozzarella add new interest in this tasty version, which is a great standby to make from pantry ingredients.

DIETITIAN'S MESSAGE

There is something from all the food groups in this recipe, which provides generous amounts of high-quality protein, niacin, vitamin A and calcium. Add some zip with Ginger Linguine (see recipe, page 188) and a green salad.

Cheesy Salmon Loaf

Preheat oven to 350°F (180°C)
9- by 5-inch (2 L) loaf pan, lightly greased

2	eggs	2
1 cup	rolled oats	250 mL
2	cans (each 7.5 oz/213 g) salmon	2
1 cup	shredded part-skim mozzarella cheese	250 mL
¼ cup	chopped onion	50 mL
1	stalk celery, chopped	1
1	large carrot, grated	1
2 tbsp	lemon juice	25 mL

1. In a large bowl, beat eggs. Stir in rolled oats, salmon, cheese, onion, celery, carrot and lemon juice until well combined. Turn salmon mixture into nonstick or lightly greased 9- by 5-inch (2 L) loaf pan. Bake in preheated oven for about 35 minutes. Let stand for 5 minutes before slicing.

PER SERVING	
Calories: 235	
Dietary Fiber: 2 g	Carbohydrate: 12 g
Fat: 10 g	Protein: 23 g

Sole with Fresh Fruit Sauce

SERVES 6 P

Fran J. Maki

1½ lb	sole fillets	750 g
1½ cups	boiling water	375 mL
⅓ cup	finely chopped onion	75 mL
2 tbsp	lemon juice	25 mL
¾ tsp	salt	4 mL
Sauce		
1 cup	orange juice	250 mL
¼ cup	water	50 mL
2 tbsp	cornstarch	25 mL
2 tbsp	liquid honey	25 mL
1 tsp	grated orange zest	5 mL
1 tsp	grated lemon zest	5 mL
1 tsp	Dijon mustard	5 mL
1 cup	fresh orange sections	250 mL
1 cup	seedless green grapes, halved	250 mL
	Fresh mint leaves	

1. Roll fish fillets and secure with toothpicks. Arrange in shallow skillet. Add boiling water, onion, lemon juice and salt. Poach, covered, over low heat for about 8 minutes. To microwave, place fish in casserole; omit water but sprinkle fish with lemon juice and salt. Cover and microwave on High for 5 to 7 minutes or until fish flakes easily when tested with a fork.

2. *Sauce:* Meanwhile, in a small saucepan, combine orange juice, water, cornstarch, honey, orange and lemon zest, and mustard. Cook over low heat, stirring constantly. Add orange sections and green grapes. Spoon sauce over drained fish fillets and garnish with mint leaves.

PER SERVING	
Calories: 161	
Dietary Fiber: 1 g	Carbohydrate: 21 g
Fat: 1 g	Protein: 17 g

Here's an intriguing and stylish recipe that is easy enough for a weeknight meal.

TIPS

Replace the sole fillets with halibut, haddock or turbot, if desired.

Add the grapes just before serving — otherwise the color will disappear and you won't notice them in the sauce.

DIETITIAN'S MESSAGE

This lower-fat fish recipe needs only rice and a colorful vegetable to complete your plate. End the meal with frozen yogurt sprinkled with fresh berries.

Steven Watson, Chef
Jane McDonald,
Dietitian

*Nothing could be easier
than this citrus-flavored
fish dish, which is ready
in less than 15 minutes.
Use snapper, sole or any
firm white fish if halibut
isn't available.*

TIP

You can use frozen fish
for this recipe, if desired.
To cook from its frozen
state, double the cooking
time to 20 minutes per
inch (2.5 cm) of thickness,
measuring the fish from
its thickest point.

DIETITIAN'S MESSAGE

Halibut is a flavorful fish.
The citrus juices add both
flavor and a nutritional
punch. Serve with rice,
Italian Broiled Tomatoes
(see recipe, page 349)
and a spinach salad to
add color. Feature all the
food groups by adding
Orange Crème Caramel
(see recipe, page 423).

South Side Halibut

Preheat oven to 400°F (200°C)
Baking dish

1	clove garlic, minced	1
⅓ cup	finely chopped onion	75 mL
1 tsp	vegetable oil	5 mL
2 tbsp	chopped fresh parsley	25 mL
½ tsp	grated orange zest	2 mL
⅛ tsp	black pepper	0.5 mL
¼ cup	orange juice	50 mL
1 tbsp	lemon juice	15 mL
4	halibut steaks (4 oz/125 g each)	4
	or 1 lb (500 g) halibut	
	or Pacific snapper fillets	

1. In a small skillet, sauté garlic and onion in oil over medium heat until tender. Remove from heat; stir in parsley, orange zest and pepper. Combine orange juice and lemon juice.

2. Arrange fish in baking dish. Spread onion mixture over fish; pour juice over top. Cover tightly with foil. Bake in preheated oven for 8 to 10 minutes or until fish flakes easily when tested with fork.

PER SERVING	
Calories: 149	
Dietary Fiber: Trace	Carbohydrate: 4 g
Fat: 4 g	Protein: 24 g

Rosemary Smoked Halibut with Balsamic Vinaigrette

Preheat oven to 425°F (220°C)
Baking dish

| 2 *or* 3 | sprigs fresh rosemary | 2 *or* 3 |
| 1½ lb | halibut fillets | 750 g |

Balsamic Vinaigrette

¼ cup	olive oil	50 mL
2 tbsp	balsamic vinegar	25 mL
¼ tsp	coarsely crushed black pepper	1 mL
⅛ tsp	salt	0.5 mL
½ cup	diced seeded tomato	125 mL
1 tsp	finely chopped shallot	5 mL

1. In a baking dish, place rosemary beside halibut; light rosemary with match (rosemary may not remain lit). Cover tightly with foil. Bake in preheated oven for 8 to 12 minutes or until fish flakes easily when tested with fork.

2. *Balsamic Vinaigrette:* Meanwhile, in a small bowl, whisk together oil, balsamic vinegar, pepper and salt; stir in tomato and shallot. Serve with halibut.

PER SERVING	
Calories: 208	
Dietary Fiber: Trace	Carbohydrate: 1 g
Fat: 12 g	Protein: 24 g

SERVES 6
....
Pamela Good, Chef
Carrie Roach, Dietitian

It's hard to believe this impressive-sounding recipe is so easy to make. Just lighting the sprigs of rosemary gives the fish a tantalizing herb flavor and aroma.

TIP

Rosemary is an aromatic herb, native to the Mediterranean. In this recipe, it is used almost like wood to add flavor to barbecued food.

DIETITIAN'S MESSAGE

The flavor and aroma of this simple dish is enhanced by using the rosemary. You can control the amount of fat by limiting the amount of vinaigrette you use.

Kris Bauchman, Chef
Elizabeth McLelan,
Dietitian

In this recipe, a tangy, fat-free marinade adds zest to swordfish, which is particularly well suited to grilling as its flesh is very dense. Since you don't need to worry about tenderizing fish, the marinating time is short.

TIP

Use a fish basket or grill, which has narrow spaces, to prevent the fish from falling through the grill onto the barbecue.

VARIATION

Grilled Halibut: Substitute halibut steaks for the swordfish.

DIETITIAN'S MESSAGE

As fish is very tender, unlike many meats, it is marinated to add flavor. Experiment with different marinades to vary the taste of this fish. For a simple meal, serve with baked potatoes and a tossed green salad.

Grilled Swordfish

1½ lb	swordfish steaks	750 g
⅓ cup	minced onion	75 mL
2 tbsp	white wine vinegar	25 mL
1 tbsp	liquid honey	15 mL
Pinch	white pepper	Pinch
	Lime wedges	

1. Cut swordfish into 6 pieces; place in plastic bag. Combine onion, vinegar, honey and pepper; pour over fish. Seal bag and marinate, refrigerated, for 30 minutes, rotating bag occasionally.

2. Remove steaks from marinade. Grill on greased grill or broil for 3 to 5 minutes per side or until fish flakes easily when tested with fork. Garnish with lime wedges.

PER SERVING	
Calories: 132	
Dietary Fiber: Trace	Carbohydrate: 2 g
Fat: 3 g	Protein: 24 g

Swordfish with Gazpacho

2 tbsp	olive oil	25 mL
2	cloves garlic, minced	2
4	swordfish *or* shark steaks (4 oz/125 g each)	4
1	small onion, chopped	1
3	tomatoes, peeled and chopped (about 2 cups/500 mL)	3
1 cup	chopped seeded peeled cucumber	250 mL
2	green onions, sliced	2
2 tbsp	lemon juice	25 mL
2 tsp	dried basil (*or* 2 tbsp/25 mL chopped fresh)	10 mL
½ tsp	ground cumin	2 mL
Pinch	each dried thyme and black pepper	Pinch

1. In a large skillet, heat oil over medium-high heat; cook garlic, stirring, for a few seconds. Add fish; lightly brown on both sides. Add onion; cook for 1 to 2 minutes.

2. Add tomatoes, cucumber, green onions, lemon juice, basil, cumin, thyme and pepper. Reduce heat and simmer until fish flakes easily when tested with fork, about 5 minutes.

PER SERVING

Calories: 219

Dietary Fiber: 2 g	Carbohydrate: 8 g
Fat: 11 g	Protein: 22 g

SERVES 4

Ronald Davis, Chef
Debra McNair, Dietitian

This recipe works well with both swordfish and shark, which are available at many seafood counters or fish shops. Gazpacho, a cold soup made with tomatoes, is given a twist as a warm topping for the fish.

TIPS

Substitute drained canned tomatoes if ripe fresh tomatoes are not available.

There are many different varieties of basil, a leafy herb known for its heady aroma. Basil goes so well with tomatoes, which is how it is used in this recipe, that it is often referred to as "the tomato herb."

DIETITIAN'S MESSAGE

Using gazpacho as a sauce is an innovative way to add vegetables to this dish. To make this dish the centerpiece of a special dinner with a Mediterranean theme, begin with Eggplant Tapas (see recipe, page 83). Serve the fish with Simple Risotto (see recipe, page 213) and steamed green beans. End the meal with Light Tiramisu (see recipe, page 422).

Alfred Fan, Chef
Leah Hawirko, Dietitian

Although it sounds quite exotic, this is a quick and easy dish with a tropical flavor that can be made from readily available ingredients if papaya and mahi mahi aren't available.

TIP

Substitute sea bass or halibut if mahi mahi is not available. If papaya is not in season, use fresh or canned pineapple or mango instead.

DIETITIAN'S MESSAGE

Try different types of fish in this recipe. The colorful, festive relish adds vitamin A. It can be made ahead of time and refrigerated until ready to serve.

Pan-Seared Mahi Mahi with Papaya Mint Relish

Papa Mint Relish

1½ cups	diced peeled papaya (1 large)	375 mL
⅓ cup	finely diced shallots *or* green onions	75 mL
3 tbsp	finely chopped fresh mint	45 mL
2 tbsp	lime juice	25 mL
Pinch	each salt, black pepper and granulated sugar	Pinch

Fish

2 tbsp	all-purpose flour	25 mL
Pinch	each salt and black pepper	Pinch
4	mahi mahi fillets (30 oz/90 g each)	4
1 tbsp	extra-virgin olive oil	15 mL

1. *Papaya Mint Relish:* In a small bowl, mix papaya, shallots, mint, lime juice, salt, pepper and sugar; set aside.

2. *Fish:* Mix together flour, salt and pepper; dip fish fillets into flour to coat both sides. In a nonstick pan, heat oil over medium-high heat; cook fish for 1½ to 3 minutes per side or until fish flakes easily when tested with fork. Serve topped with Papaya Mint Relish.

PER SERVING	
Calories: 149	
Dietary Fiber: 1 g	Carbohydrate: 11 g
Fat: 4 g	Protein: 17 g

Crunchy Fish Burgers

Preheat oven to 375°F (190°C)
Baking sheet, greased

Crunchy Coating

1 cup	crushed cornflakes	250 mL
½ tsp	garlic powder	2 mL
½ tsp	dry mustard	2 mL
¼ tsp	black pepper	1 mL

Burgers

1	egg	1
1 tbsp	water	15 mL
1 lb	fresh *or* frozen fish fillets (sole, perch *or* halibut), patted dry	500 g

Zippy Tartar Sauce

¼ cup	sweet pickle *or* dill pickle relish	50 mL
2 tbsp	light mayonnaise	25 mL
¼ tsp	horseradish	1 mL
4	6-inch (15 cm) submarine-type buns, halved	4
4	lettuce leaves	4
2	medium tomatoes, sliced	2

1. *Crunchy Coating:* In a heavy plastic bag, combine crumbs, garlic powder, mustard and pepper.
2. *Burgers:* In a shallow bowl, lightly beat together egg and water; set aside. Dip fish fillets in egg mixture and transfer, 1 piece at a time, to plastic bag; shake gently to coat. Place on baking sheet. Bake in preheated oven for 10 to 15 minutes or until fish is opaque and flakes easily when tested with fork.
3. *Zippy Tartar Sauce:* In a small bowl, blend together relish, mayonnaise and horseradish.
4. *Assembly:* Spread buns with tartar sauce; add fish fillets and top with lettuce and tomato.

PER SERVING	
Calories: 503	
Dietary Fiber: 3 g	Carbohydrate: 72 g
Fat: 9 g	Protein: 32 g

SERVES 4

Diana Stenlund-Moffat, Dietitian

These are fairly substantial burgers, so serve them with something light. For young children, half a burger will probably be enough.

TIP
Dipping the fish in an egg mixture before covering with the coating helps the crumb mixture to stick.

VARIATION
Crunchy Fried Chicken: Substitute 3 lb (1.5 kg) boneless skinless chicken for the fish. Prepare coating as for fish fillets, but bake in preheated oven for 20 to 25 minutes or until chicken is no longer pink inside.

DIETITIAN'S MESSAGE

The deep-fried fish sandwiches or burgers typically served at fast food restaurants are loaded with fat — some have more than twice that of a cheeseburger! With these fish burgers, however, the fat content is about the same as that of a plain hamburger.

In this recipe, fish is marinated with lemon and wine, then topped after baking with a tomato sauce made with yogurt.

TIPS

When using bay leaves in cooking, keep them whole or break into large pieces so that they can be easily removed before serving.

If desired, use fresh tarragon and chervil in this recipe. Double or triple the quantity, depending on your taste, and add some finely chopped leaves as a garnish.

Chervil, a herb often used in French cuisine, resembles parsley with a licorice taste. If you don't have chervil in your cupboard, add 2 tbsp (25 mL) fresh parsley to the sauce.

DIETITIAN'S MESSAGE

In this recipe, yogurt provides a creamy base for the tomato sauce without adding a lot of fat.

Poached Fish Jardinière

Preheat oven to 425°F (220°C)

1	small onion, chopped	1
6 to 8	bay leaves	6 to 8
6 to 8	portions (4 oz/125 g each) fresh *or* frozen halibut *or* haddock	6 to 8
6 to 8	thin slices lemon	6 to 8
1 cup	dry white wine	250 mL
½ cup	water	125 mL
Sauce		
4	large tomatoes, chopped	4
2	cloves garlic, minced	2
¼ cup	plain yogurt	50 mL
2 tbsp	olive oil	25 mL
2 tbsp	chopped fresh parsley	25 mL
1 tbsp	Dijon mustard	15 mL
2 tsp	each dried chervil and tarragon	10 mL
1 tsp	Worcestershire sauce	5 mL
¼ tsp	salt	1 mL
	Black pepper	

1. Spread onion on bottom of a large shallow baking dish. Place bay leaves in dish; top each with piece of fish and lemon slice. Pour wine and water over top. Cover and chill for at least 1 hour.

2. *Sauce:* In a saucepan, combine tomatoes, garlic, yogurt, oil, parsley, mustard, chervil, tarragon, Worcestershire sauce, salt, and pepper to taste; cook over low heat for 10 to 15 minutes to blend flavors. (Do not boil.)

3. Bake fish in preheated oven for 10 to 15 minutes or until fish flakes easily when tested with fork. Remove fish from liquid and arrange on plates, adding some liquid to sauce for desired consistency if necessary. Pour sauce over fish.

PER SERVING	
Calories: 204	
Dietary Fiber: 2 g	Carbohydrate: 7 g
Fat: 8 g	Protein: 26 g

Hot 'n' Spicy Turkey Burgers (page 303) ➤
Overleaf: Grilled Lamb and Vegetables with Roasted Garlic (page 265)

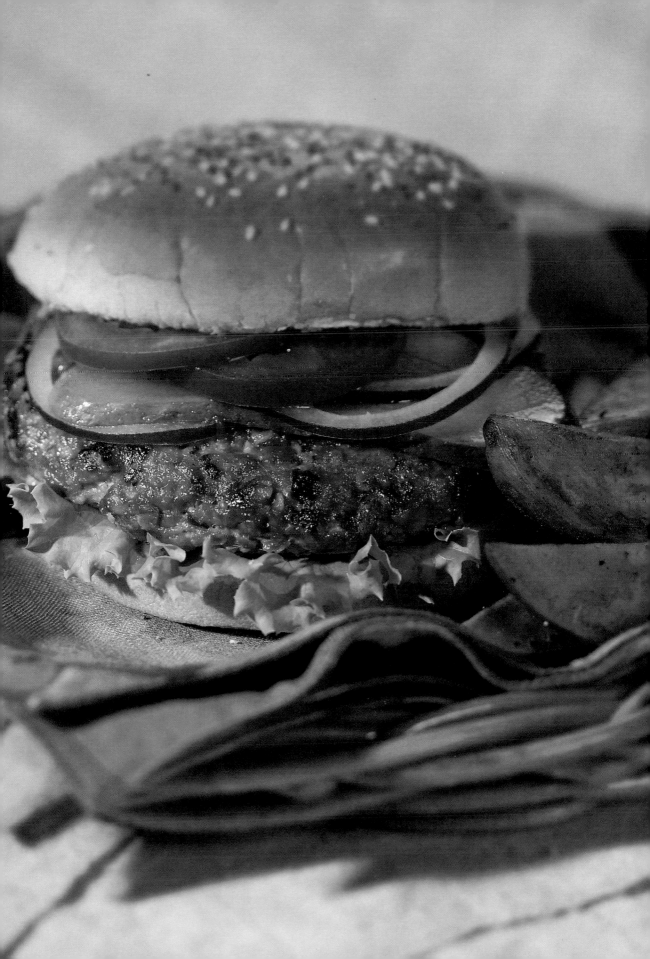

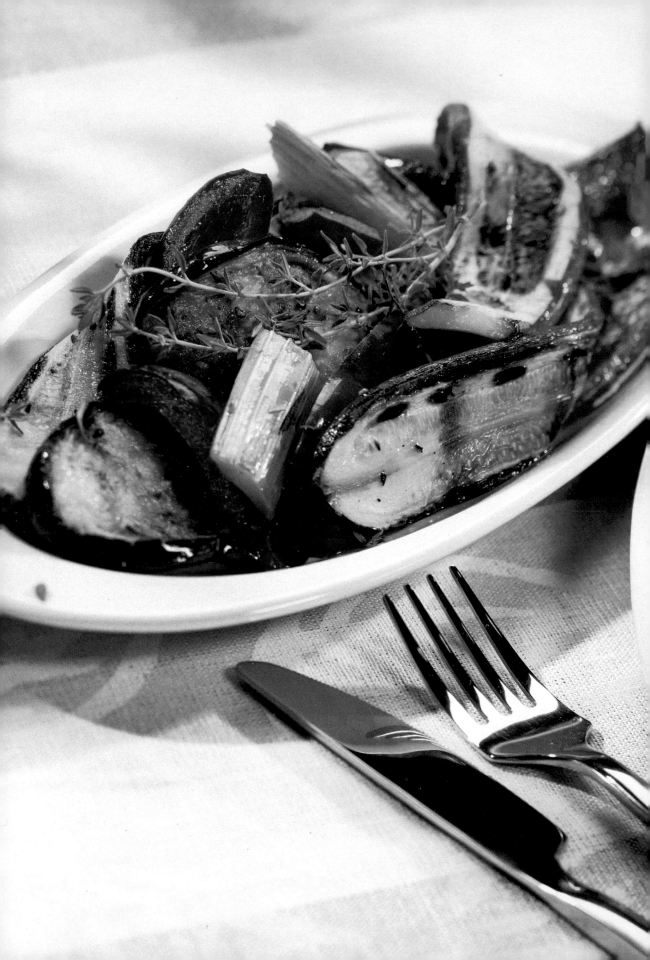

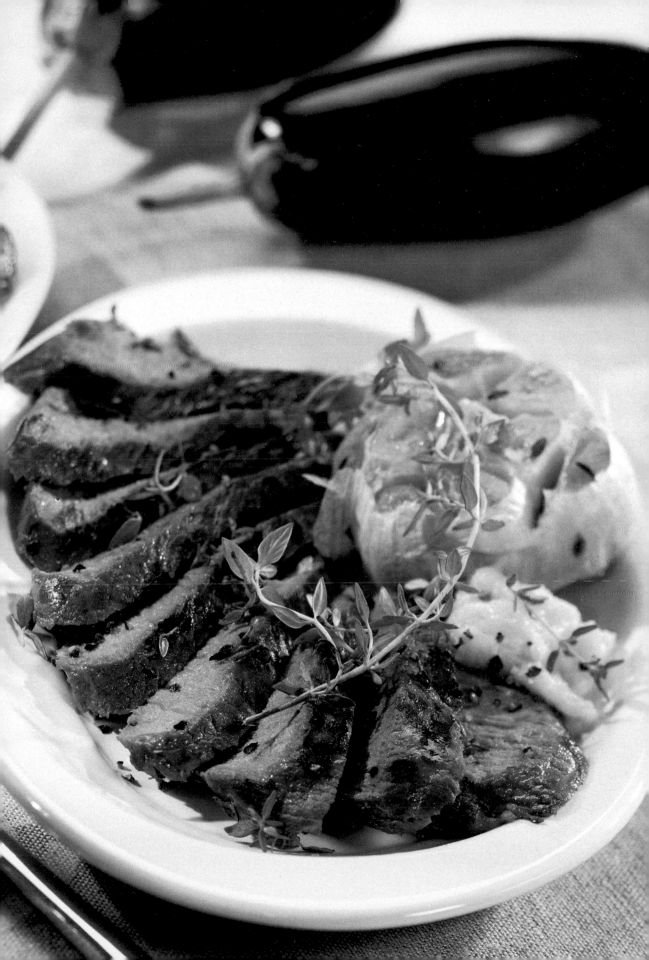

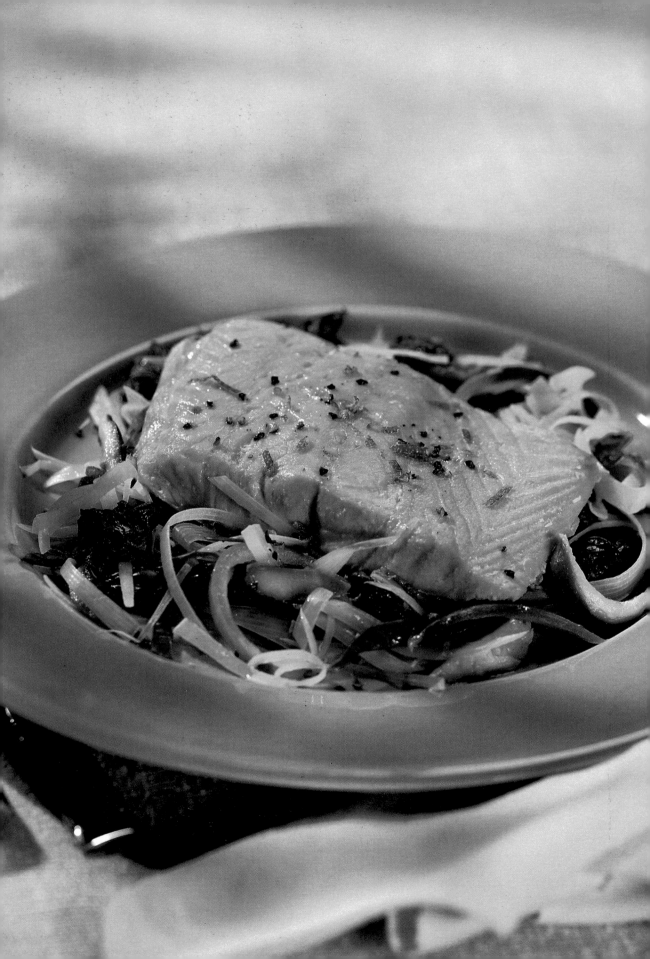

Oriental Fish Fillets

SERVES 4
....
Joanne Rankin, Dietitian

4	green onions, diagonally sliced	4
2	cloves garlic, minced	2
1 tbsp	canola oil	15 mL
4	fish fillets (turbot, cod, haddock *or* halibut)	4
1 tbsp	finely chopped ginger root	15 mL
½ cup	dry sherry	125 mL
2 tbsp	soy sauce	25 mL
¼ cup	coarsely chopped fresh cilantro	50 mL

1. In a heavy skillet over high heat, cook green onions and garlic in hot oil for about 2 minutes. Remove onion mixture and add fish to skillet.

2. Combine onion mixture, ginger root, sherry and soy sauce; pour over fish. Sprinkle with cilantro. Cook, covered, over medium heat for about 5 minutes or until fish flakes easily when tested with fork. Transfer fillets to preheated platter. Cook sauce over high heat until reduced and slightly thickened. Pour sauce over fish and serve.

PER SERVING	
Calories: 214	
Dietary Fiber: Trace	Carbohydrate: 5 g
Fat: 10 g	Protein: 25 g

In this recipe, the oriental flavors of ginger root, soy sauce and cilantro give ordinary fish fillets a new lease on life.

TIP

Don't confuse cilantro with parsley. They look similar but they are different. Cilantro is the parsley-like leaf on the coriander plant. Cilantro leaves are more tender than parsley and have a zesty, almost bitter, flavor that lingers on the tongue.

DIETITIAN'S MESSAGE

To continue the oriental theme, serve this tasty fish with plain rice. Add some crisp stir-fried vegetables for added vitamins as well as fiber.

≺ Cedar-Baked Salmon (page 305)   *Main Meals*

In combination with onions and mushrooms, spinach makes a tasty filling for fish.

TIP

If you prefer, use frozen chopped spinach to replace fresh in this recipe. Just thaw 1 pkg (10 oz/300 g), drain well and squeeze dry. Use half in this recipe and save the remainder for another use.

DIETITIAN'S MESSAGE

This recipe is a real winner in the lower-fat category. Complement the delicate blend of sole, spinach and mushrooms with a rice dish and baby carrots to add color and vitamin A.

Fish Roll-Ups

Preheat oven to 425°F (220°C)
Baking pan, lightly greased

½	pkg (10 oz/300 g) fresh spinach	½
1	small onion, chopped	1
1 tbsp	butter *or* margarine	15 mL
1 cup	chopped mushrooms	250 mL
¼ cup	whole-wheat bread crumbs	50 mL
1 lb	sole fillets	500 g
	Salt, black pepper and dried thyme to taste	
½	lemon	½
	Paprika	

1. Steam spinach until tender; drain well. In a small skillet over medium-high heat, cook onion in butter for about 5 minutes or until browned. Add mushrooms; cook for 3 minutes. In a food processor, combine spinach, mushroom mixture and bread crumbs. Process using on/off motion until coarsely chopped.

2. Season fish fillets with salt, pepper and thyme. (If fish fillets are too wide, cut in half down center.) Spoon spinach filling over each fillet; roll up and secure with toothpicks. Place fish seam side down in nonstick or lightly greased baking pan. Squeeze lemon over fish; sprinkle with paprika. Bake, uncovered, in preheated oven for 10 minutes per inch (2.5 cm) of thickness or until fish flakes easily with fork. Remove toothpicks and serve.

PER SERVING	
Calories: 144	
Dietary Fiber: 1 g	Carbohydrate: 8 g
Fat: 4 g	Protein: 19 g

Fish Fillets with Basil Walnut Sauce

SERVES 6

Betty Jane Humphrey

This easily prepared sauce, which is similar to pesto, is absolutely delicious.

Preheat broiler
Broiler or roasting pan

½ cup	fresh parsley, snipped and loosely packed	125 mL
½ cup	fresh basil, snipped and loosely packed	125 mL
3 tbsp	finely chopped walnuts	45 mL
2 tbsp	chicken broth	25 mL
2 tbsp	grated Parmesan cheese	25 mL
1 tbsp	olive oil	15 mL
1 tbsp	balsamic vinegar *or* malt vinegar	15 mL
1 tsp	granulated sugar	5 mL
1	clove garlic, minced	1
½ tsp	freshly ground black pepper	2 mL
1½ lb	fish fillets (cod, haddock *or* halibut), 1 inch (2.5 cm) thick	750 g
¼ cup	dry white wine	50 mL
½	lemon	½
1 tbsp	butter *or* margarine	15 mL
	Salt and black pepper to taste	

1. In a food processor or blender, combine parsley, basil, walnuts, chicken broth, cheese, oil, vinegar, sugar, garlic and pepper. Process until smooth; add more broth if thinner sauce is desired.

2. Arrange fish in broiler or roasting pan. Pour wine into pan; squeeze lemon juice over fish. Dot with butter; sprinkle with salt and pepper. Broil for 5 minutes. Spoon sauce over top and broil for another 4 to 5 minutes, allowing total of 10 minutes per inch (2.5 cm) of thickness, or until fish flakes easily with fork.

TIPS

This sauce, like pesto, is quite thick but it can be thinned with chicken broth, if desired.

Many people dislike walnuts because they think they have a bitter, acrid taste. In fact, fresh walnuts are quite sweet. The problem is that by the time they reach consumers, many walnuts have passed their peak. Walnuts, like all nuts, contain a high proportion of fat, which goes rancid quickly. Always buy walnuts from a natural foods store or a shop with high turnover, and taste before buying. Store walnuts in the refrigerator or, if you don't intend to use them in the near future, keep them in the freezer.

DIETITIAN'S MESSAGE

Brown rice will complement the lively sauce of fresh herbs, cheese and walnuts in this dish. It will also add a touch of fiber.

PER SERVING	
Calories: 200	
Dietary Fiber: Trace	Carbohydrate: 3 g
Fat: 9 g	Protein: 25 g

This elegant entrée is a great dish for entertaining.

TIPS

For convenience and speed, this recipe uses frozen fish fillets, but fresh fish may also be used. If you prefer a thicker fish fillet such as salmon or halibut, increase the cooking time by about 5 minutes.

If available, substitute 1 to 2 tbsp (15 to 25 mL) chopped fresh basil for the dried basil.

Remember to use dry bread crumbs in this recipe; fresh bread crumbs will make the dish too soggy.

DIETITIAN'S MESSAGE

Light-colored fish, such as haddock, halibut, sole and cod, tend to be lower in fat than darker-colored fish, such as salmon, tuna, mackerel and rainbow trout. Sautéed Spinach with Pine Nuts (see recipe, page 355) and boiled new potatoes would be great accompaniments to this dish. End the meal with a fruit dessert.

Parmesan Herb Baked Fish Fillets

Preheat oven to 400°F (200°C)
11- by 7-inch (2 L) baking dish, greased

1	pkg (1 lb/500 g) frozen fish fillets, thawed and patted dry	1
¼ cup	light mayonnaise	50 mL
¼ cup	grated Parmesan cheese	50 mL
2 tbsp	chopped green onions	25 mL
1 tbsp	chopped pimiento *or* red bell pepper	15 mL
	Cayenne pepper to taste	
½ cup	dry bread crumbs	125 mL
½ tsp	dried basil	2 mL
	Black pepper to taste	

1. Place fish fillets in a single layer in bottom of greased 11- by 7-inch (2 L) baking dish. Set aside.

2. In a small bowl, stir together mayonnaise, Parmesan cheese, onions, pimiento and cayenne. Spread mixture evenly over fish fillets.

3. In a separate bowl, combine bread crumbs, basil, and pepper; sprinkle over top of fish. Bake in preheated oven for 10 to 12 minutes or until fish is opaque and flakes easily with fork.

PER SERVING	
Calories: 216	
Dietary Fiber: Trace	Carbohydrate: 12 g
Fat: 8 g	Protein: 23 g

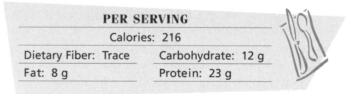

Quick Steamed Fish Fillets with Potatoes and Asparagus

SERVES 2
....
N. Schnedier

This elegant supper for 2 is simplicity itself. The entire meal is prepared in a steamer and ready in 15 minutes.

Steaming basket

1 cup	small new red potatoes, quartered	250 mL
1 cup	asparagus, cut into 1-inch (2.5 cm) pieces	250 mL
2	4-oz (125 g) fish fillets, about 1 inch (2.5 cm) thick	2
⅓ cup	julienned tomatoes (preferably roma)	75 mL
¼ to ½ tsp	dried basil *or* tarragon	1 to 2 mL
	Black pepper to taste	
1 tsp	butter	5 mL
1 tsp	lemon juice	5 mL
	Salt	

TIP

If available, substitute 1 to 2 tsp (5 to 10 mL) of your favorite fresh herbs for the dried herbs. If asparagus is out of season, use fresh green beans instead.

DIETITIAN'S MESSAGE

Steaming is a fast, efficient and low-fat way to prepare fish. It's also a great way to cook vegetables so that they stay crisp and retain their color, vitamins and minerals.

1. Salt potatoes in a large steamer set over a pot of boiling water. Cover and steam for 8 to 10 minutes or until potatoes are beginning to soften but are not yet cooked.

2. Place asparagus on top of potatoes. Place fish fillets on top of asparagus. Top with tomatoes; sprinkle with basil, and pepper. Cover and steam for 5 to 6 minutes or until fish is opaque and flakes easily when tested with fork. Dot with butter; cover and steam for 30 seconds or until butter is melted. Sprinkle with lemon juice. Season to taste with salt.

PER SERVING	
Calories: 183	
Dietary Fiber: 2 g	Carbohydrate: 14 g
Fat: 3 g	Protein: 25 g

This is a lower-fat version of fondue that uses chicken broth rather than oil to cook the seafood, tofu and vegetables. After these items have been eaten, cabbage and green onions can be added to the delicious broth that remains and the resulting mélange can be served as a soup course.

TIP
Try using extra-firm tofu in this recipe, if available. When buying tofu, read the labels carefully and look for added calcium.

DIETITIAN'S MESSAGE
This fondue is a meal on its own. It contributes ample protein from the tofu and seafood and a variety of vitamins and minerals from the vegetables. For a fun ending, serve Strawberry Apple Salsa with Cinnamon Crisps (see recipe, page 68).

Oriental Seafood Fondue

Fondue pot and forks

2½ cups	chicken broth	625 mL
¼ cup	chopped fresh cilantro	50 mL
1 tbsp	chopped ginger root	15 mL
1	small clove garlic, minced	1
¼ tsp	cayenne pepper	1 mL
1 lb	seafood (scallops, shrimp, lobster tails, cut into bite-size pieces)	500 g
12	small whole mushrooms	12
½ lb	firm tofu, drained and cut into bite-size pieces	250 g
6	green onions, cut into 2-inch (5 cm) pieces	6
2 cups	spinach leaves, trimmed	500 mL
	Cooked white rice (approx. 3 cups/750 mL)	
	Asian sweet-and-sour *or* plum sauce (available in most grocery stores)	
1 cup	finely grated cabbage	250 mL

1. In a fondue pot, bring chicken broth, cilantro, ginger, garlic and cayenne pepper to a boil.

2. Arrange seafood, mushrooms, tofu, white part of onions and spinach on large platter. Using fondue fork, dip pieces of seafood, tofu and vegetables into hot broth, cooking to desired doneness. Serve with rice and dipping sauces.

3. When all seafood and vegetables have been cooked, add cabbage and green part of onion to broth; cook for several minutes. Serve soup in individual bowls.

PER SERVING	
Calories: 113	
Dietary Fiber: 1 g	Carbohydrate: 5 g
Fat: 4 g	Protein: 16 g

Paella Valencia

SERVES 6
....

Kris Bauchman, Chef
Elizabeth McLelan,
Dietitian

Preheat oven to 350°F (180°C)
4-quart (4 L) ovenproof saucepan

12	clams	12
12	mussels	12
2 tbsp	olive oil	25 mL
6	chicken drumsticks, skinned (about 1¼ lb/625 g)	6
½ cup	diced onion	125 mL
2	cloves garlic, minced	2
1½ cups	diced mixed bell peppers (yellow, red *or* green)	375 mL
2	medium jalapeño peppers, seeded and diced	2
1½ cups	sliced mushrooms	375 mL
2 cups	long-grain rice	500 mL
¼ tsp	crushed saffron	1 mL
3 cups	chicken broth	750 mL
6 to 12	large shrimp, peeled and deveined (4 oz/125 g)	6 to 12
1½ cups	frozen peas	375 mL

1. Scrub clams and mussels; remove beards from mussels. Discard any open mussels.

2. In 4-quart (4 L) ovenproof saucepan, heat 1 tbsp (15 mL) of the oil over medium heat; brown chicken on both sides and remove. Add remaining oil; cook onion and garlic, stirring, for 2 to 3 minutes or until golden. Add bell and jalapeño peppers; cook, stirring, until softened. Add mushrooms; cook, stirring, for 1 to 2 minutes. Stir in rice and saffron; cook, stirring, for 2 to 3 minutes. Add chicken broth; bring to a boil. Return chicken to saucepan; cover and bake in preheated oven for 8 minutes.

3. Add clams; bake, covered, for 5 minutes. Nestle mussels and shrimp in rice; cook, covered, for 6 to 8 minutes or until shrimp are pink, mussels and clams open and rice is tender. Discard any mussels or clams that haven't opened. Stir in peas; let stand for 1 to 2 minutes.

PER SERVING	
Calories: 462	
Dietary Fiber: 3 g	Carbohydrate: 59 g
Fat: 9 g	Protein: 33 g

Paella is a Spanish dish made with rice and just about anything else the cook has on hand. It usually contains chicken, seafood and often pork, and the rice is highly seasoned with saffron and other spices.

TIPS

If desired, replace the saffron with less expensive turmeric. The dish will be appropriately colored but missing the saffron's pleasant bitter taste.

If clams are not available, use extra mussels and/or shrimp. Or use 4 oz (125 g) pork tenderloin, cut into 1-inch (2.5 cm) cubes. Brown and add to the casserole with the chicken.

DIETITIAN'S MESSAGE

Well-made paella is a genuine treat. It is also a great dish to include in your repertoire as part of a program of healthy eating. This winning combination of vegetables, rice, chicken and seafood, followed by Lemon Mousse (see recipe, page 388), translates into a tasty meal. The simple step of skinning the chicken helps to reduce the fat.

David Nicolson, Chef
Leslie Maze, Dietitian

This is a delicious lower-fat variation of the traditional veal or beef paupiette, which is fried or braised in wine. The lemon and orange create a bittersweet flavor that is subtly accented with fresh dill.

TIP

Dill is a herb that goes particularly well with fish. Fresh dill loses its aroma when cooked, so it is best added to recipes at the last minute, just before serving. To help to preserve the flavor, snip dill leaves with sharp scissors rather than chop them.

DIETITIAN'S MESSAGE

You don't need rich sauces to add flavor to dishes. In this recipe, the citrus and the herbs work just as well as a traditional cream sauce.

Sole and Shrimp Paupiettes

1	medium orange	1
1	lemon	1
4	sole fillets (about 8 oz/250 g total)	4
	Salt and black pepper	
8	large shrimp, peeled and deveined	8
½ cup	dry white wine	125 mL
1 cup	hot cooked rice	250 mL
2 tbsp	chopped fresh dill	25 mL
1 tbsp	butter	15 mL

1. With sharp knife, peel orange and lemon, removing all pith. Cut into segments between the membranes, discarding any seeds. Coarsely chop and set aside.

2. Season sole fillets with salt and pepper to taste. Place 2 shrimp on each fillet with tails on either side; roll up to form paupiette. Secure with toothpick.

3. In a saucepan, poach paupiettes in wine over low heat for 5 to 7 minutes or just until fish flakes easily when tested with fork. With slotted spoon, place paupiettes on bed of rice on individual plates. Remove picks. Keep warm.

4. Bring wine to a rapid boil and boil until reduced to ¼ cup (50 mL). Whisk in dill and butter; stir in orange and lemon and heat through. Spoon over fish.

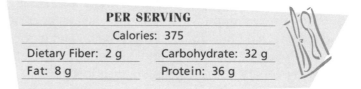

PER SERVING	
Calories: 375	
Dietary Fiber: 2 g	Carbohydrate: 32 g
Fat: 8 g	Protein: 36 g

Shrimp and Mussels with Couscous

1 tbsp	olive oil	15 mL
1 cup	sliced leeks (green and white parts)	250 mL
½ cup	diced carrots	125 mL
1	can (19 oz/540 mL) stewed tomatoes	1
1 tsp	minced garlic	5 mL
1 cup	green bell pepper strips	250 mL
1 lb	fresh mussels, cleaned and debearded	500 g
1½ cups	quick-cooking couscous	375 mL
12	large cooked shrimp	12

1. In a large saucepan or Dutch oven, heat oil over medium-high heat. Add leeks and sauté for 2 to 3 minutes. Add carrots, tomatoes and garlic; bring to a boil. Cover, reduce heat and simmer for 10 minutes.

2. Add green pepper strips and mussels; cook, covered, for about 5 minutes or until mussels have opened. Discard any mussels that haven't opened.

3. Meanwhile, cook couscous according to package directions.

4. Add shrimp to mussel mixture; cook for 2 minutes or until heated through. Serve over couscous.

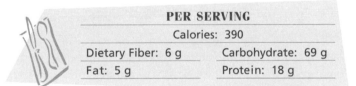

PER SERVING	
Calories: 390	
Dietary Fiber: 6 g	Carbohydrate: 69 g
Fat: 5 g	Protein: 18 g

SERVES 4

Johanne Trepanier

Here's a dish that is as delicious as it is easy to prepare! The couscous makes a great accompaniment — and it's ready in minutes.

TIP

Mussels should be rinsed in several changes of cold water to rid them of any grit. If still intact, the beard from the outer mussel shells should be removed by scrubbing with a hard brush prior to cooking. Inspect mussels before cooking and discard any with shells that are broken or any that do not close when tapped: these are not safe to eat. Likewise, discard any that have not opened after cooking.

DIETITIAN'S MESSAGE

Enjoy adding different varieties of grains to your diet. Couscous is made from hard durum semolina wheat. It is popular in Middle Eastern cooking, particularly in Moroccan cuisine, where it is traditionally served with a stew known as tagine. It is widely available in supermarkets, health food stores and specialty food shops.

Shrimp and Spinach Crêpes

6- or 7-inch (15 or 18 cm) nonstick crêpe pan

Crêpes

2	egg whites	2
6 tbsp	all-purpose flour	90 mL
1/3 cup	skim milk	75 mL

Shrimp

2 tbsp	soft margarine	25 mL
1	clove garlic, minced	1
2	green onions, sliced	2
2 cups	packed sliced trimmed spinach	500 mL
1 1/2 cups	sliced mushrooms	375 mL
1 tbsp	grated lemon zest	15 mL
1/4 cup	all-purpose flour	50 mL
1 cup	skim milk	250 mL
1/3 cup	water	75 mL
1 lb	cooked peeled deveined shrimp	500 g
1/3 cup	chopped fresh cilantro *or* parsley	75 mL
1 tbsp	lemon juice	15 mL
	Lemon pepper	

1. *Crêpes:* In a small bowl, beat egg whites with flour; gradually beat in milk. Heat pan over medium-low heat. Add 3 tbsp (45 mL) batter, swirling quickly to cover bottom. Cook until bottom is lightly browned; flip crêpe onto plate and keep warm. Repeat with remaining batter to make 6 crêpes.

2. *Shrimp:* In a large saucepan, melt margarine over medium heat; cook garlic, onions, spinach, mushrooms and lemon zest until spinach has wilted. Stir in flour. Gradually add milk and water; cook, stirring, until thickened. Stir in shrimp, cilantro and lemon juice; heat through.

3. Place crêpes on serving plates. Spoon 2 large spoonfuls of filling onto each crêpe, reserving some for garnish. Fold sides over filling. Serve remaining filling as sauce on top. Sprinkle with lemon pepper to taste.

PER SERVING	
Calories: 227	
Dietary Fiber: 2 g	Carbohydrate: 16 g
Fat: 6 g	Protein: 26 g

Shrimp and Zucchini in Buttermilk Herb Sauce

	Fish stock *or* water	
24	shrimp, peeled and deveined	24
2	medium zucchini	2
½ cup	buttermilk	125 mL
¼ cup	light sour cream	50 mL
¼ cup	lower-fat plain yogurt	50 mL
1 tbsp	each chopped fresh basil, chives and dill	15 mL
Pinch	coarsely ground black pepper	Pinch

1. In a skillet of gently simmering fish stock, poach shrimp until pink; drain and chill.

2. Cut zucchini in half lengthwise; place flat side down and slice into thin ribbons resembling fettuccine. Steam until just tender-crisp. Chill.

3. In a bowl, combine buttermilk, sour cream, yogurt, basil, chives, dill and pepper; stir in zucchini. Divide among plates; top with shrimp.

PER SERVING
Calories: 142

Dietary Fiber: 1 g	Carbohydrate: 8 g
Fat: 3 g	Protein: 21 g

SERVES 4

Judson Simpson, Chef
Violaine Sauvé, Dietitian

Here's an unusual recipe that uses thin strips of zucchini to replace pasta. Serve cold for a summer lunch, garnished with a basil leaf or sprig of dill and accompanied by French baguette slices.

DIETITIAN'S MESSAGE

Many people have the misconception that buttermilk is fattening, but, in fact, it has less fat than 2% milk! Traditionally, it came from milk that was used to make butter and that soured naturally. Today's buttermilk is artificially soured. It has a longer shelf life than regular milk because its higher acid content helps to inhibit the growth of most spoilage-causing bacteria.

*Crab cakes are a
traditional favorite at
seaside restaurants,
where the ambience and
the presentation can
range from casual to
elegant. This version
can be served as a
dinner entrée or, if you
prefer, you can reduce
the size of the cakes
to serve as a great finger-
food appetizer.*

TIP

These crab cakes will
freeze well, so use what
you need and freeze
the remainder for
another meal.

DIETITIAN'S MESSAGE

Although crab cakes are
a great treat, they are
usually high in fat. In this
version, egg whites
instead of whole eggs
bind the ingredients, and
the patties are cooked
in a skillet sprayed with
nonstick cooking spray
rather than in a
substantial quantity of
oil. Amazingly, there is
only 1 g of fat in the
entire recipe!

The Narrows Crab Cakes

1	stalk celery, finely chopped	1
¼ cup	finely chopped onion	50 mL
1 tbsp	chopped fresh parsley	15 mL
4	egg whites, lightly beaten	4
1 cup	fine dry bread crumbs, divided	250 mL
2 tsp	Worcestershire sauce	10 mL
1 tsp	dry mustard	5 mL
½ tsp	salt	2 mL
2	cans (6 oz/170 g each) crabmeat, drained and flaked	2
	Lemon wedges	

1. In a skillet sprayed with nonstick cooking spray, cook celery, onion and parsley over medium heat, stirring, until tender, about 5 minutes.

2. In a bowl, stir together egg whites, ¾ cup (175 mL) of the bread crumbs, Worcestershire sauce, mustard and salt. Stir in celery mixture and crabmeat, mixing well. Using about ⅓ cup (75 mL) crab mixture for each, shape into ½-inch (1 cm) thick patties. Coat with remaining bread crumbs.

3. Spray skillet again with cooking spray. Cook patties over medium heat for about 3 minutes per side or until golden. Serve with lemon wedges.

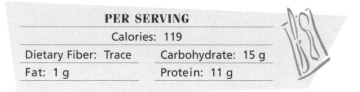

PER SERVING	
Calories: 119	
Dietary Fiber: Trace	Carbohydrate: 15 g
Fat: 1 g	Protein: 11 g

Punjabi Potato and Chickpea Curry

2 tbsp	vegetable oil	25 mL
6	cloves garlic, minced	6
1	large onion, diced	1
1 tsp	crushed red pepper flakes	5 mL
1 tsp	each turmeric and ground coriander	5 mL
1 tsp	each cumin seeds and brown *or* black mustard seeds	5 mL
2 tbsp	tomato paste	25 mL
4 cups	apple juice	1 L
2	large (unpeeled) potatoes, diced	2
1	can (19 oz/540 mL) chickpeas, drained	1
1 tbsp	brown sugar	15 mL
1	bay leaf	1
1 tbsp	lemon juice	15 mL
	Hot pepper sauce	

1. In a large skillet, heat oil over medium-high heat; cook garlic and onion, stirring, for 3 to 4 minutes or until softened. Add red pepper flakes, turmeric, coriander and cumin and mustard seeds; cook, stirring for 2 to 3 minutes.

2. Stir in tomato paste; pour in apple juice. Add potatoes, chickpeas, brown sugar, bay leaf and lemon juice; bring to a boil. Reduce heat and simmer, uncovered, for 25 to 30 minutes, stirring occasionally, or until potatoes are tender and mixture has thickened. Discard bay leaf. Add hot pepper sauce to taste.

PER SERVING	
Calories: 439	
Dietary Fiber: 6 g	Carbohydrate: 82 g
Fat: 9 g	Protein: 10 g

SERVES 4

**Stephen Ashton, Chef
Jane Thornthwaite,
Dietitian**

Explore new flavor dimensions while eating vegetables and healthy legumes in this delicious and easy-to-make dish.

TIPS

If you prefer, substitute 1 cup (250 mL) dried chickpeas, soaked, cooked and drained, for the canned.

Chickpeas offer lower-fat, high-fiber, inexpensive protein. A great-tasting and versatile legume, chickpeas are a delicious addition to spreads, soups and sauces, as well as main-course meals.

DIETITIAN'S MESSAGE

Serve this delicious curry as the centerpiece of a vegetarian meal. Add brown rice and whole-wheat chapattis. Start the meal with Carrot Soup with Raita (see recipe, page 107).

Yams, a popular ingredient in Southern dishes, take center stage in this fun-to-eat fajita recipe.

TIP

Although the true yam is different from the sweet potato, the terms tend to be used interchangeably in North America and refer to an elongated, brown-skinned tuber with an orange-colored flesh. Sweet potatoes are nutritious. Like all orange-colored vegetables, they are a good source of vitamin A. They also contain potassium, and vitamin C.

DIETITIAN'S MESSAGE

Vitamin A is plentiful in this tasty vegetarian fajita. Try serving it with Colorful Bean and Corn Salad (see recipe, page 163) and end the meal with a fruit dessert.

Roasted Yam Fajitas

Preheat oven to 350°F (180°C)
Baking sheet

Sauce

⅓ cup	orange juice	75 mL
1 tsp	grated lime zest	5 mL
2 tbsp	lime juice	25 mL
1 tbsp	olive oil	15 mL
1 tbsp	minced garlic	15 mL
1 tsp	crushed dried oregano	5 mL
1 tsp	ground cumin	5 mL
¼ tsp	red pepper flakes	1 mL
¼ tsp	black pepper	1 mL

Filling

4	medium yams *or* sweet potatoes (1½ lb/750 g)	4
2 tbsp	olive oil	25 mL
	Salt and black pepper	
1	each medium red and green bell pepper, cut into strips	1
1	medium onion, sliced	1
10	7- to 8-inch (18 to 20 cm) flour tortillas	10

Toppings

Chopped tomatoes

Shredded lettuce

Shredded cheese

Light sour cream

1. *Sauce:* In a bowl, combine orange juice, lime zest and juice, oil, garlic, oregano, cumin, red pepper flakes and pepper; cover and let stand for at least 4 hours at room temperature. (Or refrigerate overnight.)

2. *Filling:* Peel yams and cut into ½-inch (1 cm) cubes; toss with 1 tbsp (15 mL) of the oil. Place on baking sheet; sprinkle with salt and pepper to taste. Bake in preheated oven for 20 to 25 minutes or until tender but not mushy. Cool completely.

3. In a large skillet, heat remaining oil over medium-high heat; sauté red and green peppers and onions for about 5 minutes. Add yams and sauce; heat through (most of sauce will be absorbed).

4. Meanwhile, wrap tortillas in foil; bake in preheated oven for 5 to 10 minutes or until heated. (Or wrap in paper towels and microwave at High for 40 seconds.) Spoon yam filling into tortillas. Top with desired toppings.

PER SERVING	
Calories: 484	
Dietary Fiber: 6 g	Carbohydrate: 82 g
Fat: 14 g	Protein: 10 g

Monster Quesadilla

Preheat oven to 350°F (180°C)
Pizza pan or baking sheet

2 cups	lower-fat cottage cheese	500 mL
2	cloves garlic, minced	2
2 tbsp	grated Parmesan cheese	25 mL
¼ tsp	black pepper	1 mL
1	pkg (10 oz/300 g) frozen chopped spinach, thawed, moisture squeezed out	1
12	10-inch (25 cm) flour tortillas	12
1	can (14 oz/398 mL) refried beans	1
1¼ cups	mild, medium *or* hot salsa	300 mL
2	large tomatoes, sliced	2
½ cup	shredded part-skim mozzarella cheese	125 mL

1. Blend cottage cheese, garlic, Parmesan cheese and pepper until smooth. Stir into spinach.
2. Place 1 tortilla on baking sheet. Spread with ⅔ cup (150 mL) of the beans; top with a tortilla. Spread with ½ cup (125 mL) salsa; cover with tortilla. Spread with 1 cup (250 mL) spinach mixture; cover with tortilla. Starting with refried beans, repeat layers twice. Arrange sliced tomatoes and mozzarella cheese on top.
3. Bake in preheated oven for 45 to 60 minutes; cut into pie-shaped wedges to serve.

PER SERVING	
Calories: 613	
Dietary Fiber: 10 g	Carbohydrate: 95 g
Fat: 12 g	Protein: 34 g

Don Costello, Chef
Lisa Diamond, Dietitian

Layer upon layer of seasoned cheese with spinach, refried beans and salsa, topped with sliced tomatoes and mozzarella cheese, make this spectacular recipe a standout for taste and appearance. Serve with extra salsa and lower-fat sour cream.

TIP
Use whole-wheat tortillas for additional fiber. If desired, use a food processor to blend the cottage cheese mixture. Bake the quesadilla on a pizza pan, if you prefer.

DIETITIAN'S MESSAGE
This tasty dish offers a serving from all the food groups. Add a serving of sliced tomatoes sprinkled with fresh parsley or basil. For dessert, offer a selection of fruit.

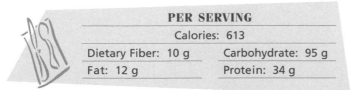

Red Pepper and Goat Cheese Pizza

Preheat oven to 400°F (200°C) if using flatbread or 450°F (230°C) if using pizza dough
Pizza pan or baking sheet

1	12-inch (30 cm) round flatbread *or* enough pizza dough for a 12-inch (30 cm) pizza	1
1 tbsp	olive oil	15 mL
1 cup	shredded mozzarella cheese	250 mL
¼ cup	soft crumbled goat cheese	50 mL
1	large red bell pepper, thinly sliced	1
1	large tomato, sliced	1
¼ cup	sliced black olives	50 mL
¼ cup	sweet Vidalia onion, sliced (optional)	50 mL
1 tsp	dried basil (*or* 2 tbsp/25 mL chopped fresh basil)	5 mL

1. Place flatbread on baking sheet. Alternatively, if using pizza dough, spread out dough on lightly greased pizza pan to make a 12-inch (30 cm) circle.
2. Brush olive oil on top of flatbread or pizza dough. Sprinkle with mozzarella cheese. Top with goat cheese, red pepper, tomato, black olives, onion, if using, and basil.
3. Bake pizza in bottom half of preheated oven for 10 to 15 minutes or until crust is golden and filling is bubbly.

PER SERVING	
Calories: 373	
Dietary Fiber: 3 g	Carbohydrate: 40 g
Fat: 18 g	Protein: 14 g

Spaghetti Squash with Mushrooms

Preheat oven to 350°F (180°C)
Baking sheet

1	spaghetti squash (about 3½ lb/1.5 kg)	1
2 tbsp	butter *or* margarine	25 mL
2 cups	sliced mushrooms	500 mL
2 cups	chopped tomatoes (4 small)	500 mL
1	green onion, sliced	1
1	small stalk celery, chopped	1
2 tbsp	all-purpose flour	25 mL
1 cup	2% milk	250 mL
½ cup	shredded Cheddar cheese	125 mL
1 tsp	dried oregano	5 mL
½ tsp	garlic powder	2 mL
½ tsp	salt	2 mL
¼ tsp	freshly ground black pepper	1 mL
	Grated Parmesan cheese	

1. Cut squash in half lengthwise. Bake cut side down on a baking sheet in preheated oven for 25 to 30 minutes or boil, cut side down and covered, in 2 inches (5 cm) of water for about 20 minutes.

2. In a skillet over medium-high heat, cook mushrooms, onion, celery and tomatoes in butter for about 5 minutes or until tender. Stir in flour; gradually add milk. Cook, stirring constantly, until thickened. Stir in Cheddar cheese and seasonings until cheese is melted.

3. Pour sauce over squash; sprinkle with Parmesan cheese and serve.

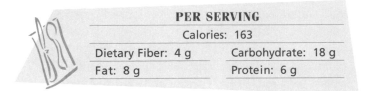

PER SERVING	
Calories: 163	
Dietary Fiber: 4 g	Carbohydrate: 18 g
Fat: 8 g	Protein: 6 g

Marlyn Ambrose-Chase

Spaghetti squash, which is most readily available from August to November, looks just like golden strands of spaghetti yet tastes like squash when cooked. Since spaghetti squash acts like both pasta and vegetable, you can serve it with your favorite spaghetti sauce.

TIPS

Spaghetti squash is easily recognized by its oblong shape and pale to bright yellow skin. It bakes and microwaves quite easily.

To keep the strands intact, be sure to cut squash in half lengthwise.

DIETITIAN'S MESSAGE

Serve this dish over brown rice for a light meal. End with a substantial dessert such as Matrimonial Cake (see recipe, page 430) and a glass of milk.

You can find everything you need in the supermarket to make this Southwestern dish.

TIP

The canned beans in this recipe can be replaced with dried black beans. Soak ¾ cup (175 mL) black beans overnight. Drain; cover with water and bring to a boil. Reduce heat and simmer until tender, about 30 minutes. Drain, rinse and use in recipe.

DIETITIAN'S MESSAGE

This fabulous dish offers a serving from all the food groups. For a terrific brunch, serve with a lightly dressed green salad and whole-grain bread. You'll provide vitamins, minerals and fiber to spare.

Beans and legumes provide protein as well as iron, zinc, calcium, vitamin B6 and fiber, and are an important source of protein in vegetarian diets. Combining grains with legumes as this recipe does (the cornmeal with the beans), creates high-quality protein. If you are serving this meal to a vegetarian, replace the chicken broth with vegetable broth.

Southwestern Torta

Preheat oven to 350°F (180°C)
10-inch (25 cm) springform pan sprayed
with nonstick vegetable spray

1	clove garlic, minced	1
½	medium onion, chopped	½
1½ tsp	vegetable oil	7 mL
3	medium tomatoes, seeded and diced	3
2 tbsp	chopped fresh cilantro	25 mL
1 tsp	chili powder	5 mL
1	can (14 oz/398 mL) black beans, drained and rinsed	1
2 cups	chicken broth	500 mL
1¼ cups	sun-dried tomatoes, diced	300 mL
½ cup	yellow cornmeal	125 mL
2 tbsp	chopped fresh basil (*or* 2 tsp/10 mL dried)	25 mL
4	10-inch (25 cm) tortillas	4
1	each medium red, yellow and green bell peppers, cut into julienne strips	1
2 tbsp	vegetable oil	25 mL
2	eggs, lightly beaten	2
⅔ cup	shredded light Monterey Jack–style cheese	150 mL
⅔ cup	shredded light medium Cheddar-style cheese	150 mL
	Salsa	

1. In a skillet, sauté garlic and onion in oil until tender. Add tomatoes, cilantro and chili powder; cook, stirring, for 3 to 5 minutes. Stir in beans. Set aside.

2. In a medium saucepan, bring broth to a boil; stir in sun-dried tomatoes, cornmeal and basil. Cook, stirring constantly, until mixture leaves side of pot. Cover and let stand for 5 minutes. Fit 1 tortilla snugly into 10-inch (25 cm) springform pan sprayed with vegetable oil. Spread with half of the cornmeal mixture. Top with second tortilla. Stir half of the remaining polenta into bean mixture; spread over tortilla. Cover with third tortilla.

3. In a skillet, sauté red, yellow and green peppers in oil until tender; stir in remaining polenta. Spread over torta. Place fourth tortilla on top.

4. Using paring knife, poke holes through all layers of torta. Slowly pour eggs over torta, allowing to run down through holes. Sprinkle with Monterey Jack–style and Cheddar-style cheeses. Bake in preheated oven for 25 to 30 minutes or until firm. Remove from pan; serve warm or cooled, accompanied with salsa.

PER SERVING

Calories: 412

Dietary Fiber: 8 g	Carbohydrate: 58 g
Fat: 11 g	Protein: 23 g

Vegetable Quinoa

1 cup	quinoa	250 mL
1 cup	boiling water	250 mL
¼ cup	diced tomatoes	50 mL
¼ cup	carrot strips	50 mL
¼ cup	chopped broccoli	50 mL
¼ cup	cauliflower florets	50 mL
¼ cup	diced zucchini	50 mL
2 tbsp	sunflower oil	25 mL
1 tbsp	soy sauce	15 mL

1. Rinse quinoa under cold water until water runs clear. In a medium saucepan, add quinoa to boiling water; cover and simmer for about 15 minutes or until tender. (Watch carefully to prevent sticking.)

2. In a skillet over medium-high heat, stir-fry tomatoes, carrot, broccoli, cauliflower and zucchini in oil for about 4 minutes. Stir vegetables and soy sauce into quinoa and serve immediately.

PER SERVING

Calories: 164

Dietary Fiber: 1 g	Carbohydrate: 25 g
Fat: 6 g	Protein: 5 g

SERVES 6

Monique Clément

Quinoa (pronounced keen-wa) is a seed-like grain available from health food stores that originates from the Andes Mountains in South America. Here, its slightly crunchy texture and nutty flavor add a new twist to a conventional stir-fry.

TIP

Quinoa is rich in plant fat and, like seeds and nuts, it spoils easily. Store in an airtight glass container no longer than a month, or in the refrigerator or freezer.

DIETITIAN'S MESSAGE

Although on their own plant sources of protein do not contain the complete array of amino acids that your body needs, vegetarians can ensure a full complement of protein every day by combining grains such as quinoa and couscous with legumes such as kidney beans and lentils.

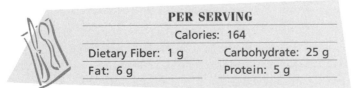

Serve this appetizing loaf as a main course at brunch or dinner. With the refreshing tang of lemon in the loaf and in the companion Lemon Tomato Sauce, this recipe will easily become a favorite.

TIP

When buying celery, look for heads that are tight. Avoid any that are discolored or cracked as they are not fresh. In this recipe, celery is used to flavor the vegetable loaf. But celery is also one of the all-time great healthy snacks. Keep plenty on hand as it keeps well refrigerated.

DIETITIAN'S MESSAGE

This unusual recipe contains both Milk Products and eggs. It makes an excellent meal choice for lacto-ovo vegetarians. Add fiber to the meal with whole-grain bread and broccoli.

Vegetable Cheese Loaf with Lemon Tomato Sauce

Preheat oven to 350°F (180°C)
9- by 5-inch (2 L) loaf pan

¾ cup	finely chopped onion	175 mL
3 tbsp	butter *or* margarine	45 mL
¾ cup	finely chopped celery	175 mL
2	medium carrots, peeled and grated	2
2 cups	small-curd cottage cheese	500 mL
2 cups	fresh bread crumbs	500 mL
2	eggs, well beaten	2
	Lemon zest and juice of ½ a lemon	
1 tsp	salt	5 mL
½ tsp	black pepper	2 mL
¼ tsp	dried basil	1 mL
Sauce		
2½ cups	tomato juice, divided	625 mL
1	medium onion, cut in half	1
4	fresh parsley sprigs	4
1	bay leaf	1
1	whole clove	1
½ tsp	dried basil	2 mL
½ tsp	granulated sugar	2 mL
⅓ cup	butter *or* margarine	75 mL
¼ cup	all-purpose flour	50 mL
½	lemon, squeezed	½

1. In a medium skillet over medium heat, cook onion in melted butter for about 5 minutes or until tender. Add celery and carrots; cook for 1 minute.

2. In a large bowl, combine cottage cheese, bread crumbs, eggs, lemon zest and juice, and seasonings. Add vegetable mixture; stir.

3. Place in nonstick or lightly greased 9- by 5-inch (2 L) baking pan. Bake in preheated oven for 35 to 40 minutes or until knife inserted in center comes out clean. Remove loaf from pan.

4. *Sauce:* In a medium saucepan, combine 1½ cups (375 mL) tomato juice, onion, parsley, seasonings and sugar. Bring to a boil, reduce heat and simmer for 15 to 20 minutes. Press mixture through sieve. Reserve sieved tomato mixture.

5. In a small saucepan, melt butter and blend in flour; cook for 1 to 2 minutes. Gradually add remaining tomato juice. Cook, stirring constantly, for 4 to 5 minutes or until smooth and thickened. Add reserved tomato mixture and lemon juice. Reheat to serving temperature. To serve, slice loaf; pour sauce over slices.

PER SERVING	
Calories: 319	
Dietary Fiber: 1 g	Carbohydrate: 23 g
Fat: 19 g	Protein: 15 g

Stir-Fried Vegetables with Tofu

2 tbsp	vegetable oil	25 mL
1	large onion, cut into wedges	1
3	medium carrots, sliced diagonally	3
3	celery stalks, sliced diagonally	3
¼	small cabbage, sliced thinly	¼
1 cup	snow peas, trimmed	250 mL
1 cup	sliced mushrooms	250 mL
1 cup	firm tofu, cubed	250 mL
½ cup	chicken broth	125 mL
1 tbsp	cornstarch	15 mL
1 tsp	finely chopped ginger root (or ½ tsp/2 mL ground ginger)	5 mL
¼ tsp	black pepper	1 mL

1. In a wok or large heavy skillet, heat oil over high heat. When oil is very hot, add onion, carrot and celery; cover and steam for 5 minutes. Add cabbage, snow peas, mushrooms and tofu; steam, covered, for 5 minutes longer.

2. Mix together chicken broth, cornstarch, ginger and pepper; pour over vegetable mixture. Stir-fry for 1 minute or until sauce thickens. Serve over hot rice.

PER SERVING	
Calories: 151	
Dietary Fiber: 4 g	Carbohydrate: 12 g
Fat: 8 g	Protein: 9 g

SERVES 6

Marilyn Peters

Ginger root adds zest to this tasty dish.

TIP
Tofu, a source of protein and some calcium, is made from soy milk, in much the same way that cheese is made from animal milk. Tofu is best stored in water in a covered container in the refrigerator. Change the water daily to keep tofu fresh for 1 week.

DIETITIAN'S MESSAGE
Vegetarians are generally described according to the foods they include in their diets, from a lacto-ovo vegetarian, who includes milk and eggs, to a vegan, who avoids all foods of animal origin. Tofu is a popular protein choice for most types of vegetarians. If you are serving this meal to a vegetarian, replace the chicken broth with vegetable broth, tomato juice or vegetable juice cocktail.

Teriyaki Tofu Stir-Fry

1⅓ cups	diced firm tofu	325 mL
½ cup	teriyaki sauce	125 mL
1 tsp	brown sugar	5 mL
1 tsp	cornstarch	5 mL
1 tbsp	water	15 mL
2 tsp	olive oil	10 mL
½ cup	diced onion	125 mL
1 cup	diced green bell peppers	250 mL
1 cup	diced red bell peppers	250 mL
1 tsp	minced garlic	5 mL
1 tsp	grated ginger root	5 mL
2 cups	roughly chopped vegetables (see Variation, at left, for suggestions)	500 mL
3 cups	cooked rice	750 mL
1 to 2 tbsp	chopped fresh cilantro *or* parsley (optional)	15 to 25 mL

1. In a medium bowl, gently toss tofu with teriyaki sauce and brown sugar until well coated. Cover and refrigerate for 10 minutes or for up to several hours.

2. In a small bowl, whisk together cornstarch and water. Set aside.

3. In a large nonstick skillet, heat oil over medium-high heat. Add onion, green peppers, red peppers, garlic and ginger; stir-fry for 3 minutes. Stir in vegetables of your choice and stir-fry for 3 to 4 minutes or until vegetables are tender-crisp.

4. Add tofu mixture and cornstarch mixture. Stir for 3 to 4 minutes or until thickened and heated through. Serve over rice. Sprinkle with cilantro, if using.

PER SERVING	
Calories: 287	
Dietary Fiber: 3 g	Carbohydrate: 49 g
Fat: 5 g	Protein: 12 g

Puffed Tofu and Vegetables

SERVES 4
....

Jon Paudler, Chef
Leslie Maze, Dietitian

	Vegetable oil for frying	
1	medium soft tofu cake (about 10 oz/300 g)	1
1 tbsp	vegetable oil	15 mL
1	clove garlic, crushed	1
½ tsp	crushed red pepper flakes	2 mL
1	small carrot, sliced	1
1	medium onion, cut into wedges	1
½	small cucumber, peeled and sliced	½
1½ cups	sliced bok choy	375 mL
8	snow peas	8
¼ cup	water	50 mL
1 tbsp	dry sherry	15 mL
Sauce		
¼ cup	water	50 mL
1 tsp	tamari *or* soy sauce	5 mL
1 tsp	cornstarch	5 mL
Pinch	granulated sugar	Pinch

Tofu is frequently used in Asian cuisine. In this recipe, it's fried first to give it a golden brown color, then stir-fried with garlic and vegetables.

TIP
Don't judge tofu by how it tastes on its own. Tofu is bland almost to the point of being tasteless. However, it has a remarkable affinity for other foods and spices and takes on their flavors when combined in cooking.

DIETITIAN'S MESSAGE

This is a tasty and inexpensive vegetarian meal. Serve as a side dish or add rice to make into a meal.

1. Heat ¼ inch (5 mm) oil in a wok or skillet. Cut tofu into 4 slices; fry until light golden brown. Transfer to paper towel–lined plate to drain excess oil. Place in hot water for 5 minutes; drain again on paper towel–lined plate.

2. In same wok or skillet, heat 1 tbsp (15 mL) oil; stir-fry garlic and tofu pieces. Remove garlic. Sprinkle tofu with red pepper flakes; remove from wok and keep warm.

3. Stir-fry carrot and onion for 2 minutes. Add cucumber, bok choy and snow peas; stir-fry for 2 minutes. Add water and sherry; cover and cook for 1 to 2 minutes.

4. *Sauce:* Combine water, tamari sauce, cornstarch and sugar; add to wok and cook until thickened. Transfer to serving dish and top with tofu.

PER SERVING	
Calories: 159	
Dietary Fiber: 3 g	Carbohydrate: 9 g
Fat: 11 g	Protein: 8 g

This is a great lower-fat vegetarian version of a Greek classic. The rich cream sauce normally used in moussaka has been replaced with a tofu mixture that gives all the taste with a fraction of the fat!

TIP

To vary the flavors in this tasty dish and transform it into a great party pleaser, add grilled peppers and zucchini to the eggplant layer.

DIETITIAN'S MESSAGE

Here's a great vegetarian dish that can be the centerpiece for even the most elegant buffet. If serving as a meal, add a green salad tossed with Raspberry Basil Vinaigrette (see recipe, page 130) and some crusty bread.

Vegetable Moussaka

Preheat oven to 350°F (180°C)
Baking sheets, greased
13- by 9-inch (3.5 L) baking pan, greased

2	medium eggplants	2
1 tsp	salt	5 mL
1	medium onion, chopped	1
1	clove garlic, minced	1
1	can (19 oz/540 mL) chickpeas, drained and rinsed	1
1	can (28 oz/796 mL) tomatoes	1
1 tbsp	each dried oregano and basil	15 mL
½ tsp	each ground cinnamon and black pepper	2 mL
¼ cup	grated Parmesan cheese	50 mL
Topping		
1 lb	tofu	500 g
1	medium onion, quartered	1
2	egg whites	2
Pinch	ground nutmeg	Pinch

1. Slice eggplants lengthwise into ¼-inch (5 mm) thick slices; sprinkle with salt. Drain in colander for 30 minutes. Bake in preheated oven for 15 minutes. Turn and bake for 15 minutes longer.

2. In a nonstick skillet sprayed with nonstick cooking spray, cook onion and garlic, stirring, for 2 minutes. Add chickpeas, mashing slightly. Stir in tomatoes, oregano, basil, cinnamon, pepper and ½ tsp (2 mL) salt; bring to a boil. Reduce heat and simmer, uncovered, for 20 minutes, stirring occasionally. Process in food processor until mixture resembles coarse meal.

3. In greased baking pan, layer half of the eggplant, then all of the chickpea mixture, half of the Parmesan, then remaining eggplant.

4. *Topping:* Purée ingredients for topping; spread over moussaka. Sprinkle with remaining cheese. Bake in preheated oven for 30 minutes.

PER SERVING	
Calories: 187	
Dietary Fiber: 6 g	Carbohydrate: 26 g
Fat: 5 g	Protein: 12 g

Spinach and Mushroom Pizza Pie

Preheat oven to 375°F (190°C)
12-inch (30 cm) pizza pan or baking sheet, greased

1½ lb	prepared pizza dough	750 g
1 tbsp	olive oil	15 mL
2 tsp	minced garlic	10 mL
½ cup	chopped onion	125 mL
2 cups	sliced mushrooms	500 mL
1	pkg (10 oz/300 g) frozen chopped spinach, thawed and squeezed dry	1
⅛ tsp	ground nutmeg	0.5 mL
¼ tsp	black pepper	1 mL
2 cups	shredded old Cheddar cheese	500 mL

1. Divide dough into 2 pieces; 1 piece (bottom) should be slightly larger than the second (top) piece. Shape the larger piece of dough into a 12-inch (30 cm) circle and place on prepared pizza pan. Set aside.

2. In a large nonstick skillet, heat oil over medium heat. Add garlic, onion and mushrooms; cook, stirring constantly, for 5 to 6 minutes or until mixture is lightly browned. Add spinach and cook, stirring constantly, until all liquid has evaporated and mixture is quite dry. Stir in nutmeg and pepper. Spread mixture evenly over dough; sprinkle with cheese.

3. Roll out top portion of dough and place on top of pizza. Lightly moisten edges and pinch edges together, sealing well. Prick top of pizza all over with a fork. Bake in bottom half of preheated oven for 25 to 35 minutes or until bottom is browned and top is crispy and golden. Cool for 5 minutes and cut into wedges.

PER SERVING

Calories: 496

Dietary Fiber: 3 g	Carbohydrate: 59 g
Fat: 20 g	Protein: 19 g

SERVES 6

Mary Persi

Here's a quick and easy pizza recipe that is bound to become a favorite of all family members.

TIPS

Make sure that the filling is sautéed until all of the moisture has evaporated; otherwise, the bottom crust will be soaked with liquid. Sprinkling cornmeal over the crust before adding the filling will also help to absorb any liquid.

To make the crust crispier, use a perforated pizza pan.

MAKE AHEAD

Pizza can be made 1 day ahead and reheated in a 375°F (190°C) oven. Do not reheat in a microwave or the crust will become soggy.

DIETITIAN'S MESSAGE

As this pizza is relatively high in fat, serve it with a romaine lettuce salad tossed with a lower-fat dressing and offer fruit for dessert.

Vegetables

In this chapter, you'll find some great vegetable side dishes that will add variety and nutrients to any meal. Some, such as Honey-Glazed Carrots and Deluxe Peas, will become family favorites. Others, such as Sautéed Spinach with Pine Nuts and Braised Red Cabbage, may be saved for special occasions. We hope this chapter encourages you to eat more vegetables and to think of them not only as foods that are good for you but ones you thoroughly enjoy.

veggie me up!

Vegetables are an amazing and versatile food. Not only do they add color, texture and taste to any dish or meal, they are delicious on their own, cooked or raw. Like an artist painting a picture, a good chef will use a variety of different vegetables in an array of colors to create delicious dishes with maximum eye appeal.

Even more importantly, vegetables, like fruit, are full of wonderful things called nutrients. As the word implies, nutrients nourish our bodies and help to make us strong and healthy. Vegetables are nutrient-dense, packing a variety of vitamins and minerals into a minimum of calories. They are an important source of dietary fiber and, in most cases, are virtually fat-free. The few calories found in vegetables come mainly from carbohydrates, which provide our bodies with energy. Another plus to eating lots of vegetables is that they contain substances known as phytochemicals and antioxidants. Both compounds are thought to have strong health benefits. (See page 12 for more details.) Although our knowledge of the healthful properties of vegetables has increased dramatically in recent years, scientists have really only begun to investigate all the magical things these foods contain and how they help to keep us healthy and strong.

vegetables and longevity

Did you know that some of the oldest people in the world come from an island in the south of Japan? Okinawa is home to the highest percentage of centenarians (people at least 100 years old or older) anywhere, and they have the lowest rate of heart disease and cancer in the world. Although scientists are still studying the population there, they theorize that their longevity is due to active lifestyles and healthy diets. Most Okinawans eat at least seven servings of nutrient-dense vegetables daily, plus grains, soy products and fish. Makes you want to reach for a crunchy carrot, doesn't it? It's no wonder we recommend eating five to ten servings of vegetables and fruit daily and suggest choosing dark green and orange varieties more often.

vitamin A

Carrots are an excellent source of beta-carotene. Beta-carotene is an antioxidant and a member of a group of pigments known as carotenoids, which are responsible for the bright, warm colors in vegetables and fruit. Our bodies convert beta-carotene to vitamin A as we need it. Unlike most vegetables, cooked carrots are actually more nutritious than raw carrots because cooking breaks down the stiff cell walls, allowing the nutrients to become more easily absorbed by our bodies.

vary vegetable choices

It's important to eat a variety of vegetables, because no single vegetable provides all the nutrients that our bodies need. Challenge your family to try a new vegetable every month. If you find one you don't like right away, don't worry. Sometimes it takes two or three trials before our taste buds get accustomed to an unusual flavor and texture. Or try cooking it in a different way.

fresh, frozen or canned?

Whether you choose fresh, frozen or canned vegetables, you are essentially getting the same nutrients with only minor variations. Differences depend on the length of time between harvesting and freezing or canning. In fact, vegetables that are frozen or canned hours after they have been harvested may contain more vitamins than fresh ones that have been stored and transported over a period of time. One consideration with canned vegetables is that salt is added during processing, making them higher in sodium than fresh or frozen varieties.

You can prepare these stuffed vegetables earlier in the day, then cover and chill until you are ready to heat and serve. For best flavor and texture, don't make them the day before.

TIP

When making the Mushroom Stuffing in this recipe, experiment with the many varieties of mushrooms that are now readily available.

DIETITIAN'S MESSAGE

Use this recipe to take advantage of fresh tomatoes or zucchini when these vegetables are in season. It is an easy and delicious way to add to the 5 to 10 recommended daily servings of vegetables and fruit in your diet.

Stuffed Tomatoes or Zucchini

Preheat oven to 350°F (180°C)
Baking pan

6	small tomatoes *or* 2 large zucchini	6
Provençale Stuffing		
2	medium onions, finely chopped	2
2	cloves garlic, finely chopped	2
2 cups	packed fresh parsley, finely chopped	500 mL
1 tbsp	olive oil	15 mL
3	slices white bread, crusts removed	3
⅓ cup	grated Parmesan cheese	75 mL
Mushroom Stuffing		
1	medium onion, finely chopped	1
1 tbsp	butter	15 mL
½ lb	mushrooms, chopped (about 15)	250 g
½ cup	beef broth	125 mL
1 tbsp	chopped fresh dill (*or* 1 tsp/5 mL dried dillweed)	15 mL
3	slices white bread, crusts removed	3
	Salt and black pepper	

1. Halve tomatoes and hollow out using small spoon or melon baller. Slice each zucchini into six 1-inch (2.5 cm) pieces; hollow out, leaving bottom ¼ inch (5 mm) thick. (If desired, before slicing zucchini, use vegetable peeler to cut lengthwise strips down zucchini to give striped effect.) Stuff with 1 of the stuffing mixtures.

2. *Provençale Stuffing:* In a skillet, sauté onions, garlic and parsley in olive oil for about 3 minutes; remove from heat. Finely chop bread; add to onion mixture. Stir in cheese. Fill vegetables; place in baking pan. Bake in preheated oven for 10 to 15 minutes or until heated through and lightly browned.

3. *Mushroom Stuffing:* In a skillet, sauté onion in butter for 2 minutes. Add mushrooms; cook for about 2 minutes longer. Stir in beef broth and dill; bring to a boil, stirring until slightly thickened. Remove from heat. Finely chop bread; stir into mushroom mixture. Season with salt and pepper to taste. Fill vegetables; place in baking pan. Bake in preheated oven for 10 to 15 minutes or until heated through.

Stuffed Tomatoes

PER SERVING
Calories: 112

Dietary Fiber: 3 g	Carbohydrate: 14 g
Fat: 4 g	Protein: 5 g

Stuffed Zucchinis

PER SERVING
Calories: 62

Dietary Fiber: 1 g	Carbohydrate: 9 g
Fat: 2 g	Protein: 2 g

Italian Broiled Tomatoes

Preheat broiler
Shallow baking pan

2	large tomatoes	2
Pinch	garlic powder	Pinch
1 tbsp	chopped fresh parsley	15 mL
1 tsp	dried basil	5 mL
½ tsp	dried oregano	2 mL
	Freshly ground black pepper to taste	
2 tbsp	bread crumbs	25 mL

1. Cut tomatoes in half crosswise. Place cut side up on rack in shallow baking pan. Sprinkle lightly with garlic powder. Combine parsley, seasonings and bread crumbs. Divide mixture over surface of tomato halves.

2. Place pan about 6 inches (15 cm) below broiler. Broil for 3 to 4 minutes until tomatoes are heated through, or cook on barbecue along with meat being grilled.

PER SERVING
Calories: 30

Dietary Fiber: 1 g	Carbohydrate: 4 g
Fat: 1 g	Protein: 2 g

SERVES 4

Helen Haresign, Dietititan

Serve this often during tomato season to accompany broiled or barbecued meat.

TIP
Fresh tomatoes in season are a real treat. Store underripe tomatoes, unwashed, at room temperature away from sunlight until slightly soft. Room temperature tomatoes will have more flavor than cold ones.

DIETITIAN'S MESSAGE
Red and orange fruits and vegetables are a source of carotenoids, which are being investigated for their benefit in reducing the risk of cancer. Serve this colorful vegetable with fish dishes. Or, for a treat, sprinkle with crumbled Roquefort or any other good blue cheese and serve with grilled steak.

Ralph Graham, Chef
Rosanne E. Maluk,
Dietitian

*In this tasty recipe,
tomatoes serve as the
container for an unusual
fruit-and-nut filling. Serve
at room temperature, or
chilled if desired.*

TIPS

Toasting nuts and seeds
helps to bring out their
flavor. To toast, preheat
oven (350°F/180°C) and
spread nuts or seeds on
a baking sheet. Place in
oven and roast, shaking
pan occasionally, for
5 to 6 minutes. Or toast
in a nonstick skillet
over medium heat,
shaking pan often. Watch
carefully.

Sultanas are usually larger
and paler than most
raisins and have a slightly
higher acid content. If
you can't find sultanas,
use any other variety of
raisin instead.

DIETITIAN'S MESSAGE

These unusual
tomatoes make a great
accompaniment for
barbecued meat and
will add vitamin C to
your diet.

Sweet Baked Tomatoes

Preheat oven to 325°F (160°C)
Baking dish

4	medium tomatoes	4
¼ cup	sultana raisins	50 mL
¼ cup	currants	50 mL
2 tbsp	liquid honey	25 mL
1 tbsp	lemon juice	15 mL
¼ tsp	ground cinnamon	1 mL
¼ tsp	ground ginger	1 mL
¼ cup	chopped walnuts *or* pecans, lightly toasted (see Tip, at left)	50 mL
	Salt	
½ cup	apple cider *or* juice	125 mL
	Grated orange zest *or* 4 mint leaves	

1. Slice tops off tomatoes; seed, scoop out pulp and reserve. Invert tomato shells on paper towels to drain for at least 15 minutes.

2. In a bowl, coarsely mash tomato pulp; stir in raisins, currants, honey, lemon juice, cinnamon and ginger. Refrigerate for 1 hour to allow flavors to blend. Stir in nuts.

3. Sprinkle inside of each tomato shell lightly with salt; evenly spoon in raisin mixture. Place in small baking dish or pie plate; drizzle cider over and around tomatoes. Bake in preheated oven for 15 to 20 minutes or just until soft.

4. With slotted spoon, transfer tomatoes to serving dish or small individual dishes, reserving juice. Cover tomatoes and juice; refrigerate for at least 2 hours or until thoroughly chilled. At serving time, drizzle some juice over each tomato and garnish with orange zest or mint.

PER SERVING	
Calories: 177	
Dietary Fiber: 3 g	Carbohydrate: 34 g
Fat: 5 g	Protein: 3 g

Oven-Dried Tomatoes

Preheat oven to 200°F (100°C)
Wire rack
Baking pan

2 tbsp	dried basil	25 mL
2 tbsp	dried parsley	25 mL
	Salt and black pepper	
12	plum tomatoes, halved	12

1. Mix together basil, parsley, and salt and pepper to taste; sprinkle on tomatoes. Place cut side up on wire rack over baking pan. Bake in preheated oven for 6 hours.

PER SERVING	
Calories: 26	
Dietary Fiber: 2 g	Carbohydrate: 6 g
Fat: Trace	Protein: 1 g

**SERVES 6 AS
A SIDE DISH**

**Wayne Fagan, Chef
Mary Margaret Laing,
Dietitian**

These tasty tomatoes can be used as a substitute for sun-dried tomatoes.

DIETITIAN'S MESSAGE

No one food is the proverbial magic bullet that will produce good health. Eating a mixed and balanced diet rich in nutrients and fiber is the real key to healthy living.

Orange Broccoli

2 tbsp	orange juice	25 mL
2 tsp	lemon juice	10 mL
1 tbsp	vegetable oil	15 mL
1½ tsp	granulated sugar	7 mL
½ tsp	crushed dried basil	2 mL
¼ tsp	coarsely ground black pepper	1 mL
¼ tsp	Dijon mustard	1 mL
1	bunch broccoli florets, blanched	1
2 tbsp	unsalted shelled sunflower seeds, toasted	25 mL

1. Whisk first 7 ingredients until blended.

2. Drizzle mixture over broccoli. Cover and heat until warm. Sprinkle with sunflower seeds.

PER SERVING	
Calories: 57	
Dietary Fiber: 2 g	Carbohydrate: 4 g
Fat: 4 g	Protein: 2 g

SERVES 6

**Murray Henderson, Chef
Carole Doucet Love,
Dietitian**

Citrus juice, mustard, herbs and spices give broccoli a new taste

TIP

If you don't have sunflower seeds on hand, substitute toasted nuts such as pine nuts, walnuts or almonds. See page 151 for instructions on blanching vegetables.

DIETITIAN'S MESSAGE

The snappy combination of broccoli and fruit juices is rich in folic acid as well as vitamin C. Serve with Party-Style Lamb (see recipe, page 270) for an elegant meal.

Top potatoes and broccoli with nippy Cheddar cheese for a comforting and homey casserole.

TIP
Don't throw away broccoli stems. Peel off the outer coat and slice thinly. Cook as for florets.

DIETITIAN'S MESSAGE
This creamy, fiber-rich casserole can be served with plainer meats such as grilled chicken. Made with cheese and milk, it is a great way to add calcium to your diet. If you are lactose-intolerant, use lactose-reduced milk or a fortified soy beverage.

Cheesy Broccoli and Potato Casserole

Preheat oven to 350°F (180°C)
8-cup (2 L) baking dish, lightly greased

6	medium potatoes, cubed	6
¼ cup	2% milk	50 mL
1 tsp	butter *or* margarine	5 mL
½ tsp	white pepper	2 mL
½ tsp	dried parsley	2 mL
2 cups	broccoli florets	500 mL
1	small onion, sliced	1
1 cup	shredded old Cheddar cheese	250 mL

1. In a large saucepan, cook potatoes in boiling water until tender; drain well. Mash potatoes with milk, butter and seasonings.

2. Meanwhile, steam broccoli and onion until barely tender, or microwave on High for 5 to 8 minutes.

3. Spread potato mixture in lightly greased 8-cup (2 L) baking dish; top with broccoli, onion and cheese. Bake, covered, in preheated oven for 10 minutes; remove cover and bake for 5 minutes longer or until cheese is melted. Or microwave, covered, on High for about 8 minutes.

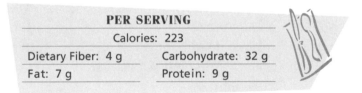

PER SERVING	
Calories: 223	
Dietary Fiber: 4 g	Carbohydrate: 32 g
Fat: 7 g	Protein: 9 g

Quick Steamed Fish Fillets with ➤
Potatoes and Asparagus (page 325)

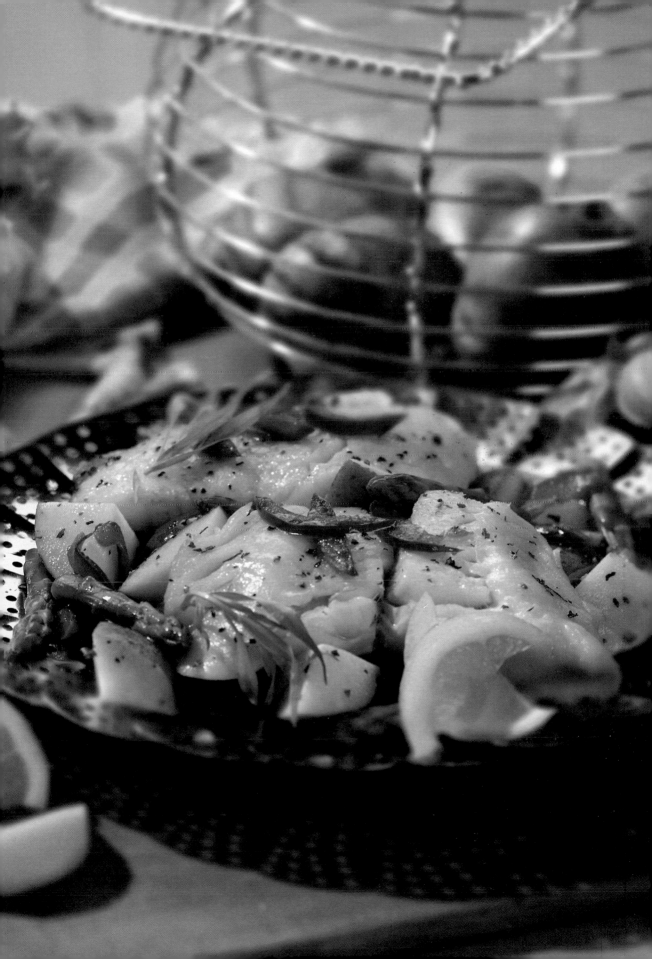

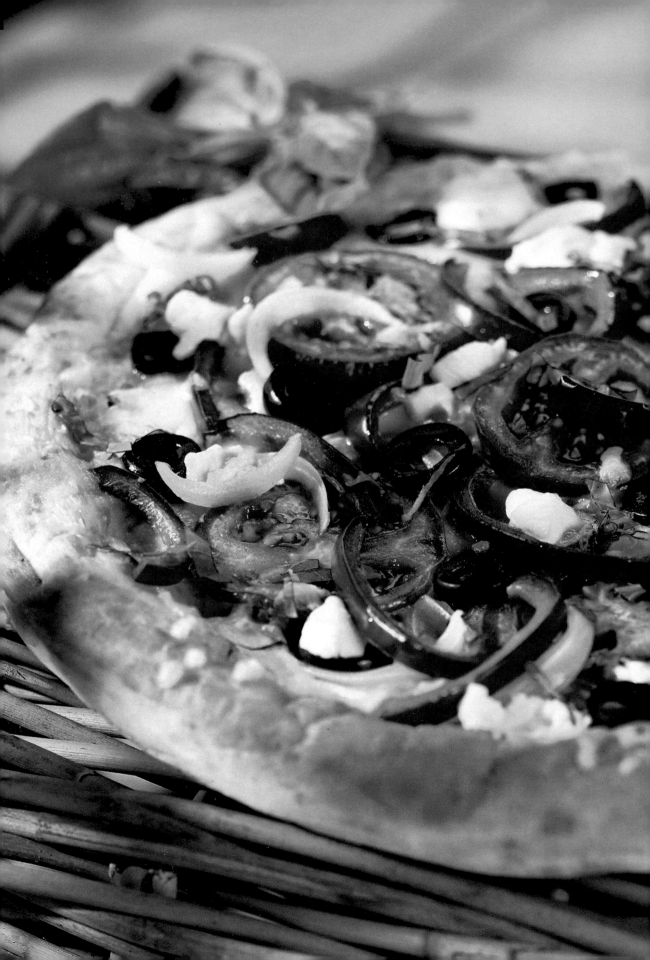

Cauliflower Casserole

Preheat oven to 375°F (190°C)
11- by 7-inch (2 L) shallow baking dish, greased

6 cups	cauliflower florets	1.5 L
1 tbsp	butter	15 mL
2 tbsp	all-purpose flour	25 mL
½ tsp	dry mustard	2 mL
1¼ cups	milk	300 mL
1 cup	shredded Swiss *or* Cheddar cheese	250 mL
¼ tsp	salt	1 mL
¼ tsp	black pepper	1 mL
½ cup	cornflakes crumbs	125 mL
2 tsp	butter, melted	10 mL

1. In a large saucepan, cook cauliflower in boiling water for 3 to 4 minutes or until just barely tender-crisp; drain and place in prepared baking dish.

2. In another saucepan, melt butter over medium heat; stir in flour and mustard. Whisk in milk and cook, stirring constantly, until mixture boils and thickens. Remove from heat; stir in cheese. Add salt and pepper. Pour mixture evenly over cauliflower.

3. In a small bowl, combine crumbs and butter; sprinkle over top of cauliflower mixture. Bake in preheated oven for 10 to 15 minutes or until heated through.

PER SERVING	
Calories: 193	
Dietary Fiber: 2 g	Carbohydrate: 18 g
Fat: 10 g	Protein: 10 g

SERVES 6
....
Dairy Farmers of Canada

This casserole is simple to prepare yet elegant enough for entertaining.

TIP
Replace the cauliflower with broccoli or use a combination of broccoli and cauliflower, if desired.

MAKE AHEAD
Casserole can be made up to 1 day ahead and refrigerated. Remove from fridge 30 minutes before baking and increase baking time by about 5 minutes.

DIETITIAN'S MESSAGE
When cooking vegetables, use as little water as possible or steam them. Water-soluble vitamins are lost in cooking water. You can also use the water in which you cooked vegetables to make soups. Serve this side dish with Sesame Steak (see recipe, page 251) for a protein-rich meal.

Spinach Fancy

No one will have to tell you to eat your spinach anymore! You will be more than willing to enjoy this tasty dish, which is particularly good with fish.

TIP

Use fresh herbs to replace any of the dried herbs in this recipe, but double or triple the amounts as the drying process intensifies the flavor of herbs.

DIETITIAN'S MESSAGE

Like all dark, leafy greens, spinach is a source of vitamin A, folic acid and non-heme iron. When consuming foods that contain iron, avoid drinking caffeinated beverages, such as coffee, tea or cola, for at least an hour as caffeine can reduce the body's ability to absorb iron.

1	pkg (10 oz/300 g) fresh spinach	1
3 tbsp	raisins	45 mL
Pinch	dried mint	Pinch
Pinch	ground fennel	Pinch
Pinch	dried oregano	Pinch
1 tbsp	butter *or* margarine	15 mL
2 tbsp	water	25 mL
1 tsp	lemon juice	5 mL
½ tsp	salt	2 mL
Pinch	black pepper	Pinch
	Lemon slices	

1. Wash spinach and dry thoroughly; remove stems and chop.

2. In a large skillet over medium heat, cook raisins, mint, fennel and oregano in butter. Add spinach and water; cover and steam for 2 to 3 minutes or until wilted. Drain liquid. Sprinkle with lemon juice, salt and pepper; toss well. Serve with lemon slices.

PER SERVING	
Calories: 50	
Dietary Fiber: 1 g	Carbohydrate: 7 g
Fat: 2 g	Protein: 2 g

Sautéed Spinach with Pine Nuts

2 tsp	olive oil	10 mL
¼ cup	pine nuts	50 mL
1	pkg (10 oz/300 g) fresh spinach, trimmed	1
1 tsp	minced garlic	5 mL
1 tsp	lemon juice	5 mL
⅛ tsp	ground nutmeg	0.5 mL
	Black pepper	

1. In a large nonstick skillet, heat 1 tsp (5 mL) of the oil over medium heat. Add pine nuts and cook, stirring constantly, for 2 to 3 minutes or until golden. Remove pine nuts from pan and set aside.

2. Add remaining oil to pan. Add spinach in several bunches (it will cook down quickly), stirring constantly. Add garlic and cook for 1 to 2 minutes. Stir in lemon juice and nutmeg. Season with pepper to taste. Add reserved pine nuts. Cook until heated through.

PER SERVING	
Calories: 90	
Dietary Fiber: 3 g	Carbohydrate: 4 g
Fat: 8 g	Protein: 4 g

SERVES 4
....
Bev Callaghan, Dietitian

This is an easy way to add flavor to spinach. You can substitute Swiss chard, kale, rapini or mustard greens for the spinach. If you don't have pine nuts, try pecans or walnuts.

TIP

Stir-frying vegetables is a great way to preserve nutrients. When boiled, vegetables can lose up to 45% of vitamin C compared with losing only 5% when stir-fried.

DIETITIAN'S MESSAGE

Women who are pregnant or thinking of becoming pregnant need more iron and folic acid. Serve this dish with Beef Stroganoff (see recipe, page 250) and noodles, and both nutrients will be present in spades.

Here's a great way to turn a family favorite into company fare.

TIP

Try this with other frozen vegetables such as mixed vegetables or green beans. If desired, use 1 tbsp (15 mL) chopped fresh dill instead of the dried; stir in with the water chestnuts and pimiento.

DIETITIAN'S MESSAGE

Consuming the recommended amount of fiber can be a challenge. One serving of this side dish provides only 3 g of the 25 to 35 g that are recommended daily. Serve with a main course such as a legume to increase fiber.

Deluxe Peas

1 tbsp	butter *or* margarine	15 mL
1 tsp	chicken bouillon powder	5 mL
2 tbsp	water	25 mL
1½ cups	sliced mushrooms	375 mL
1 cup	diagonally sliced celery	250 mL
½ tsp	dried dillweed	2 mL
¼ tsp	curry powder	1 mL
2 cups	frozen peas	500 mL
¾ cup	sliced water chestnuts	175 mL
2 tbsp	chopped pimiento *or* red bell pepper (optional)	25 mL

1. In a large skillet over medium heat, melt butter; stir in chicken bouillon powder, water, mushrooms, celery and seasonings; cook for about 6 minutes or until vegetables are almost tender. Stir in peas; cook, covered, for 2 minutes. Add water chestnuts and pimiento, if using; cook, stirring occasionally, for about 1 minute or until heated through.

PER SERVING	
Calories: 83	
Dietary Fiber: 3 g	Carbohydrate: 13 g
Fat: 2 g	Protein: 3 g

Apple-Stuffed Squash

Preheat oven to 375°F (190°C)
Shallow baking pan

2	acorn squash	2
2 cups	unsweetened applesauce	500 mL
½ cup	raisins	125 mL
¼ cup	liquid honey *or* molasses	50 mL
¼ cup	chopped walnuts	50 mL
1 tbsp	butter *or* margarine	15 mL
1 tbsp	grated lemon zest	15 mL
2 tsp	lemon juice	10 mL
¼ tsp	ground cinnamon	1 mL

1. Cut squash in half; remove seeds. Combine applesauce, raisins, honey and walnuts. Fill squash with mixture; dot each squash with butter. Sprinkle with lemon zest, juice and cinnamon.

2. Place filled squash in shallow baking pan; pour in hot water to ¼-inch (1 cm) depth. Bake, covered, in preheated oven for 30 minutes; uncover and bake for another 20 minutes or until squash is tender.

PER SERVING	
Calories: 323	
Dietary Fiber: 6 g	Carbohydrate: 68 g
Fat: 8 g	Protein: 4 g

SERVES 4
....
Irene Mofina

Squash, a favorite fall vegetable, makes a wonderful container for rice, meats or fruit. This version is particularly tasty served with pork.

TIP
Have you ever wrestled with a large hard-shelled squash trying to cut it into pieces? Here's a technique that simplifies the chore. First, split off the stem. Then, using a large, sharp knife, pierce the skin of the squash where you want to cut it. Insert the knife slightly into the squash and tap it several times with a hammer or meat mallet. The squash should split open. Alternatively, place the squash in the microwave and cook on High for 2 minutes. Then cut.

DIETITIAN'S MESSAGE
Squash is rich in beta-carotene, a form of vitamin A, which promotes healthy tissues and cells.

·······················

Hans Hartman, Chef
Donna Antonishak,
Dietitian

In this tasty and unusual recipe, thin slices of zucchini double for spaghetti and are topped with both white and tomato sauces.

TIPS

If available, substitute 1 tbsp (15 mL) chopped fresh basil for the dried. You may also use 1 cup (250 mL) homemade tomato sauce, such as Versatile Tomato Sauce (see recipe, page 179), if desired.

Replace the wine with chicken stock, if you prefer.

DIETITIAN'S MESSAGE

This recipe is a great way to get kids — and adults — to eat their recommended daily servings from the Vegetables and Fruit group. Make this a meal with whole-grain bread, a selection of cheeses and fruit for dessert.

Saucy Zucchini Spaghetti

4	medium zucchini, trimmed	4
1 tbsp	butter	15 mL
White Sauce		
1 tbsp	butter	15 mL
½ cup	finely chopped carrots	125 mL
¼ tsp	crushed dried thyme	1 mL
1	bay leaf	1
½ cup	dry white wine	125 mL
1 tbsp	all-purpose flour	15 mL
1½ cups	2% milk	375 mL
1 tbsp	lemon juice	15 mL
1 tsp	chopped fresh chives *or* green onion	5 mL
¼ tsp	each salt and black pepper	1 mL
Tomato Sauce		
1	can (7½ oz/213 mL) tomato sauce	1
1 tsp	dried basil	5 mL

1. Cut zucchini lengthwise into very thin slices; cut into thin spaghetti-like strands. Set aside.

2. *White Sauce:* In a skillet, melt butter over medium heat; add carrots, thyme and bay leaf. Cover and cook for 3 to 5 minutes, stirring occasionally. Add wine; simmer, uncovered, until wine is reduced by half. Dissolve flour in milk; stir into skillet and bring to a boil. Simmer until slightly thickened. Remove bay leaf. Pour into food processor and blend until smooth. Add lemon juice, chives, salt and pepper; keep warm.

3. *Tomato Sauce:* In a small saucepan, gently bring tomato sauce and basil to a boil; keep warm.

4. In a large skillet, melt butter over medium-high heat; sauté zucchini for about 2 minutes or until slightly softened. Do not overcook. Drain off any liquid.

5. To serve, divide zucchini among 4 plates; swirl with fork. Top with white sauce; drizzle with tomato sauce.

PER SERVING	
Calories: 161	
Dietary Fiber: 4 g	Carbohydrate: 18 g
Fat: 8 g	Protein: 5 g

Carrot Rolls

Preheat oven to 350°F (180°C)
Baking sheet, lightly greased

8 cups	sliced carrots	2 L
3 cups	fresh bread crumbs	750 mL
2 cups	shredded Cheddar cheese	500 mL
	Salt, black pepper and ground nutmeg to taste	
2	egg whites	2
1 cup	crushed cornflakes (about 3 cups/750 mL cornflakes)	250 mL
	Fresh parsley sprigs	

1. Steam carrots for about 10 minutes or until soft. Drain and mash well. Add bread crumbs, cheese and seasonings.

2. Beat egg whites until stiff; fold into carrot mixture. Shape mixture into twenty-four 2-inch (5 cm) long rolls. Roll in crushed cornflakes. Place on nonstick or lightly greased baking sheet. Bake in preheated oven for about 20 minutes or until browned. Serve garnished with parsley.

PER SERVING

Calories: 159	
Dietary Fiber: 2 g	Carbohydrate: 18 g
Fat: 7 g	Protein: 7 g

SERVES 12
Makes 24 rolls

Laura M. Hawthorn

P

Here's a simple and appealing way to dress up an everyday vegetable. Potatoes work equally well in this recipe, so try a potato version for a change.

TIP

This recipe makes 24 rolls, a large quantity, but they freeze very well. So make lots and keep them on hand for busy evenings.

DIETITIAN'S MESSAGE

Kids will love this simple but delicious transformation of the lowly carrot. If you are concerned about fat, look for cheese with 20% M.F. or less. The M.F. represents the milk fat in the cheese.

Honey-Glazed Carrots

1 lb	carrots, cut into 1-inch (2.5 cm) pieces	500 g
1 tbsp	liquid honey *or* brown sugar	15 mL
1 tbsp	orange juice	15 mL
2 tsp	butter *or* margarine	10 mL
½ tsp	ground ginger	2 mL
½ tsp	grated orange zest (optional)	2 mL

1. In a medium saucepan over high heat, boil carrots until tender-crisp; drain. Add honey, orange juice, butter, ginger and, if using, orange zest. Quickly stir for 2 to 3 minutes or until glaze forms.

PER SERVING	
Calories: 77	
Dietary Fiber: 2 g	Carbohydrate: 16 g
Fat: 2 g	Protein: 1 g

Sweet Potato "Fries"

Preheat oven to 375°F (190°C)
Nonstick baking sheet

1 lb	sweet potatoes, each cut lengthwise into 6 wedges	500 g
2 tsp	vegetable oil	10 mL
¼ tsp	paprika	1 mL
⅛ tsp	garlic powder	0.5 mL
	Black pepper	

1. Place potatoes in a bowl. Add oil, paprika and garlic powder. Season with pepper to taste. Toss to coat. Transfer to baking sheet. Bake in preheated oven for 25 minutes or until tender and golden, turning once.

PER SERVING	
Calories: 105	
Dietary Fiber: 2 g	Carbohydrate: 20 g
Fat: 2 g	Protein: 1 g

Parsnip Scallop

Preheat oven to 375°F (190°C)
Shallow baking dish, lightly greased

1½ lb	parsnips, cut into coins, *or* combination of sliced parsnips and carrots	750 g
¼ cup	chopped onion	50 mL
3 tbsp	butter *or* margarine	45 mL
3 tbsp	all-purpose flour	45 mL
1 tsp	granulated sugar	5 mL
½ tsp	dried basil	2 mL
½ tsp	salt	2 mL
Pinch	black pepper	Pinch
2 cups	tomato juice	500 mL
½ cup	dried bread crumbs	125 mL
1 tbsp	melted butter *or* margarine	15 mL

1. Cook parsnips in boiling water for 5 to 10 minutes or just until tender (do not overcook as they fall apart and become mushy); drain well.

2. In a skillet over medium-high heat, cook onion in butter for about 5 minutes. Blend in flour, sugar and seasonings. Gradually add tomato juice; cook, stirring constantly, for about 5 minutes or until thickened.

3. Combine parsnips and tomato sauce in lightly greased casserole. Mix bread crumbs and melted butter; sprinkle over parsnips. Bake in preheated oven for 15 minutes or until browned.

PER SERVING	
Calories: 225	
Dietary Fiber: 5 g	Carbohydrate: 37 g
Fat: 8 g	Protein: 4 g

SERVES 6
Irene Ferguson

This scallop of parsnips is equally good using a combination of parsnips and carrots. The addition of the small amount of sugar heightens the natural sweetness of the vegetables.

TIP
Peel parsnips before using in this recipe. Parsnips perform best when they are precooked, then finished in a sauce.

DIETITIAN'S MESSAGE
The creamy sauce used in this recipe makes it a higher-fat vegetable choice. Balance this selection with Fish Roll-Ups (see recipe, page 322) for protein, and brown rice and green peas to add dietary fiber.

The maple syrup in this recipe makes sweet-tasting vegetables that even children will enjoy.

FOOD FAST
For a quick vegetable fix, cut a fresh tomato in half; sprinkle with dry bread crumbs, dried herbs and Parmesan cheese. Bake in 350°F (180°C) oven for 20 minutes as you prepare the rest of dinner.

DIETITIAN'S MESSAGE
Not only does roasting vegetables add a sweet smoky taste, more nutrients are preserved than when they are boiled. Serve these delicious winter vegetables with Fish Fillets with Basil Walnut Sauce (see recipe, page 323) and end the meal with Lemon Pudding (see recipe, page 425).

Roasted Carrots and Parsnips

Preheat oven to 400°F (200°C)
13- by 9-inch (3 L) baking dish, greased

1 lb	parsnips, peeled and cut into 1-inch (2.5 cm) pieces	500 g
1 lb	carrots, peeled and cut into 1-inch (2.5 cm) pieces	500 g
1	large onion, cut into wedges	1
2 tbsp	vegetable oil	25 mL
1 tsp	dried thyme	5 mL
2 tbsp	maple syrup	25 mL
1 tbsp	Dijon mustard	15 mL

1. Place parsnips, carrots, onions, oil and thyme in prepared baking dish; toss until vegetables are well coated with oil. Roast in preheated oven for 30 minutes.

2. Meanwhile, in a small bowl, combine maple syrup and mustard. Pour over vegetables; toss to coat. Roast for another 20 to 25 minutes or until vegetables are tender and golden, stirring once.

PER SERVING	
Calories: 113	
Dietary Fiber: 3 g	Carbohydrate: 20 g
Fat: 4 g	Protein: 1 g

Sautéed Vegetables

¼ cup	sliced onion	50 mL
1 tbsp	olive oil	15 mL
1 cup	broccoli florets	250 mL
1 cup	cauliflower florets	250 mL
1 cup	cubed zucchini	250 mL
½ cup	chopped raw beets	125 mL
1 cup	chicken broth	250 mL
1 cup	chopped Swiss chard *or* spinach (optional)	250 mL
1 cup	chopped tomatoes	250 mL
2 tbsp	water	25 mL
2 tsp	cornstarch	10 mL
	Salt and black pepper to taste	

1. In a large skillet over medium-high heat, cook onion in hot oil for about 5 minutes. Add broccoli, cauliflower, zucchini, beets and chicken broth. Cook, covered, for about 3 minutes or until tender-crisp.

2. Stir in chard, if using, and tomatoes. Mix together water, cornstarch and seasonings; stir into vegetable mixture. Cook for about 2 minutes or until thickened.

PER SERVING	
Calories: 53	
Dietary Fiber: 2 g	Carbohydrate: 6 g
Fat: 3 g	Protein: 2 g

SERVES 6

Jeanette Snowden

Chopped beets add an attractive rosy red color to this dish. Serve this colorful mix of vegetables over white rice.

TIPS

Fresh beets are delicious steamed or cold in salads. To maximize flavor and nutrition, cut the green tops from beets, leaving at least 1 inch (2.5 cm) attached. Don't remove the root end. This prevents the beet color and vitamins from being lost in the cooking water. Once the beets are cooked, rinse under cold water and slide off the skins, using rubber gloves if desired.

If the beet greens are fresh and crisp, they make a great addition to salads.

DIETITIAN'S MESSAGE

This colorful array of vegetables will add eye appeal to many dishes while providing lots of fiber, vitamins and minerals. The vitamin C in this recipe will enhance the absorption of iron from non-meat sources. Try serving this tasty mélange over whole-wheat pasta for a fiber-rich main course.

Raymond Colliver, Chef
Dani Flowerday,
Dietitian

*Stir-fries are a great
solution for busy
weeknights. Not only are
they quick and easy, you
can mix and match
vegetables to suit
whatever is in your crisper.*

TIP

You'll find shiitake
mushrooms in the
produce or specialty
section of most
supermarkets. If using
dried mushrooms,
rehydrate for 15 minutes
in 1 cup (250 mL) boiling
water. Discard the stems
before slicing. Strain the
soaking liquid and use it
instead of chicken or
vegetable broth in the
recipe, if desired.

DIETITIAN'S MESSAGE

Stir-frying is an easy way
to enjoy an abundance of
vegetables that provide
us with valuable vitamins,
minerals and antioxidants.
In addition to adding
flavor without fat,
garlic and some other
seasonings are thought
to have disease-fighting
properties. To make this
recipe into a meal, serve
with steamed rice and
South Side Halibut (see
recipe, page 314).
Complete the meal with
a choice from the Milk
Products food group,
such as frozen yogurt.

Stir-Fried Mixed Vegetables

12 oz	Chinese cabbage *or* bok choy	375 g
2 tbsp	vegetable oil	25 mL
2	cloves garlic, minced	2
3 to 4 tsp	grated ginger root	15 to 20 mL
2 cups	carrots, julienned	500 mL
8	black Chinese *or* shiitake mushrooms, sliced	8
1	can (5½ oz/156 mL) sliced bamboo shoots (optional)	1
1	can (14 oz/398 mL) baby corn cobs, drained and halved	1
4	green onions, sliced diagonally	4
1 cup	chicken *or* vegetable broth	250 mL
2 tbsp	sodium-reduced soy sauce	25 mL
4 tsp	cornstarch	20 mL
2 tbsp	cold water	25 mL

1. Trim cabbage, cutting center rib into 2-inch (5 cm) chunks; slice leaves into strips.

2. In a large wok or skillet, heat oil over medium-high heat; cook garlic and ginger root, stirring, for 30 seconds. Add cabbage ribs and carrot; stir-fry for 2 to 3 minutes. Add mushrooms, bamboo shoots, if using, corn and green onions; stir-fry for 2 minutes. Add sliced cabbage leaves, broth and soy sauce; cook, stirring, for 1 to 2 minutes or until vegetables are tender-crisp. Mix cornstarch with water; slowly add to broth, stirring constantly until thickened.

PER SERVING	
Calories: 113	
Dietary Fiber: 3 g	Carbohydrate: 15 g
Fat: 5 g	Protein: 4 g

Fried Chinese Mushrooms

SERVES 4
....
Jon Paudler, Chef
Leslie Maze, Dietitian

4	green onions	4
10	large dried shiitake mushrooms	10
½ cup	water	125 mL
4 tsp	cornstarch	20 mL
1 tsp	granulated sugar	5 mL
1 tsp	rice vinegar	5 mL
3½ tsp	tamari sauce *or* soy sauce	17 mL
¼ tsp	sesame oil	1 mL
Pinch	5-spice powder	Pinch
	Vegetable oil for frying	
1	slice ginger root	1
½	head iceberg lettuce, shredded	½

1. Cut green portion of onions lengthwise into slivers, without detaching from white part. Soak in bowl of water until slivers have curled. Soak mushrooms in medium bowl of water until soft, about 30 minutes.

2. Meanwhile, in a small saucepan, combine water, 1 tsp (5 mL) of the cornstarch, sugar, vinegar, ½ tsp (2 mL) of the tamari sauce and sesame oil. Bring to a boil and cook until thickened; set aside.

3. Drain and rinse mushrooms; squeeze out excess water. Discard stems; slice caps into strips. Toss with 3 tsp (15 mL) of the tamari sauce; sprinkle with 5-spice powder and toss to coat. Roll mushrooms in remaining cornstarch.

4. In a wok or frying pan, heat ¼ inch (5 mm) oil to 350°F (180°C). Fry ginger root until lightly browned; discard. In small batches, fry mushroom strips until crisp, gently stirring with fork to prevent sticking. Drain on paper towels.

5. Place bed of lettuce on 4 individual plates. Rewarm sauce, then toss mushroom strips in sauce. Place strips on lettuce; drizzle with sauce. Garnish with curled green onion.

In this recipe, slices of meaty Chinese mushrooms are coated with seasoning and cornstarch, then fried in oil until brown. This dish can be served as an appetizer or as a tasty accompaniment to grilled meat.

TIP

Five-spice powder is available in Asian markets or the specialty foods section of some supermarkets. Although dried shiitake mushrooms are available in most supermarkets, they are much more economical if purchased in Asian markets.

DIETITIAN'S MESSAGE

The secret to low-fat deep-frying is proper coating with cornstarch. If all of the mushroom is coated, very little fat will penetrate the food.

PER SERVING	
Calories: 79	
Dietary Fiber: 2 g	Carbohydrate: 12 g
Fat: 3 g	Protein: 2 g

Souvlaki usually consists of cubes of lamb or pork that are grilled on skewers then served on a bun. For a light luncheon, serve this vegetable version with rice and pita bread. The Feta Tzatziki provides more than a hint of garlic!

TIPS
Soak bamboo skewers in water for 30 minutes before using to prevent them from burning.

Vegetables tend to slip when placed on skewers. Try using 2 skewers for each kebab to provide good balance and make turning easier when grilling. To ensure even cooking, allow some space between the vegetables when threading them on the skewers. Cook over medium-low heat and turn frequently to prevent the tomatoes from bursting open.

DIETITIAN'S MESSAGE

This vegetable souvlaki is a tasty way to boost your intake of fiber and provide some bone-building calcium. The Feta Tzatziki is an interesting variation on the Greek dip. Garlic, which may have disease-fighting properties, adds loads of flavor without fat.

Vegetable Souvlaki with Feta Tzatziki

12 bamboo skewers

24	each cherry tomatoes and mushrooms	24
1	each large red and green bell pepper, cut into 1-inch (2.5 cm) squares	1
2	red onions, cut into wedges	2
1	can (14 oz/398 mL) artichoke hearts, drained and halved	1

Marinade

½ cup	olive oil	125 mL
2 tbsp	lemon juice	25 mL
1 tbsp	minced garlic	15 mL
2 tsp	crushed dried oregano	10 mL
1 tsp	crushed dried mint	5 mL
1 tsp	black pepper	5 mL
Pinch	red pepper flakes	Pinch

Feta Tzatziki

1½ cups	lower-fat plain yogurt	375 mL
½ cup	grated English cucumber	125 mL
½ cup	crumbled feta cheese	125 mL
1	large clove garlic, minced	1
2 tbsp	lemon juice	25 mL

1. Dividing evenly and alternating vegetables, thread tomatoes, mushrooms, red and green peppers, onions and artichoke hearts onto 12 bamboo skewers.

2. *Marinade:* In a large shallow nonmetallic dish, combine oil, lemon juice, garlic, oregano, mint, pepper and red pepper flakes; add skewers, turning to coat well. Chill for 3 to 6 hours, turning occasionally.

3. *Feta Tzatziki:* In a serving bowl, combine yogurt, cucumber, feta, garlic and lemon juice; refrigerate.

4. Remove souvlaki from marinade. Grill over medium heat for 10 minutes. Or bake on greased baking sheet in 425°F (220°C) oven for 15 minutes. Serve with Feta Tzatziki.

PER SERVING	
Calories: 262	
Dietary Fiber: 7 g	Carbohydrate: 31 g
Fat: 13 g	Protein: 10 g

Golden Mushroom Sauté

1 tsp	olive oil	5 mL
1	medium onion, chopped	1
2	cloves garlic, minced	2
1¼ lb	chanterelle *or* portobello mushrooms, sliced	625 g
½ lb	small button mushrooms	250 g
3	sun-dried tomatoes, softened and chopped	3
¾ cup	chicken broth	175 mL
½ cup	dry white wine	125 mL
2 tbsp	lemon juice	25 mL
1 tbsp	sweet Hungarian paprika	15 mL
½ tsp	caraway seeds	2 mL
	Salt and black pepper	
2 tbsp	chopped fresh parsley	25 mL

1. In a large skillet, heat oil over medium heat; cook onion, stirring, for 2 minutes. Add garlic, chanterelle and button mushrooms and tomatoes; cook for 2 to 3 minutes.

2. Add chicken broth, wine, lemon juice, paprika and caraway seeds; bring to a boil. Simmer over low heat for about 15 minutes or until slightly thickened, stirring occasionally. Season with salt and pepper to taste. Sprinkle with parsley.

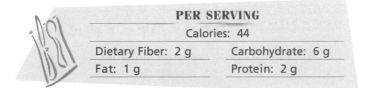

PER SERVING

Calories: 44

Dietary Fiber: 2 g	Carbohydrate: 6 g
Fat: 1 g	Protein: 2 g

SERVES 8 AS A SIDE DISH

Hans Anderegg, Chef
Cheryl Turnbull-Bruce, Dietitian

This sauté has a great mix of herbs and spices, and the result is spectacular flavor with little fat. Serve either as a side dish or on rice as a main dish.

TIP
To soften sun-dried tomatoes, cover with boiling water and let stand for 10 minutes. Drain well.

DIETITIAN'S MESSAGE
For a special meal, serve this delicious sauté with Aphrodite's Pasta (see recipe, page 188).

Turnip Soufflé

The idea, prevalent in many circles, that soufflés are difficult to make is a bit of a myth. Just ensure that the egg whites are stiff, and don't open the oven to peek until you're certain the dish is almost done. Cooked turnip and squash are both excellent in this delicately flavored dish, which is almost a meal in itself.

TIP

For best results when beating egg whites, bring them to room temperature and beat them in a copper or ceramic bowl. Make sure that there is no yolk in the bowl as even a speck will prevent the whites from forming peaks.

DIETITIAN'S MESSAGE

To make this delicious soufflé the centerpiece of a lunch or light meal, serve with Tomato Mozzarella Salad (see recipe, page 148) and crusty bread.

Preheat oven to 375°F (190°C)
6-cup (1.5 L) baking dish, lightly greased

½ cup	chopped onion	125 mL
1 tbsp	melted butter *or* margarine, divided	15 mL
3 cups	cooked mashed turnip	750 mL
2	eggs, separated	2
¼ cup	skim milk	50 mL
3 tbsp	all-purpose flour	45 mL
1 tbsp	baking powder	15 mL
½ tsp	salt	2 mL
¼ tsp	ground nutmeg	1 mL
Pinch	freshly ground black pepper	Pinch
½ cup	whole-wheat bread crumbs	125 mL

1. Cook onion in a nonstick skillet in 1 tsp (5 mL) butter until tender. Add to mashed turnip.

2. Beat egg whites until stiff; set aside. Beat egg yolks with milk; stir in flour, baking powder and seasonings. Stir egg yolk mixture into mashed turnip. Fold in beaten egg whites.

3. Turn into lightly greased 6-cup (1.5 L) baking dish. Combine bread crumbs and remaining melted butter. Sprinkle over turnip. Bake in preheated oven for about 30 minutes.

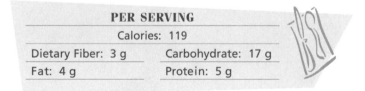

PER SERVING	
Calories: 119	
Dietary Fiber: 3 g	Carbohydrate: 17 g
Fat: 4 g	Protein: 5 g

Vegetable Hodgepodge

12	small red-skinned potatoes (unpeeled)	12
16	baby carrots	16
1 cup	snow peas	250 mL
1 cup	yellow wax beans	250 mL
1 tbsp	all-purpose flour	15 mL
1 cup	2% milk *or* 2% evaporated milk	250 mL
½ tsp	salt	2 mL
¼ tsp	black pepper	1 mL
1 tsp	butter	5 mL

1. In a skillet with small amount of boiling water, cook potatoes, covered, for 10 to 15 minutes or until almost tender. Add carrots; cook for 5 minutes longer. Add snow peas and beans; cook for 3 minutes longer or until all vegetables are tender. Drain.

2. Dissolve flour in milk; stir into vegetables until thickened. Add salt, pepper and butter.

PER SERVING	
Calories: 349	
Dietary Fiber: 7 g	Carbohydrate: 74 g
Fat: 3 g	Protein: 10 g

SERVES 4
....

Howard Selig, Chef
Tricia Cochrane, Dietitian

Hodgepodge is traditionally served as a main dish in Nova Scotia's Annapolis Valley, made with vegetables fresh from the garden.

TIPS
You can substitute frozen peas for the snow peas and green beans for the yellow wax beans.

Although any fresh vegetable can be used in this recipe, traditional hodgepodge uses "early" vegetables.

DIETITIAN'S MESSAGE
To make this hearty one-pot vegetable stew the centerpiece of a meal, add other food groups. Start the meal with Hummus with Tahini (see recipe, page 72) with whole-wheat pita for a serving from the Grain Products group and finish with fruit and yogurt.

Vegetable Stew

1	large onion, quartered and thinly sliced	1
1 tbsp	olive oil	15 mL
8	cloves garlic, chopped	8
2 cups	sliced small zucchini	500 mL
1 cup	diced fresh fennel	250 mL
1	each medium green and red bell pepper, cut into julienne strips	
1	can (28 oz/796 mL) tomatoes, diced	1
1 tsp	fennel seeds	5 mL
1 tsp	salt	5 mL
¼ tsp	black pepper	1 mL

1. In a Dutch oven, sauté onion in oil until tender. Stir in garlic, zucchini, fennel, green and red peppers, tomatoes and fennel seeds; simmer, uncovered, until desired consistency and vegetables are tender, about 15 minutes. Season with salt and pepper.

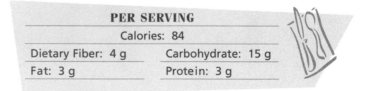

PER SERVING	
Calories: 84	
Dietary Fiber: 4 g	Carbohydrate: 15 g
Fat: 3 g	Protein: 3 g

Leek and Potato Pancakes

Preheat oven to 375°F (180°C)
Baking sheet, greased

4	large baking potatoes, cooked and chilled	4
1 tbsp	butter	15 mL
3	bunches leeks (white part only), coarsely chopped	3
½ cup	water	125 mL
2	eggs, lightly beaten	2
½ tsp	salt	2 mL
¼ tsp	white pepper	1 mL
Pinch	ground nutmeg	Pinch

1. Peel chilled potatoes; grate coarsely.

2. In a skillet, melt butter over medium heat; cook leeks, stirring, for 3 minutes. Add water and bring to a boil; simmer for 2 to 3 minutes. Drain.

3. In a bowl, gently mix together potatoes, leeks, eggs, salt, pepper and nutmeg. Spoon onto greased baking sheet, forming 16 mounds; flatten to ¼-inch (5 mm) thickness. Bake in preheated oven for 10 to 15 minutes or until golden.

PER SERVING	
Calories: 124	
Dietary Fiber: 2 g	Carbohydrate: 22 g
Fat: 3 g	Protein: 4 g

SERVES 8
Makes 16 pancakes
....
Richard Franz, Chef
Susan Sutherland, Dietitian

Pancakes are not just for breakfast. They can be made from many vegetables and, like this savory combination, make a delicious accompaniment to many foods.

TIP

The secret to making these delicious pancakes is cooking the potatoes the day before in their skins, then refrigerating overnight.

DIETITIAN'S MESSAGE

Because they are baked rather than fried, these pancakes are lighter tasting and lower in fat than traditional potato pancakes. They make a very tasty accompaniment to grilled meat or fish, such as Barbecued Butterflied Leg of Lamb (see recipe, page 267) or Cedar-Baked Salmon (see recipe, page 305). Complete the meal with a green salad and serve fruit for dessert.

**Larry DeVries, Chef
Jackie Kopilas, Rachel
Barkley and Heather
Duncan, Dietitians**

*Eight cloves of garlic may
seem overpowering, but
when roasted, garlic
assumes a mellow and
gentle flavor, which
complements the
subtle taste of the
potatoes. The herbs add
additional flavor to this
tasty mixture.*

TIPS

If desired, use 1 tsp (5 mL)
fresh tarragon instead of
the dried.

When mashing potatoes,
be sure to use a potato
masher or a ricer, not a
food processor. A
food processor quickly
over processes the
potatoes, breaking
down their starch content
and producing an
unappetizing, gluey result.

DIETITIAN'S MESSAGE

Don't fall for the myth
that potatoes are
fattening. It is usually the
topping or sauce that
adds calories and fat to
potatoes. These Garlic
Mashed Potatoes will
complement roast
chicken or turkey, or any
grilled or roasted meat.

Garlic Mashed Potatoes

Preheat oven to 350°F (180°C)
Small ovenproof dish

8	cloves garlic	8
½ tsp	olive oil	2 mL
4	medium potatoes (russet, Yukon Gold)	4
½ cup	2% evaporated milk	125 mL
2 tsp	chopped fresh parsley	10 mL
1 tsp	chopped fresh chives (*or* green onions)	5 mL
¼ tsp	crumbled dried tarragon	1 mL
½ tsp	salt	2 mL
¼ tsp	white pepper	1 mL

1. In a small ovenproof dish, toss garlic with olive oil; roast in preheated oven for 20 to 25 minutes or until lightly browned.

2. Peel potatoes; boil or microwave until tender. Mash potatoes with garlic. Add milk, parsley, chives, tarragon, salt and pepper; mash until soft and creamy. (Add more milk if necessary for desired consistency.)

PER SERVING	
Calories: 105	
Dietary Fiber: 1 g	Carbohydrate: 21 g
Fat: 1 g	Protein: 3 g

Colorful Potato Pie

Preheat oven to 350°F (180°C)
8-inch (2 L) square baking dish, lightly greased

4	slices side bacon, diced	4
2	large onions, finely chopped	2
½	green bell pepper, finely chopped	½
1	stalk celery, finely chopped	1
3	large potatoes, peeled and coarsely chopped	3
2	tomatoes, coarsely chopped	2
1 cup	shredded old Cheddar cheese	250 mL
2	eggs, separated	2
1 tbsp	2% milk	15 mL
¼ tsp	salt	1 mL
¼ tsp	black pepper	1 mL

1. In a skillet, cook bacon until almost crisp; remove and drain on paper towel. Add onions, green pepper and celery to skillet; cook over medium-high heat for about 5 minutes; drain fat.

2. Partially cook potatoes in boiling water for 10 minutes; drain well. In a nonstick or lightly greased 8-inch (2 L) square baking dish, layer half of the potatoes, tomatoes, bacon and onion mixture, and cheese; repeat layers.

3. Whisk together egg yolks and milk. Beat egg whites, salt and pepper until foamy. Fold egg whites into egg yolk mixture; pour over vegetables. Bake in preheated oven for about 40 minutes or until mixture has set.

PER SERVING	
Calories: 233	
Dietary Fiber: 3 g	Carbohydrate: 24 g
Fat: 11 g	Protein: 11 g

SERVES 6
Rose Telfer

Here's a tasty and easy-to-prepare potato-based vegetable casserole that is perfect as part of a buffet or at a barbecue.

TIP

Green potatoes? Greening is an undesirable but normal change caused by a substance called solenine and occurs when a potato is exposed to light. It also occurs in the eye when the potato sprouts. Besides the bitter flavor, eating large quantities of green potatoes can make you sick. To prevent greening, store your potatoes in the dark. And unless you want to get sick, don't eat green potatoes.

DIETITIAN'S MESSAGE

This calcium-rich pie is both colorful and economical. Serve with a hearty soup such as Beef Barley Soup (see recipe, page 123) for an easy and nutritious family meal.

These are the easiest, most delicious scalloped potatoes you will ever make!

TIP

For a change, try using Swiss instead of Cheddar cheese, or cream of mushroom instead of cream of celery soup.

FOOD FAST

Want to bake potatoes in a hurry? Use your microwave! A medium potato (6 to 8 oz/175 to 250 g) takes only 3 to 4 minutes to cook on High. Pierce with a fork before cooking. Let stand for 2 minutes to soften before serving. Alternatively, you can start baked potatoes in the microwave and crisp them up in a toaster oven or on the barbecue.

DIETITIAN'S MESSAGE

When cooking with milk, whenever possible choose the lower-fat varieties — skim, 1% or 2%. You will be getting the same nutrients and taste, minus the fat.

Easy Scalloped Potatoes

Preheat oven to 325°F (160°C)
13- by 9-inch (3 L) baking dish, greased

1	can (10 oz/285 mL) condensed cream of celery soup	1
1¼ cups	milk (1 full soup can)	300 mL
½ cup	sliced onion	125 mL
3 cups	potatoes, cut into ¼-inch (5 mm) thick slices	750 mL
½ cup	shredded Cheddar cheese	125 mL
	Black pepper	
	Paprika	

1. In a large bowl, stir together soup, milk, onion and potatoes. Pour into prepared baking dish; sprinkle with cheese. Season with pepper and paprika to taste. Bake in preheated oven for 65 to 75 minutes or until potatoes are tender.

PER SERVING	
Calories: 149	
Dietary Fiber: 1 g	Carbohydrate: 22 g
Fat: 5 g	Protein: 5 g

Braised Curried Potatoes

1	medium onion, chopped	1
2 tbsp	vegetable oil	25 mL
1 tbsp	curry powder	15 mL
½ tsp	granulated sugar	2 mL
3	medium potatoes, cut into wedges, slices *or* cubes	3
¾ cup	water	175 mL
	Salt	

1. In a skillet or wok over medium heat, stir-fry onion in oil until tender. Add curry and sugar; stir-fry for 1 minute, ensuring curry doesn't burn. Add potatoes; stir-fry until coated, about 2 minutes.

2. Add water and bring to a boil; cover, reduce heat and simmer for 8 to 10 minutes or until potatoes are tender. Uncover and simmer until liquid evaporates. Season with salt to taste.

PER SERVING
Calories: 174

| Dietary Fiber: 2 g | Carbohydrate: 26 g |
| Fat: 7 g | Protein: 3 g |

SERVES 4 **P**

Jon Paudler, Chef
Leslie Maze, Dietitian

This great make-ahead recipe makes a wonderful accompaniment to an Indian meal, as well as to grilled fish or meat.

TIP

Try making this recipe with tiny new potatoes, in season. Leave them whole and increase the cooking time.

DIETITIAN'S MESSAGE

Easy to make, this delicious side dish is even better the next day when reheated. To reheat, cover and microwave at Medium until hot, or bake in a covered casserole in a 350°F (180°C) oven for 20 minutes. Serve with Yogurt-Marinated Chicken (see recipe, page 277) and rice. Add a tossed green salad and complete the meal with fresh fruit.

Braised Cabbage

TIP

When cooking cabbage, discard the tough outer leaves and remove the hard core at the base. And don't overcook; cabbage should be tender but firm.

DIETITIAN'S MESSAGE

This recipe uses back bacon as a lower-fat alternative to side bacon. It adds a delicious flavor to cabbage, which is low in calories and high in vitamin C.

3	slices back bacon, diced	3
1	small onion, sliced	1
¼ cup	finely diced carrot	50 mL
4 cups	grated cabbage	1 L
1	bay leaf	1
Pinch	dried thyme	Pinch
¼ cup	chicken broth	50 mL
	Freshly ground black pepper	

1. In a large skillet over low heat, cook bacon and onion for about 5 minutes, stirring frequently.

2. Add carrot; cover and cook for 1 minute. Stir in cabbage, bay leaf, thyme and chicken broth. Cook, covered, over low heat for about 10 minutes or until tender-crisp, stirring occasionally. Season with pepper to taste. Remove bay leaf before serving.

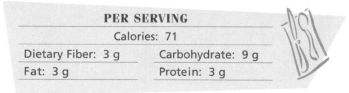

PER SERVING	
Calories: 71	
Dietary Fiber: 3 g	Carbohydrate: 9 g
Fat: 3 g	Protein: 3 g

Braised Red Cabbage

Preheat oven to 325°F (160°C)
8-cup (2 L) baking dish

1	small red cabbage (about 1½ lb/750 g)	1
⅓ cup	red wine vinegar	75 mL
1 tbsp	granulated sugar	15 mL
1 tsp	salt	5 mL
1	slice bacon, chopped *or*	1
1 tbsp	olive oil	15 mL
⅓ cup	chopped onion	75 mL
2	Granny Smith apples, peeled, cored and cut into eighths	2
1	whole clove	1
1	small onion	1
1	bay leaf	1
½ cup	boiling water	125 mL
2 tbsp	dry red wine (optional)	25 mL

1. Remove outer leaves of cabbage and discard. Cut cabbage into quarters; trim off excess white heart. Shred about ⅛ inch (3 mm) thick to make 6 cups (1.5 L). Place in bowl; toss with vinegar, sugar and salt.

2. In a large skillet, brown bacon; remove bacon, reserving drippings in pan. Set bacon aside. Add chopped onion; cook, stirring, for 2 minutes. Add apples; cook for 5 minutes.

3. Push clove into onion; add to skillet along with cabbage mixture, bay leaf, boiling water and bacon. Mix well. Pour into 8-cup (2 L) baking dish. Cover and bake in preheated oven for 2 hours, stirring occasionally. (If it becomes dry, add more water.) Remove onion and bay leaf. Stir in wine, if desired.

PER SERVING	
Calories: 44	
Dietary Fiber: 2 g	Carbohydrate: 8 g
Fat: 1 g	Protein: 1 g

SERVES 10
....
Alastair Gray, Chef
Mary Margaret Laing, Dietitian

Long, slow cooking develops the flavors in this fabulous fall or winter dish. It will reheat well and may be stored for 1 week in the refrigerator.

TIP
The apple and the red wine vinegar in this recipe add acid, which helps the cabbage keep its rich red color.

DIETITIAN'S MESSAGE
Here is an outstanding oven-baked dish. Vegetables, fruit and herbs create mouthwatering aromas and tastes while they gently bake together. Serve this delicious casserole with Turkey Hazelnut Roll (see recipe, page 301) and Pumpkin Custard (see recipe, page 427) for a great fall meal.

Desserts

The recipes in this chapter are proof that you can indulge your sweet tooth as part of a healthy and balanced diet. Tantalize your family and friends with these delicious recipes. Some are ideal for everyday or informal family gatherings, and others will impress your guests at more elaborate meals. Remember, you can choose foods from *Canada's Food Guide to Healthy Eating* to make desserts — custards, bread pudding and fresh fruit are great choices. Many recipes, such as Apricot Bread Pudding, Cinnamon Baked Pears, Autumn Crumble and Pumpkin Custard, demonstrate how easy it is to include food groups in your dessert selections.

plan for *indulgences*

A key point to remember is that all foods fit into a healthy lifestyle, as long as you use moderation and balance in your food choices. Clearly, with a little planning, you can enjoy many different kinds of desserts.

By planning ahead, you can balance your food choices to get the nutrients you need while controlling fat and maintaining energy intake. Don't deprive yourself of your favorite food just because it may be high in fat. Remember, it's not necessary to balance every meal. Instead, you need to look at your total dietary needs and intake over a few days. A treat here and there won't make or break a balanced diet.

make **healthy** dessert choices

Planning requires know-how and education. If you are looking for ways to make healthier dessert choices, here are some suggestions.

- Use lower-fat dairy foods more often.
- When baking, use purées, such as applesauce, pumpkin or zucchini, to replace three-quarters of the fat in quick-bread recipes such as muffins and coffee cakes.
- Use nonstick baking sheets and pans rather than greased ones.
- Mind the serving size. Sometimes a smaller but sweeter chocolate truffle satisfies a craving just as well as a larger chocolate dessert.
- Use fruit more often. For refreshing, nutritious desserts, it's hard to beat fresh fruit — almost anything goes, so let your imagination work its wonders. Try different combinations, such as melon and grapes, strawberries and pears, melon and blueberries. Serve fruit plain or dressed with frozen yogurt, custard sauce or vanilla pudding. To make it look more festive, use low-fat meringue shells as serving dishes.

pleasure is healthy

Picture yourself at the dining room table surrounded by family and friends. You've just finished a delicious and satisfying meal. The room is filled with laughter as you enjoy the occasion. Flickering candles illuminate the happy faces, the glasses of wine and the mouthwatering dessert.

Pleasure, relaxation and a sense of well-being are all part of a healthy lifestyle. And so is dessert. Dessert provides the opportunity to relax, linger and savor the pleasure of a good meal and enjoyable company. Occasional indulgences in rich desserts are OK as long as you balance those occasions with lighter desserts such as fruit or yogurt, or the decision not to have dessert at all.

Strawberries in Phyllo Cups

Preheat oven to 350°F (180°C)
8-cup muffin tin

4 cups	strawberries, cut into quarters	1 L
⅓ cup	peach schnapps *or* peach juice	75 mL
5	sheets phyllo pastry	5
3 tbsp	soft margarine, melted	45 mL
¾ cup	lower-fat peach yogurt	175 mL
2 tsp	icing (confectioner's) sugar	10 mL
	Fresh mint	

1. In a bowl, combine strawberries and peach schnapps; cover and refrigerate for 3 to 4 hours.

2. Place 1 phyllo sheet on work surface, keeping remaining phyllo covered with damp towel to prevent drying out. Brush with margarine, covering all edges. Top with second sheet; brush with margarine. Repeat with remaining phyllo. Brush top of last sheet. Cut stack into 8 pieces. Place in muffin tins, margarine side down, forming cup. Bake in preheated oven for 10 to 12 minutes or until golden brown. Cool in tins, then remove.

3. At serving time, divide yogurt among 8 dessert plates. Place phyllo cups on top, pressing gently into yogurt so that cup sits firmly. Fill cups with strawberries; sieve icing sugar over top. Garnish with mint.

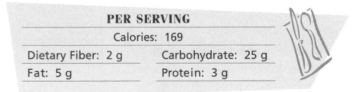

PER SERVING	
Calories: 169	
Dietary Fiber: 2 g	Carbohydrate: 25 g
Fat: 5 g	Protein: 3 g

Almond Shells with Fresh Fruit

Preheat oven to 350°F (180°C)
Parchment paper
Baking sheet

	Raspberry Coulis (see recipe, page 401)	
2²⁄₃ cups	frozen vanilla yogurt	650 mL
2 cups	diced mixed fresh fruit	500 mL
Almond Shells		
½ cup	sliced almonds	125 mL
²⁄₃ cup	icing (confectioner's) sugar	150 mL
¼ cup	all-purpose flour	50 mL
1	large egg white	1
3 tbsp	2% milk	45 mL

1. *Almond Shells:* In a food processor with steel blade, pulse almonds until finely chopped. Add sugar and flour; process until very finely chopped. With motor running, add egg white and milk through feed tube, mixing until well blended.

2. Line baking sheet with parchment paper; draw four 4-inch (10 cm) circles on paper. Place about 4 tsp (20 mL) mixture in each circle, spreading to cover circle. Bake in preheated oven until light golden and slightly brown at edges, about 10 minutes. Remove immediately with lifter or peel away paper; place each on inverted small custard cup, fruit nappy or glass. Mold slightly with hand or place second dish on top to form fluted edge. Let cool; remove and turn upright. Repeat with remaining mixture.

3. Spoon Raspberry Coulis onto each plate. Top with almond shell. Spoon frozen yogurt into each shell; arrange fruit on top.

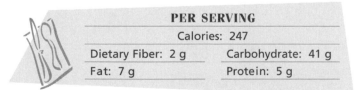

PER SERVING	
Calories: 247	
Dietary Fiber: 2 g	Carbohydrate: 41 g
Fat: 7 g	Protein: 5 g

SERVES 8
....
Donald Pattie, Chef
Joan Rew, Dietitian

Here's an impressive dessert that is not too difficult to make. Using parchment paper ensures that the shells will be easily removed from the baking sheet.

TIPS
Do not make more than 2 or 4 shells at a time since they are fragile and become difficult to mold if too crisp. If too crisp, return to oven for a few seconds to reheat.

Make the crisp shells up to 2 weeks in advance and store in an airtight container until ready to use.

DIETITIAN'S MESSAGE
These elegant pastry shells are one way to showcase fresh fruit. Because the crust contains almonds, it has more vitamins and fiber than conventional pastry.

*Meringue circles may
take a little time but not
much effort. They are the
perfect "dish" for sliced
fruit topped with this
tasty version of crème
fraîche: a mixture of
sour cream and sugar
flavored with cinnamon
and vanilla.*

TIPS

When beating egg
whites, separate the
yolks from the whites
while still cold, then
allow 10 minutes for the
whites to come to
room temperature
before beating.

If you don't have fruit
or berry sugar, pulse
granulated sugar a few
times in a food processor.

DIETITIAN'S MESSAGE

Meringues have minimal
fat and can be used with
whatever fruits are
available. You can use a
variety of fresh, frozen
or canned fruit — all will
contribute fiber and other
important nutrients.

Fruit Meringues with Cinnamon Crème Fraîche

Preheat oven to 275°F (140°C)
Baking sheet
Parchment paper or aluminum foil
Piping bag (optional)

2	large egg whites	2
¼ tsp	cream of tartar	1 mL
½ cup	instant dissolving (fruit *or* berry) sugar	125 mL
¼ tsp	vanilla	1 mL
Fruit Filling		
2 cups	sliced fruit	500 mL
2 tbsp	granulated sugar	25 mL
2 tbsp	orange liqueur *or* orange juice	25 mL
Crème Fraîche		
2 tbsp	granulated sugar	25 mL
½ tsp	ground cinnamon	2 mL
½ cup	light sour cream *or* lower-fat plain yogurt	125 mL
1 tsp	vanilla	5 mL

1. Line baking sheet with parchment paper or foil. In a small bowl, beat egg whites with cream of tartar until soft peaks form; gradually beat in sugar, beating until stiff shiny peaks form. Beat in vanilla.

2. Using piping bag or spoon, pipe meringue into 4 circles on prepared pan, building up sides to form shells. Bake in preheated oven for 50 to 60 minutes or until lightly browned. Turn off oven and let meringues stand in oven for 1 hour.

3. *Fruit Filling:* Toss fruit with sugar and liqueur; chill.

4. *Crème Fraîche:* Mix sugar and cinnamon; stir in sour cream and vanilla. Chill.

5. To serve, place meringues on dessert plates; fill with fruit and top with crème fraîche.

PER SERVING	
Calories: 257	
Dietary Fiber: 2 g	Carbohydrate: 54 g
Fat: 2 g	Protein: 4 g

Spicy Fruit Compote

3 tbsp	granulated sugar	45 mL
3 tbsp	brown sugar	45 mL
4 tsp	unsalted butter	20 mL
3 tbsp	lemon juice	45 mL
1 cup	orange juice	250 mL
1 tsp	each ground cinnamon and ginger	5 mL
½ tsp	ground cardamom	2 mL
Pinch	ground nutmeg	Pinch
⅓ cup	dark rum	75 mL
2	each medium apples and pears (unpeeled), cut into wedges	2
2	medium peaches, peeled and cut into wedges	2
2	kiwi fruit, peeled and cut into wedges	2
2	bananas, sliced	2
2 cups	strawberries, sliced	500 mL
3 tbsp	each lightly toasted sliced almonds (for technique see page 389) and coconut	45 mL

1. In a large skillet, combine granulated and brown sugars, butter, lemon juice, orange juice, cinnamon, ginger, cardamom and nutmeg; heat, stirring constantly, until boiling. Cook until reduced by half and thickened and glossy.

2. Stir in rum, apples, pears and peaches; simmer until barely tender. Remove from heat. Stir in kiwi fruit, bananas and strawberries just until heated. Serve warm in individual dishes; sprinkle with almonds and coconut.

PER SERVING	
Calories: 213	
Dietary Fiber: 5 g	Carbohydrate: 42 g
Fat: 5 g	Protein: 2 g

SERVES 8

Margaret Carson, Chef
Pam Lynch, Dietitian

This delicious compote may be made in advance, but don't stir in the kiwi, bananas and strawberries until serving time. Serve with a scoop of vanilla frozen yogurt or a slice of angel food cake.

TIP

This spicy syrup can be used with different varieties of fruit. In the winter months, try adding dried fruits such as apricots, apples and pears. Soak them in the rum and a bit of warm water to cover before adding to the syrup.

DIETITIAN'S MESSAGE

Compotes are an easy solution to the problem of what to have for dessert. They are delicious and versatile enough to complete any meal. They also provide a simple method for increasing your daily intake of fruit.

**John Higgins, Chef
Susan Iantorno,
Dietitian**

*Here's a simple but
elegant twist on fruit
salad that can be made
using any seasonal
fresh fruit.*

TIPS

Asking kids to help with
threading fruit onto the
skewers is one way to
get them involved in
food preparation. For
presentation, cut fruit
into cubes about the
same size as strawberries.

Although pepper is a
spice not often used in
dessert, in this recipe it
helps to bring out the
flavor of the fruit.

DIETITIAN'S MESSAGE

The elegance of this
dessert suggests that it
is complicated to prepare,
but it is actually very
simple. Another excellent
idea for adding fruit
to your diet, it is a
perfect finish to a stylish
summer meal.

Sumptuous Fruit Brochettes

8 bamboo skewers

8	medium whole strawberries (*or* 4 halved large)	8
8	cubes each peeled cantaloupe, honeydew melon and pineapple	8
24	seedless grapes	24
	Mint springs	

Fruit Coulis

1 cup	fresh *or* thawed frozen berries	250 mL
¼ cup	apple juice	50 mL
Pinch	freshly crushed black *or* white peppercorns	Pinch

Minted Orange Cream

¼ cup	lower-fat plain yogurt	50 mL
2 tbsp	finely chopped fresh mint	25 mL
1½ tsp	liquid honey	7 mL
1 tsp	frozen orange juice concentrate, thawed	5 mL

1. Alternately thread strawberries, cantaloupe, honeydew melon, pineapple and grapes onto 8 wooden skewers; cover or place in plastic bag and chill.

2. *Fruit Coulis:* In a food processor or blender, purée berries, apple juice and pepper; cover and chill.

3. *Minted Orange Cream:* In a bowl, mix together yogurt, mint, honey and orange juice concentrate; cover and chill.

4. To serve, spoon ¼ cup (50 mL) fruit coulis onto each of 4 dessert plates; spoon about 1 tbsp (15 mL) minted orange cream into middle of coulis and swirl with point of knife. Top with 2 fruit brochettes; garnish with mint sprigs.

PER SERVING	
Calories: 106	
Dietary Fiber: 3 g	Carbohydrate: 25 g
Fat: 1 g	Protein: 2 g

Vegetable Souvlaki with ➤
Feta Tzatziki (page 366)

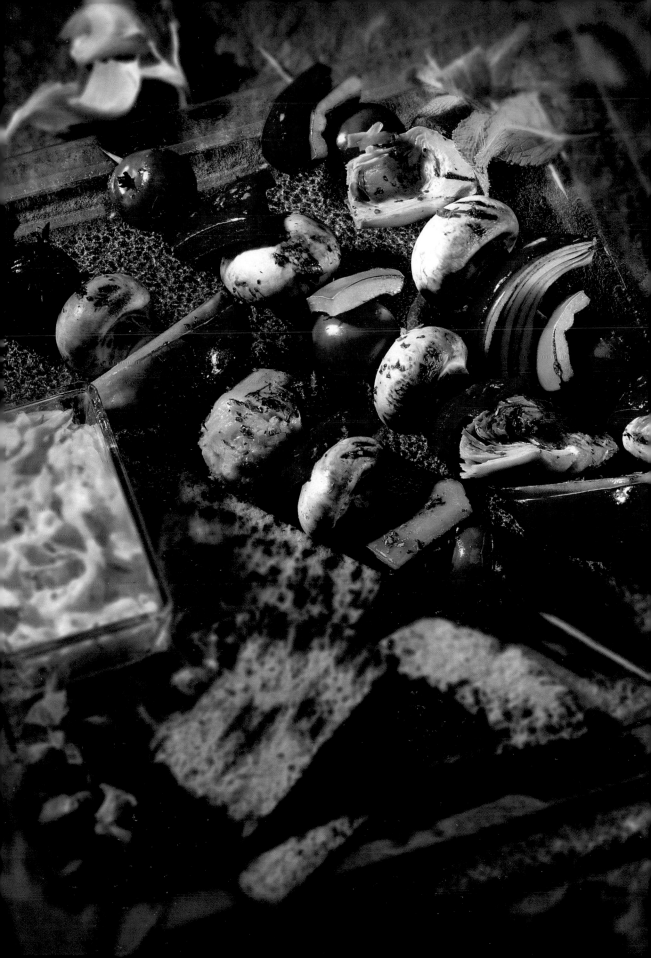

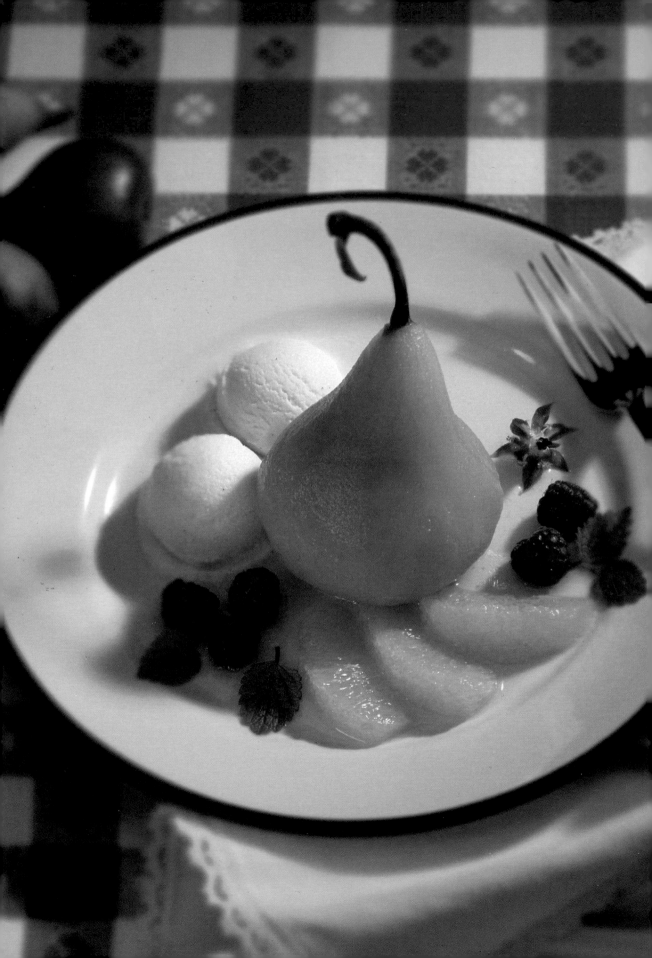

Cinnamon Baked Pears

Preheat oven to 350°F (180°C)
Baking dish

4	medium pears	4
½ cup	blueberries	125 mL
½ cup	water	125 mL
2 tbsp	brown sugar	25 mL
1 tbsp	lemon juice	15 mL
¼ tsp	ground cinnamon	1 mL

Yogurt Sauce

½ cup	lower-fat plain yogurt	125 mL
1 tbsp	brown sugar	15 mL
½ tsp	ground cinnamon	2 mL
½ tsp	vanilla	2 mL

1. Peel pears and cut in half lengthwise; scoop out core. Place cut side down in shallow baking dish. Sprinkle blueberries around pears.

2. Combine water, brown sugar, lemon juice and cinnamon; pour over pears. Bake, covered, in preheated oven for about 45 minutes or until pears are tender, basting occasionally with pan juices.

3. *Yogurt Sauce:* In a small bowl, combine yogurt, brown sugar, cinnamon and vanilla. Serve pears with pan juices; spoon a dollop of yogurt sauce over cooked pear halves.

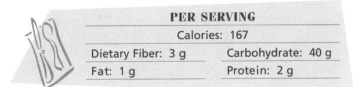

PER SERVING	
Calories: 167	
Dietary Fiber: 3 g	Carbohydrate: 40 g
Fat: 1 g	Protein: 2 g

SERVES 4
....
Christine Cauch

Here's another easy and delicious way to serve fruit. Try poaching peaches, nectarines, apples, fresh pineapple or oranges in this manner.

TIP
Most pears are shipped before they are fully ripe in order to avoid damage. If your pears are overly firm, store them in a cool place to ripen before using in this recipe.

DIETITIAN'S MESSAGE
For added fiber, leave the skin on pears, apples, peaches and nectarines when serving.

◄ Poached Pears with
  Tea Ice Cream (page 396)

Desserts

Fruit Plate with Creamy Dip

| 4½ cups | Fresh pineapple cubes; watermelon, cantaloupe *or* honeydew balls; red *or* green grapes; blueberries, raspberries *or* strawberries | 1.125 L |

Dip

½ cup	unsweetened pineapple juice	125 mL
¼ cup	granulated sugar	50 mL
1 tbsp	cornstarch	15 mL
1 tbsp	lemon juice	15 mL
1	egg, beaten	1
4 oz	light cream cheese	125 g
	Fresh mint leaves	

1. Refrigerate fruit.

2. *Dip:* In a small saucepan over medium heat, cook pineapple juice, sugar, cornstarch and lemon juice, stirring constantly, for about 5 minutes or until clear and thickened. Slowly stir some of the hot mixture into beaten egg. Return to saucepan and cook over low heat until mixture thickens slightly. Cool for 5 minutes. Whisk in cream cheese until smooth. Refrigerate for at least 2 hours or until very cold before serving with fresh fruits. Garnish with mint.

Dip (1 tbsp/15 mL)

PER SERVING	
Calories: 39	
Dietary Fiber: 0 g	Carbohydrate: 5 g
Fat: 2 g	Protein: 1 g

Fruit and Dip (¾ cup/175 mL)

PER SERVING	
Calories: 156	
Dietary Fiber: 1 g	Carbohydrate: 26 g
Fat: 5 g	Protein: 4 g

Desserts

Fresh Fruit
with Yogurt Dressing

1 cup	lower-fat plain yogurt	250 mL
1 tbsp	liquid honey	15 mL
1 tbsp	freshly squeezed orange juice	15 mL
4 cups	cubed assorted fresh fruits	1 L
	Shredded coconut	

1. Stir together yogurt, honey and orange juice. Place fruit in a large bowl; pour yogurt mixture over fruit. Refrigerate until serving time. Sprinkle with coconut.

Dressing

PER SERVING
Calories: 36

Dietary Fiber: 0 g	Carbohydrate: 6 g
Fat: 1 g	Protein: 2 g

Dressing with Fruit

PER SERVING
Calories: 93

Dietary Fiber: 2 g	Carbohydrate: 20 g
Fat: 1 g	Protein: 3 g

SERVES 6
· ·
Elaine Watton

This refreshing and light dressing can be used with a fruit salad plate and it can also be drizzled over assorted fresh fruits for a dessert. Use any variety of seasonal fruits — oranges, apples, bananas, cantaloupe, mangoes, pineapple, peaches, pears or blueberries.

TIP
Mangoes are ready to eat when their skins have turned yellow-orange or red and they are soft to the touch.

DIETITIAN'S MESSAGE
This delightful combination of yogurt and fresh fruit provides a clean, fresh taste to balance a heavy meal. The recipe allows you to use fruits in season, making it a year-round dessert.

Lower-fat evaporated milk replaces whipping cream in this melt-in-your-mouth lemon mousse.

TIP

This delicious mousse uses an Italian meringue, which adds a hot sugar syrup to beaten egg whites. It is a little more work than regular meringue, but it's worth it.

DIETITIAN'S MESSAGE

Serve fresh berries in season alongside this refreshing mousse for a spectacular dessert. This lower-fat version of a traditional mousse uses evaporated milk and gelatin instead of whipping cream.

Lemon Mousse

¼ cup	2% evaporated milk	50 mL
1 tsp	unflavored gelatin	5 mL
1½ tsp	grated lemon zest	7 mL
⅓ cup	lemon juice	75 mL
	Yellow food coloring (optional)	
½ cup	granulated sugar	125 mL
⅓ cup	water	75 mL
2	egg whites	2
	Fresh berries	
	Mint leaves (optional)	

1. Pour evaporated milk into a small bowl; chill in freezer along with beaters.

2. In a small saucepan, sprinkle gelatin over lemon zest and juice; heat over low heat until dissolved. Add a few drops of food coloring, if desired. Cool.

3. In another small saucepan, cook sugar and water over high heat until candy thermometer reaches 234° to 240°F (112° to 116°C) or soft ball stage (syrup dropped into cold water forms soft ball).

4. In a bowl and using electric mixer, beat egg whites until soft peaks form; gradually pour in syrup, beating constantly. Beat until cool and very stiff. Fold in gelatin mixture.

5. Beat evaporated milk until soft peaks form; fold into egg white mixture. Pour into 5 dessert glasses. Refrigerate for 3 to 4 hours or until set. Serve topped with fresh berries, and mint leaves, if desired.

PER SERVING	
Calories: 101	
Dietary Fiber: Trace	Carbohydrate: 23 g
Fat: Trace	Protein: 3 g

Cold Maple Mousse

SERVES 10

Ingrid Ermanovics

6-cup (1.5 L) soufflé dish

1 tbsp	unflavored gelatin (1 pkg)	15 mL
2 tbsp	cold water	25 mL
1 cup	maple syrup	250 mL
1	egg, beaten	1
⅛ tsp	salt	0.5 mL
2 cups	whipping cream	500 mL
½ cup	toasted slivered almonds, optional (see Tip, at right)	125 mL

1. In a small bowl, soak gelatin in cold water.

2. Meanwhile, in a double boiler over medium-low heat, whisk together maple syrup, egg and salt; cook, stirring constantly, for 5 to 8 minutes or until slightly thickened. Remove from heat and whisk in gelatin. Refrigerate mixture until cool.

3. In a bowl and using electric mixer, whip cream until stiff. Add one-third of the cream to maple mixture; beat until well blended. (This gives the mousse a bit more volume.) Gently fold in the remaining cream. Pour into soufflé dish. Chill until set. Garnish with almonds, if using.

PER SERVING	
Calories: 244	
Dietary Fiber: 0 g	Carbohydrate: 21 g
Fat: 17 g	Protein: 2 g

This tasty dessert is particularly good served with fresh fruit.

TIP

To toast almonds: In a nonstick skillet over medium heat, toast almonds, stirring constantly, for 3 to 4 minutes or until golden brown. Alternatively, microwave on High for 3 to 5 minutes, stirring at 1-minute intervals.

DIETITIAN'S MESSAGE

This rich dessert is an indulgence. Keep your serving size small or serve after a lighter meal. Remember, it's not necessary to balance every meal but to look at your total intake over a few days.

Baked Alaska Volcano

Ralph Graham, Chef
Rosanne E. Maluk,
Dietitian

Flambé this impressive dessert, if desired. Or for an easier finish, decorate with sparklers.

TIPS

Make sure your egg whites are at room temperature to achieve maximum volume when beaten.

Purchase the ice cream in a pint (500 mL) carton for convenience.

DIETITIAN'S MESSAGE

This dramatic dessert is definitely worth the effort. Your guests will be complimenting you long after the presentation. For a lower-fat choice, replace the ice cream with your favorite flavor of frozen yogurt.

Baking sheet

4	egg whites	4
¼ tsp	cream of tartar	1 mL
½ cup	granulated sugar	125 mL
1	angel food cake	1
2 cups	Neapolitan ice cream	500 mL
Sauce		
2 cups	fresh *or* frozen sliced strawberries	500 mL
⅓ cup	granulated sugar, divided	75 mL
1 tbsp	cornstarch	15 mL
2 tbsp	sweet sherry	25 mL
	Red food coloring (optional)	

1. In a medium bowl, beat egg whites with cream of tartar until soft peaks form; gradually beat in sugar until stiff shiny peaks form.

2. Slice cake in half crosswise. Slice ice cream in ¼-inch (5 mm) thick slices; cover bottom part of cake. Replace top of cake. Place on baking sheet. Spread egg mixture evenly over entire cake, sealing well. Freeze until serving time.

3. *Sauce:* Combine strawberries with 2 tbsp (25 mL) of the sugar; refrigerate overnight. In a small saucepan, combine remaining sugar and cornstarch. Drain liquid from strawberries into measuring cup; add enough cold water to measure 1 cup (250 mL). Add to saucepan; cook, stirring, over medium heat until boiling. Reduce heat and simmer for 1 minute. Remove from heat; stir in sherry. Add food coloring, if desired. Cool and stir into strawberries.

4. At serving time, bake cake in 450°F (230°C) oven for 3 to 5 minutes or just until browned. Drizzle some of sauce over edge of cake like lava of volcano. Serve remaining sauce separately with cake.

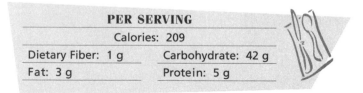

PER SERVING	
Calories: 209	
Dietary Fiber: 1 g	Carbohydrate: 42 g
Fat: 3 g	Protein: 5 g

Grapefruit Sorbet

8-inch (2 L) square metal baking pan

1 tsp	unflavored gelatin	5 mL
¾ cup	cold water	175 mL
½ cup	granulated sugar	125 mL
1 cup	grapefruit juice	250 mL
¼ cup	orange juice	50 mL
2 tbsp	lemon juice	25 mL
Pinch	salt	Pinch
1	egg white, lightly beaten	1

1. Sprinkle gelatin over ¼ cup (50 mL) of the water; set aside. In a small saucepan, combine remaining ½ cup (125 mL) water and sugar; bring to a boil. Reduce heat and simmer for 10 minutes; stir in softened gelatin until dissolved. Remove from heat. Stir in grapefruit, orange and lemon juices, and salt.

2. Pour into 8-inch (2 L) square metal pan. Freeze until slushy, about 1 hour. Pour into food processor or blender along with egg white; process until well blended. Return to pan; cover and freeze until firm. To serve, spoon into dessert glasses.

PER SERVING	
Calories: 68	
Dietary Fiber: Trace	Carbohydrate: 216 g
Fat: Trace	Protein: 1 g

SERVES 8
....

**David Powell, Chef
Rosanne E. Maluk,
Dietitian**

Smooth and light — this sorbet is the perfect ending to a meal, or simply a treat when you are trying to beat the summer heat. Sorbet, which is basically fruit juice combined with a syrup and frozen, is usually served as a dessert. However, it has long been used in Europe to refresh the palate between courses in an elaborate meal.

DIETITIAN'S MESSAGE

This sorbet provides a refreshing end to a heavier meal. To add nutrition, serve with seasonal fruits.

Cranberries, water, honey and lemon juice are simmered, then puréed and frozen to make this beautiful granita, which, like sorbet, is a type of fruit ice. You'll notice subtle changes in flavor depending on the type of honey you use. Buckwheat honey will have the strongest flavor.

TIP

Granita is a type of water ice that usually has a more granular texture than a sorbet.

DIETITIAN'S MESSAGE

This is a dessert with flair. It provides a refreshing contrast of tastes, with beautiful rich color. It will also supply your daily requirement of vitamin C and is fat-free. What a great way to end a heavier meal!

Cranberry Honey Granita with Papaya Coulis

9- by 5-inch (2 L) loaf pan

1	pkg (12 oz/340 g) cranberries	1
1/2 cup	water	125 mL
1/3 cup	(approx) buckwheat, wild flower *or* regular liquid honey	75 mL
1 tbsp	lemon juice	15 mL
	Fresh mint	

Papaya Coulis

1	medium papaya	1
2 tbsp	granulated sugar	25 mL
1 tsp	lemon juice	5 mL

1. In a saucepan, combine cranberries, water, honey and lemon juice; bring to a boil. Reduce heat and simmer for 10 minutes; cool slightly. Press through sieve to remove skins. Taste juice and add 2 tbsp (25 mL) honey if sweeter flavor is desired.

2. Pour into 9- by 5-inch (2 L) metal loaf pan. Freeze for about 1 hour or until partially frozen. Pour into food processor; process until well blended. Return to pan; cover and freeze until firm, 3 to 4 hours.

3. *Papaya Coulis:* Peel and seed papaya. In a food processor, process papaya, sugar and lemon juice until smooth. Refrigerate until serving time.

4. To serve, let granita stand at room temperature for 10 minutes. Pour coulis onto dessert plates; scoop granita on top. Garnish with fresh mint.

PER SERVING	
Calories: 129	
Dietary Fiber: 3 g	Carbohydrate: 34 g
Fat: Trace	Protein: 1 g

Cranberry Surprise

Preheat oven to 325°F (160°C)
12- by 8-inch (3 L) baking dish

Crust

2 cups	graham cracker crumbs	500 mL
½ cup	butter *or* margarine, melted	125 mL

Filling

2 cups	2% milk	500 mL
1	pkg (4-serving size) vanilla pudding (not instant, see Note, at right)	1
2 cups	fresh *or* frozen cranberries, chopped	500 mL
1	large banana, mashed	1
½ cup	granulated sugar	125 mL
¼ cup	chopped nuts (walnuts, pecans *or* almonds)	50 mL

1. *Crust:* Combine graham cracker crumbs and butter. Press two-thirds of crumb mixture onto bottom of 12- by 8-inch (3 L) baking pan. Bake in preheated oven for 10 minutes. Remove pan from oven and let cool on rack.

2. *Filling:* Cook milk and vanilla pudding according to package directions; cool for about 15 minutes.

3. Combine cranberries, banana and sugar; set aside.

4. Spread cooked pudding over crumb base. Top with cranberry mixture. Sprinkle with remaining crumbs and chopped nuts. Refrigerate for 4 to 5 hours.

PER SERVING	
Calories: 240	
Dietary Fiber: 1 g	Carbohydrate: 34 g
Fat: 11 g	Protein: 3 g

SERVES 12

Laura M. Hawthorn

This yummy combination of vanilla pudding, cranberries and banana on a graham cracker crust is sure to become a family favorite.

NOTE

If you don't have a vanilla pudding mix on hand, you can substitute the custard filling used in Strawberry Coconut Supreme (see recipe, page 394) in this recipe. Omit the coconut and add vanilla, not coconut extract.

DIETITIAN'S MESSAGE

It is good news that cranberries are becoming increasingly popular in desserts, as they are packed with vitamin C and antioxidants.

Here's an elegant dessert that features fresh fruit and coconut, and which can be made ahead of time.

DIETITIAN'S MESSAGE

This appealing chilled dessert is a delicious way to finish a meal, but remember to plan for it as it contains a significant amount of fat and calories. It is best served after a lower-fat meal.

Strawberry Coconut Supreme

Preheat oven to 325°F (160°C)
8-inch (2 L) square baking pan

Crust

1 cup	graham cracker crumbs	250 mL
3 tbsp	melted butter *or* margarine	45 mL

Custard Filling

2 cups	2% milk, divided	500 mL
1/3 cup	granulated sugar	75 mL
1	egg, lightly beaten	1
1/3 cup	finely shredded coconut	75 mL
3 tbsp	cornstarch	45 mL
1 tsp	coconut extract *or* vanilla	5 mL

Topping

1 1/2 cups	sliced strawberries	375 mL

1. *Crust:* Combine graham cracker crumbs and butter. Press onto bottom of 8-inch (2 L) square baking pan. Bake in preheated oven for 10 minutes. Remove pan from oven and let cool on rack.

2. *Custard Filling:* In a medium saucepan over medium heat, bring 1 1/2 cups (375 mL) milk, sugar, egg and coconut to a boil, stirring occasionally. Combine cornstarch with remaining milk; stir into hot milk. Cook, stirring constantly, until mixture is thickened. Remove from heat; stir in coconut extract. Cool for 10 to 15 minutes and pour over crumb mixture. Refrigerate for at least 1 1/2 hours.

3. *Topping:* At serving time, arrange sliced strawberries over pudding.

PER SERVING	
Calories: 258	
Dietary Fiber: 3 g	Carbohydrate: 35 g
Fat: 11 g	Protein: 5 g

Coupe Bircher

SERVES 8
....

Anton Koch, Chef
Kim Arrey, Dietitian

½ cup	quick-cooking rolled oats	125 mL
¼ cup	raisins	50 mL
1 tbsp	each sliced hazelnuts and almonds	15 mL
½ cup	1% milk	125 mL
1¼ cups	lower-fat plain yogurt	300 mL
3 tbsp	granulated sugar	45 mL
2 tbsp	liquid honey	25 mL
1 tsp	lemon juice	5 mL
1 tsp	vanilla	5 mL
2 cups	sliced strawberries	500 mL
2 cups	cubed peeled cantaloupe	500 mL
	Mint leaves	

Use a variety of fruits, such as apples, oranges, bananas, raspberries or blueberries, in this elegant muesli-based dessert.

DIETITIAN'S MESSAGE

Oats and fruit provide soluble fiber, which can help to lower blood cholesterol levels and control blood sugar levels in people with diabetes. This delicious dessert can also be served as a breakfast alternative to hot oatmeal.

1. In a bowl, soak oats, raisins, hazelnuts and almonds in milk for 1 hour in refrigerator. Stir in yogurt, sugar, honey, lemon juice and vanilla.

2. Reserve about ½ cup (125 mL) each of the strawberries and cantaloupe; fold remaining fruit into yogurt mixture. Refrigerate for several hours or overnight.

3. Serve in dessert glasses topped with reserved fruit and mint leaves, if desired.

PER SERVING	
Calories: 138	
Dietary Fiber: 2 g	Carbohydrate: 26 g
Fat: 3 g	Protein: 4 g

John Cordeaux, Chef
Kim Arrey, Dietitian

The poached pears in this recipe are good enough to serve on their own with a seasonal fruit garnish. But if you have time, make the Earl Grey Tea Ice Cream, then sit back and wait for the applause!

TIPS

Use medium-ripe pears in this recipe.

To ripen fruit, place in a brown paper bag, loosely closed, and leave in a warm spot.

DIETITIAN'S MESSAGE

Ice cream lovers, take heart — this unusual homemade ice cream is high in taste and lower in fat. The pears, which add fiber and vitamin C, can be left unpeeled for additional fiber.

Poached Pears with Tea Ice Cream

Shallow metal pan

Tea Ice Cream

⅔ cup	1% milk	150 mL
3 tbsp	Earl Grey tea leaves	45 mL
¾ cup	granulated sugar	175 mL
¼ cup	liquid honey	50 mL
2 tbsp	skim-milk powder	25 mL
4 oz	light cream cheese	125 g
1 cup	lower-fat plain yogurt	250 mL
½ cup	light sour cream	125 mL

Pears

2 cups	water	500 mL
⅓ cup	liquid honey	75 mL
2 tbsp	lemon juice	25 mL
1 tsp	vanilla	5 mL
6	pears, peeled but stems attached	6
	Seasonal fruit (raspberries, strawberries, orange slices, kiwi fruit slices)	

1. *Tea Ice Cream:* In a saucepan, slowly heat milk and tea. Add sugar, honey and skim-milk powder, stirring, until dissolved. Cool. Strain. Whisk in remaining ingredients until smooth. Refrigerate for at least 2 hours.

2. Pour into metal pan; cover and freeze for 2 hours or until almost firm. Transfer in chunks to food processor; purée until smooth. Return to pan; cover and freeze until firm.

3. *Pears:* In a saucepan, combine water, honey, lemon juice and vanilla; bring to a boil. Add pears, cover and reduce heat; simmer for 10 to 12 minutes or until tender, turning once. Transfer mixture to a bowl; cover and chill.

4. To serve, let Tea Ice Cream stand at room temperature for 10 minutes. Place each pear on dessert plate; drizzle with 1 tbsp (15 mL) syrup. Add scoop of ice cream and fruit.

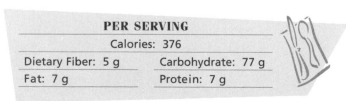

PER SERVING	
Calories: 376	
Dietary Fiber: 5 g	Carbohydrate: 77 g
Fat: 7 g	Protein: 7 g

Desserts

Chocolate Mousse and Lemon Loaf

Preheat oven to 375°F (190°C)
8- by 4-inch (1.5 L) loaf pan

1 cup	yogurt cheese (see technique, page 154)	250 mL

Cake

3	eggs	3
¾ cup	granulated sugar	175 mL
1 tbsp	grated lemon zest	15 mL
2 tsp	vanilla	10 mL
1 cup	sifted all-purpose flour	250 mL

Mousse

1 oz	semisweet chocolate, melted	30 g
¼ cup	cocoa powder	50 mL
3	egg whites	3
¼ cup	granulated sugar	50 mL

1. *Cake:* In a bowl, beat eggs, sugar, lemon zest and vanilla until pale and slightly thickened; gradually fold in flour. Pour into prepared pan. Bake in preheated oven for 25 to 30 minutes or until golden and firm to the touch. Cool in pan for 10 minutes. Remove from pan and cool on rack.

2. *Mousse:* In a bowl, whisk cocoa into yogurt cheese; stir in melted chocolate. Set aside.

3. Place egg whites in bowl over saucepan of simmering water; beat with electric mixer until foamy. Gradually beat in sugar until medium-soft peaks form; fold one-third at a time into yogurt mixture.

4. Trim top off cake; cut cake lengthwise into 3 layers. Clean pan and line with plastic wrap extending over sides. Pour in one-third of the mousse; top with 1 cake layer. Repeat twice. Cover with plastic wrap. Refrigerate until firm, about 3 hours. Turn out onto serving tray; remove plastic wrap carefully. Garnish, if desired. Slice to serve.

PER SERVING	
Calories: 233	
Dietary Fiber: 2 g	Carbohydrate: 42 g
Fat: 4 g	Protein: 7 g

SERVES 8

John Schroder, Chef
Susie Langley, Dietitian

Here's a dessert that sounds decadent enough to please even the sweetest tooth. Be sure to chill the assembled cake until it's firm before serving. For an additional flourish, garnish with chocolate shavings, slivered almonds or hazelnuts.

TIP

If time is short, purchase a light pound cake to substitute for the homemade cake in this recipe.

DIETITIAN'S MESSAGE

The chocolate mousse in this recipe owes its deceptively decadent taste to the clever combination of lower-fat ingredients — yogurt, cocoa powder, egg whites and sugar — with a small amount of semisweet chocolate.

Strawberry Sorbet

8-inch (2 L) square pan

1½ cups	fresh *or* frozen unsweetened strawberries	375 mL
2 cups	unsweetened apple juice	500 mL
¼ cup	granulated sugar	50 mL
¼ tsp	ground cinnamon	1 mL
2 tbsp	cold water	25 mL
4 tsp	cornstarch	20 mL

1. Wash and hull fresh strawberries or thaw frozen strawberries. In a blender or food processor, blend strawberries and apple juice until almost smooth.

2. In a medium saucepan over medium heat, cook strawberry mixture, sugar and cinnamon, stirring frequently, for about 5 minutes or until sugar is dissolved. Combine water and cornstarch; stir into hot mixture. Cook for about 3 minutes or until thickened and clear. Chill for 1 hour. Pour into 8-inch (2 L) square pan; cover and freeze for about 3 hours or until firm.

3. Break frozen mixture into chunks; beat with electric mixer at medium speed until fluffy. Transfer to an airtight container and freeze until firm. Transfer from freezer to refrigerator about 15 minutes before serving.

PER SERVING	
Calories: 85	
Dietary Fiber: 1 g	Carbohydrate: 21 g
Fat: 0 g	Protein: 0 g

Lemon Sherbet

SERVES 8
....
Joan Gallant

8 small custard cups

½ cup	granulated sugar	125 mL
⅓ cup	lemon juice	75 mL
2 tsp	grated lemon zest	10 mL
2	eggs, separated	2
⅔ cup	skim-milk powder	150 mL
⅔ cup	cold water	150 mL

1. Whisk together sugar, lemon juice, zest and egg yolks; set aside.

2. With an electric mixer, beat egg whites, skim-milk powder and water on high speed for 3 to 5 minutes or until stiff peaks form. Fold in lemon mixture. Pour into 8 small custard cups; cover and freeze for about 3 hours or until firm. Transfer from freezer to refrigerator about 15 minutes before serving.

PER SERVING	
Calories: 88	
Dietary Fiber: 0 g	Carbohydrate: 16 g
Fat: 1 g	Protein: 3 g

This is similar to a frozen soufflé but is lighter and lower in calories.

DIETITIAN'S MESSAGE

Because of the risk of salmonella poisoning, raw eggs should be used with caution. Cracked eggs should be avoided. Recipes calling for raw eggs should be prepared as close to serving time as possible and kept well refrigerated.

Make this light, lower-calorie, low-fat dessert a staple in your recipe repertoire. Not only does it complement any meal, it is rich in vitamins C and A as well as in calcium from the skim-milk powder.

SERVES 8
•••••••••••••••••••••••••

Antony Nuth, Chef
Lynda Chadwick,
Dietitian

*Be sure to use freshly
squeezed lemon juice in
this recipe to get a real
lemony taste.*

TIPS

Refrigerating the pastry
before rolling it out
relaxes a protein in the
flour called gluten,
making it easier to roll.
Once the crust has been
placed in the pan,
freezing it for 15 minutes
before baking will help
to set the edge and
ensure flakiness.

Use the Raspberry Coulis
as a sauce for ice cream
or vanilla yogurt.

DIETITIAN'S MESSAGE

This tart is a lemon lover's
delight. A refreshing
end to any meal, it is,
however, a higher-fat
choice, so serve it with a
lower-fat meal.

Lemon Tart with Raspberry Coulis

Preheat oven to 400°C (200°F) • 9-inch (23 cm) flan pan

Pastry

1 cup	all-purpose flour	250 mL
½ cup	icing (confectioner's) sugar	125 mL
⅓ cup	cold unsalted butter, cut into 1-inch (2.5 cm) cubes	75 mL
1	egg, lightly beaten with 2 tbsp (25 mL) whipping cream	1

Filling

1 tsp	grated lemon zest	5 mL
¾ cup	lemon juice	175 mL
5	eggs	5
1 cup	granulated sugar	250 mL
⅔ cup	whipping cream	150 mL
	Raspberry Coulis (see recipe, page 401)	

1. *Pastry:* In a food processor, combine flour and icing sugar; add butter and process until mixture resembles coarse crumbs. Add to egg mixture with machine running and process until dough starts to clump together. Form into ball; wrap in plastic wrap and chill for 1 hour.

2. On lightly floured surface, roll out pastry to fit 9-inch (23 cm) flan pan, leaving 1-inch (2.5 cm) overhang. Fold overhang inside flan pan and press to make even 1-inch (2.5 cm) thick edge. Line shell neatly with foil large enough to lift out easily; fill evenly with dried beans or rice. Bake in preheated oven for 15 minutes or until edges are golden. Remove foil with beans; bake for 4 minutes or until uniformly golden. Let cool.

3. *Filling:* In a bowl, whisk together lemon zest and juice, eggs, sugar and whipping cream. Place baked shell in oven; carefully pour in filling right to rim. Reduce temperature to 300°F (150°C) and bake until firm around edge and almost set in center, 20 to 25 minutes. Cool on rack. Cut into wedges. Serve with Raspberry Coulis.

PER SERVING WITH COULIS	
Calories: 402	
Dietary Fiber: 1 g	Carbohydrate: 55 g
Fat: 20 g	Protein: 7 g

Creamy Fruit Crêpes

3 cups	1% plain yogurt	750 mL
	Zest and juice of 1 lemon	
¼ cup	granulated sugar	50 mL
¼ tsp	ground nutmeg	1 mL
¼ tsp	vanilla	1 mL
8	crêpes (about 8 inches/20 cm)	8
4 cups	blackberries (*or* other seasonal berries)	1 L
	Raspberry Coulis (see recipe, below)	
	Icing (confectioner's) sugar	
	Mint leaves	

Raspberry Coulis

| 1 cup | fresh or frozen unsweetened raspberries (thawed if frozen) | 250 mL |
| ½ cup | icing (confectioner's) sugar | 125 mL |

1. In a coffee filter–lined strainer placed over a bowl, cover and drain yogurt overnight in refrigerator. Discard liquid.
2. In another bowl, combine drained yogurt, lemon zest and juice, sugar, nutmeg and vanilla. Spread over each crêpe.
3. Lightly mash berries with fork; spread evenly over yogurt mixture. Tightly roll up each crêpe; place on tray. Cover and refrigerate for several hours.
4. *Raspberry Coulis:* In a food processor or blender, purée raspberries; press through sieve to remove seeds. Stir in icing sugar. Cover and refrigerate until chilled. (Makes 1 cup/250 mL).
5. To serve, slice each crêpe into 4 pinwheels. Spoon Raspberry Coulis onto each plate; top with crêpes. Sprinkle with icing sugar and garnish with mint.

PER SERVING WITH COULIS	
Calories: 186	
Dietary Fiber: 4 g	Carbohydrate: 34 g
Fat: 3 g	Protein: 8 g

SERVES 8

Stephen Ashton, Chef
Leah Hawirko, Dietitian

These delicious fruit-filled crêpes are an elegant finish to any meal. If you use prepared crêpes and thick yogurt, they are so easy to make you will want to have them with weeknight meals.

TIPS

If you're short of time, instead of making your own yogurt cheese, use thick yogurt, now available in stores — no draining necessary.

Premade crêpes are available in the refrigerated produce section of many grocery stores. You can also make your own using the recipe on page 61.

DIETITIAN'S MESSAGE

Yogurt cheese, which is yogurt drained of liquid, is easy to make and is a good substitute for cream cheese in many recipes because it is lower in fat.

SERVES 8

• •

Don Costello, Chef
Lisa Diamond, Dietitian

Here's a crumble with a difference. Acorn squash and carrots, instead of fruit, provide the base for the crumble topping. Serve as a dessert with ice milk or frozen yogurt, or as a side dish with pork chops.

TIP

Try using cooked pumpkin or canned pumpkin purée instead of squash in this recipe.

DIETITIAN'S MESSAGE

This unusual variation on the traditional fruit crumble delivers more than great taste: the grains and fruit add dietary fiber, and the orange vegetables add vitamin A. This is a delicious way to end a fall meal.

Autumn Crumble

Preheat oven to 350°F (180°C)
8-inch (2 L) square baking pan, greased

2 cups	mashed cooked acorn squash (1 large)	500 mL
⅓ cup	packed brown sugar	75 mL
¼ cup	all-purpose *or* whole-wheat flour	50 mL
1	egg	1
1 tbsp	milk	15 mL
1 tsp	vanilla	5 mL
1 tsp	each ground cinnamon and nutmeg	5 mL
¼ tsp	ground cloves	1 mL
2	large apples, peeled and chopped	2
1	large carrot, grated	1
½ cup	raisins	125 mL
Topping		
½ cup	quick-cooking rolled oats	125 mL
¼ cup	natural wheat bran	50 mL
¼ cup	packed brown sugar	50 mL
2 tbsp	all-purpose *or* whole-wheat flour	25 mL
2 tbsp	soft margarine	25 mL
1 tsp	ground cinnamon	5 mL

1. With electric mixer or in food processor, blend squash, brown sugar, flour, egg, milk, vanilla, cinnamon, nutmeg and cloves until smooth; stir in apples, carrot and raisins. Spread in greased 8-inch (2 L) square baking pan.

2. *Topping:* Combine rolled oats, wheat bran, sugar, flour, margarine and cinnamon until crumbly; sprinkle over squash mixture. Bake in preheated oven for 30 to 35 minutes or until golden brown. Serve warm.

PER SERVING	
Calories: 241	
Dietary Fiber: 6 g	Carbohydrate: 51 g
Fat: 4 g	Protein: 4 g

Peach Cobbler

Preheat oven to 350°F (180°C)
8-inch (2 L) square baking dish, greased

Filling

1	can (28 oz/796 mL) sliced peaches, drained, reserving ½ cup (125 mL) juice	1
2 tbsp	granulated sugar	25 mL
2 tsp	cornstarch	10 mL
1 tsp	lemon juice	5 mL

Topping

1 cup	biscuit baking mix	250 mL
⅛ tsp	ground nutmeg	0.5 mL
⅓ cup	milk	75 mL

1. *Filling:* Place peaches in 8-inch (2 L) square baking dish. In a bowl, combine sugar and cornstarch; whisk in reserved peach juice. Stir in lemon juice. Pour mixture over peaches. Set aside.

2. *Topping:* In a medium bowl, combine baking mix and nutmeg; stir in milk to form a sticky dough. Drop dough by the spoonful on top of the peach mixture. (Not all of the filling will be covered.) Bake in preheated oven for 40 to 45 minutes or until crust is lightly browned.

PER SERVING	
Calories: 158	
Dietary Fiber: 1 g	Carbohydrate: 32 g
Fat: 3 g	Protein: 3 g

SERVES 6 P

Margie Armstrong

Prepare this easy-to-make cobbler and let it bake in the oven while you are eating dinner. Enjoy while still warm, served with vanilla ice cream or frozen yogurt.

TIPS

When fresh peaches are in season, use 3 cups (750 mL) peeled sliced peaches and omit the canned peaches and juice. Stir the peaches a bit (to release some juices) and sprinkle the sugar mixture over them. Add the lemon juice and stir to blend.

To peel fresh peaches, immerse them in a pot of rapidly boiling water for about 3 minutes. Rinse under cold water. The skins should lift off easily.

DIETITIAN'S MESSAGE

Make this dessert when you need to add to your daily servings of grains and fruit.

SERVES 4
. . . .
Marilynn Small, Dietitian
Post Cereals

This dessert is equally delicious made with fresh or frozen berries.

TIP

For an all-apple version, omit berries and add an extra sliced apple.

DIETITIAN'S MESSAGE

This variation on a traditional crisp uses shredded wheat-type biscuits instead of rolled oats. Packed with fruit and whole grains, each serving supplies 2 servings from the Vegetables and Fruit group as well as plenty of fiber.

Country Apple Berry Crisp

Preheat oven to 375°F (190°C)
4-cup (1 L) baking dish with lid, greased

3	large baking apples, cored and thinly sliced	3
2 cups	mixed berries	500 mL
1 tbsp	cornstarch	15 mL
3	large shredded wheat–type biscuits, crumbled	3
½ cup	packed brown sugar	125 mL
¼ cup	butter *or* margarine	50 mL
1 tsp	ground cinnamon	5 mL

1. In a bowl, combine apples, berries and cornstarch.

2. In another bowl, combine crumbled biscuits, brown sugar, butter and cinnamon. Rub with fingers until crumbly. Set aside 1 cup (250 mL) of the crumble mixture.

3. Toss remaining crumble mixture with fruit. Place fruit mixture in greased baking dish. Sprinkle remaining crumb mixture over top.

4. Cover and bake in preheated oven for 20 minutes. Remove cover and bake for 10 minutes or until apples are tender. Serve warm.

PER SERVING	
Calories: 405	
Dietary Fiber: 9 g	Carbohydrate: 76 g
Fat: 13 g	Protein: 3 g

Winter Fruit Crisp

Preheat oven to 400°F (200°C)
Shallow baking pan

3	large apples, peeled and sliced	3
2	large pears, peeled and sliced	2
½ cup	cranberries, fresh *or* frozen	125 mL
2 tbsp	granulated sugar	25 mL
1 cup	large-flake rolled oats	250 mL
¼ cup	packed brown sugar	50 mL
¼ cup	natural wheat bran	50 mL
½ tsp	ground cinnamon	2 mL
⅓ cup	butter *or* margarine	75 mL

1. Place apples, pears and cranberries in a shallow baking pan. Sprinkle with sugar.
2. In a medium bowl, combine oats, brown sugar, bran and cinnamon. With pastry blender or 2 knives, cut in butter until crumbly. Sprinkle over fruit mixture. Bake in preheated oven for about 40 minutes or until mixture is bubbling and fruit is barely tender.

PER SERVING

Calories: 293

Dietary Fiber: 6 g	Carbohydrate: 49 g
Fat: 11 g	Protein: 3 g

SERVES 6
....
Laurie A. Wadsworth, Dietitian

Using several fruits instead of just one makes a crisp more colorful and adds flavor. Depending on the natural sweetness of each fruit, more or less sugar may be required. Large-flake rolled oats give this crisp a deliciously old-fashioned crunchy topping.

TIP
If desired, replace the cranberries in this recipe with 2 tbsp (25 mL) dried cranberries that have been soaked in 1 tbsp (15 mL) orange juice for 10 to 15 minutes.

DIETITIAN'S MESSAGE
This crisp offers lots of nutrients, and the bran and rolled oats make it a good source of fiber.

SERVES 12
....

Alain Mercier, Chef
Fabiola Masri, Dietitian

Serve this easy-to-make cake warm for best results. If desired, substitute your favorite fruit for blueberries.

TIPS

If you reheat the cake a day later or after freezing, drizzle or brush an additional ¼ cup (50 mL) maple syrup over it to glaze.

Since blueberries have fragile skins, be gentle when folding them into any batter. Otherwise, the skins will break and the blueberries will leak their blue color into the cake.

DIETITIAN'S MESSAGE

Talk about low-fat! This recipe is a great way to serve fruit and still satisfy a sweet tooth. Add fresh blueberries when serving.

Blueberry Semolina Cake

Preheat oven to 325°F (160°C)
8-inch (2 L) square baking pan, lightly greased

1½ cups	small semolina	375 mL
1 tsp	baking soda	5 mL
1 cup	lower-fat plain yogurt	250 mL
1 cup	fresh *or* frozen blueberries	250 mL
1 tsp	vanilla	5 mL
½ cup	maple syrup	125 mL

1. In a medium bowl, mix semolina and baking soda. Combine yogurt, blueberries and vanilla; stir into dry ingredients just until moistened. Do not overmix.

2. Spoon into lightly greased 8-inch (2 L) square baking pan. Bake in preheated oven for 45 to 50 minutes or until tester inserted in center comes out clean. Remove cake from oven; pour syrup on top. Serve warm.

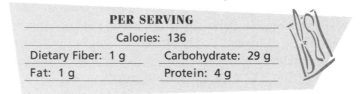

PER SERVING	
Calories: 136	
Dietary Fiber: 1 g	Carbohydrate: 29 g
Fat: 1 g	Protein: 4 g

Peachy Upside-Down Cake

SERVES 10
....
Lois Eggert

Preheat oven to 350°F (180°C)
9-inch (23 cm) round cake pan lined with waxed paper

1	can (14 oz/398 mL) sliced peaches, drained *or*	1
2 cups	sliced peeled fresh peaches	500 mL
1/3 cup	soft butter *or* margarine	75 mL
3/4 cup	lightly packed brown sugar	175 mL
3	eggs	3
1 1/2 cups	grated carrots	375 mL
3/4 cup	whole-wheat flour	175 mL
1 1/4 cups	high-fiber bran cereal	300 mL
1 tsp	baking powder	5 mL
1/2 tsp	baking soda	2 mL
1/2 tsp	ground cinnamon	2 mL
3/4 cup	raisins	175 mL

1. Drain peach slices thoroughly on absorbent paper. Arrange in bottom of 9-inch (23 cm) round cake pan lined with waxed paper. Set aside.

2. In a large bowl, cream butter and sugar. Add eggs, 1 at a time, beating well after each addition. Stir in grated carrots.

3. In a second bowl, combine flour, cereal, baking powder, baking soda, cinnamon and raisins. Stir into carrot mixture. Spread evenly over peach slices. Bake in preheated oven for about 35 minutes or until tester inserted in center comes out clean. Let stand for 30 minutes before turning out onto serving plate. Serve warm or cold.

PER SERVING	
Calories: 251	
Dietary Fiber: 6 g	Carbohydrate: 45 g
Fat: 8 g	Protein: 5 g

Here's a great way to add fiber to your diet. This cake keeps well in the refrigerator for up to 4 days.

TIP
For variety, make this using pineapple or pears. Or scatter a few blueberries between the sliced peaches.

DIETITIAN'S MESSAGE
The fruits and carrots in this recipe are a great source of vitamin A as well as other vitamins and minerals. The whole-wheat flour and high-fiber bran cereal contribute dietary fiber.

TIP

Kiwi fruit is available year-round. Buy unripened fruit and leave at room temperature for ripening within 3 to 5 days.

DIETITIAN'S MESSAGE

Nuts are the main source of fat in this recipe, but they are also rich in fiber. Keep the total amount of fat you consume in balance with your other menu choices.

Geraldine's Almond Cake

Preheat oven to 350°F (180°C)
8-inch (20 cm) round cake pan, lightly greased

4	eggs, separated	4
¾ cup	granulated sugar, divided	175 mL
¾ cup	rusk cracker crumbs (about 5 rusk crackers)	175 mL
¾ cup	ground almonds	175 mL
1 tsp	vanilla	5 mL
½ tsp	baking powder	2 mL
2 cups	seasonal fruit (kiwi fruit, blueberries, strawberries, raspberries, pineapple)	500 mL

1. In a large bowl, beat egg whites until soft peaks form. Gradually beat in ¼ cup (50 mL) sugar, beating well after each addition until sugar is dissolved and egg whites hold stiff, shiny peaks.

2. In a second bowl, beat egg yolks with remaining sugar at medium speed until thick. Stir rusk crumbs, almonds, vanilla and baking powder into egg yolk mixture. Fold in beaten egg whites; pour into lightly greased 8-inch (20 cm) round cake pan. Bake in preheated oven for about 35 minutes or until cake springs back when touched. Let stand for 10 minutes; remove cake from pan. Let cool on wire rack. Serve topped with fresh fruit.

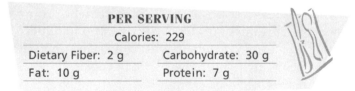

PER SERVING	
Calories: 229	
Dietary Fiber: 2 g	Carbohydrate: 30 g
Fat: 10 g	Protein: 7 g

Fluffy Pumpkin Cheesecake

9-inch (2.5 L) springform pan

Crust

1½ cups	gingersnaps crumbs	375 mL
⅓ cup	melted butter *or* margarine	75 mL
3 tbsp	brown sugar	45 mL

Filling

1 cup	unsweetened apple juice	250 mL
⅔ cup	granulated sugar	150 mL
½ tsp	salt	2 mL
1 tbsp	unflavored gelatin (1 pkg)	15 mL
3	eggs, separated	3
½ tsp	vanilla	2 mL
8 oz	cream cheese	250 g
1 tbsp	lemon juice	15 mL
¾ cup	whipping cream	175 mL
¼ tsp	each ground cloves, cinnamon and ginger	1 mL
1 cup	cooked mashed pumpkin	250 mL
	Semisweet chocolate curls (optional)	

1. *Crust:* Combine gingersnap crumbs, butter and brown sugar. Press on bottom and sides of pan. Refrigerate.

2. *Filling:* In a saucepan, combine juice, sugar and salt. Sprinkle with gelatin and stir over low heat until dissolved.

3. Beat egg yolks slightly. Gradually stir in hot liquid; return to saucepan. Cook on medium, stirring constantly, until thickened. Stir in vanilla.

4. Beat cream cheese and lemon juice. Add gelatin mixture, beating until smooth. Chill until mixture is consistency of unbeaten egg whites, about 30 minutes.

5. Beat egg whites until stiff. In a separate bowl, combine cream and spices; beat until stiff. Fold whipped cream, pumpkin and egg whites into gelatin mixture. Pour into pan; chill until firm. Garnish with chocolate before serving, if desired.

PER SERVING	
Calories: 296	
Dietary Fiber: Trace	Carbohydrate: 27 g
Fat: 19 g	Protein: 5 g

SERVES 12

Judy Koster

You can make this creamy, mellow cheesecake year-round using canned pumpkin. The spicy gingersnap crust and an optional chocolate garnish complete the mouthwatering flavors.

TIPS

If using canned pumpkin for this recipe, make sure you purchase pumpkin purée, not pumpkin pie filling, which has additional spices.

To make your own pumpkin purée, bake or steam the pumpkin, as you would a squash, then purée the cooked pumpkin in a food processor or blender. A 5-lb (2.5 kg) pumpkin will yield about 3½ cups (875 mL) of purée.

When using raw eggs in recipes, choose clean, uncracked, Grade A eggs. Keep cheesecake refrigerated until serving.

DIETITIAN'S MESSAGE

This tasty dessert is a decadent way to serve pumpkin, which is rich in vitamin A.

**Mary Sue Waisman,
Dietitian**

*This old-fashioned
family dessert is real
comfort food.*

TIP
The baking soda in this
recipe is not used as a
leavening agent but
rather to aid in browning.

DIETITIAN'S MESSAGE
Serve this gingerbread
warm with a lemon
sauce, a light custard
sauce or unsweetened
applesauce for a great
family dessert.

Hot Water Gingerbread

Preheat oven to 350°F (180°C)
8-inch (2 L) square baking pan, lightly greased

1½ cups	all-purpose flour	375 mL
1 tsp	baking soda	5 mL
1 tsp	ground ginger	5 mL
½ tsp	ground cinnamon	2 mL
¼ tsp	salt	1 mL
1	egg	1
½ cup	packed brown sugar	125 mL
½ cup	molasses	125 mL
½ cup	boiling water	125 mL
⅓ cup	melted butter *or* margarine	75 mL

1. In a large bowl, combine flour, baking soda
   and seasonings.

2. In a second bowl, beat egg, brown sugar, molasses and
   boiling water. Stir molasses mixture and melted butter
   into flour mixture until well blended. Pour into lightly
   greased or nonstick 8-inch (2 L) square baking pan. Bake
   in preheated oven for about 35 minutes.

PER SERVING	
Calories: 224	
Dietary Fiber: 1 g	Carbohydrate: 37 g
Fat: 7 g	Protein: 3 g

Lazy Daisy Cake

SERVES 9 P

Camille Morris

Preheat oven to 350°F (180°C)
8-inch (2 L) round baking pan, lightly greased

2	eggs	2
1 cup	granulated sugar	250 mL
1 tsp	vanilla	5 mL
1 cup	all-purpose flour	250 mL
1 tsp	baking powder	5 mL
Pinch	salt	Pinch
½ cup	2% milk	125 mL
2 tsp	butter *or* margarine	10 mL

1. In a medium bowl, beat together eggs, sugar and vanilla until light and fluffy.

2. Combine flour, baking powder and salt; set aside.

3. Scald milk; stir in butter until melted. Add to egg mixture alternately with flour mixture, beginning and ending with flour. Pour batter into lightly greased or nonstick 8-inch (2 L) round baking pan. Bake in preheated oven for about 35 minutes or until tester inserted in center comes out clean. Let cool on wire rack for 10 minutes before removing from pan.

PER SERVING

Calories: 163

Dietary Fiber: Trace	Carbohydrate: 33 g
Fat: 2 g	Protein: 3 g

This light, sponge-style cake is a traditional favorite. Prepare and store in the freezer for last-minute desserts or as the base for peach, raspberry or strawberry shortcake.

TIP

When baking cakes, be sure your pan is the same size as the one called for in the recipe. If your pan is larger, the cake will bake more quickly and will not rise as well. In a smaller pan, the batter may overflow.

DIETITIAN'S MESSAGE

Using this light, spongy cake as a base for shortcake is a delicious way to add fresh fruit to your diet.

The glaze poured over this fabulous cake makes it extra moist and delicious.

TIPS

This recipe is a great way to use over-ripe bananas. If you can't use bananas that are becoming ripe, pop them into a resealable plastic bag and freeze them. They will turn black, but once they are thawed and the skins are removed, they will be perfect for this recipe.

This recipe makes about 2 cups (500 mL) of glaze.

DIETITIAN'S MESSAGE

Serve this cake as a finish to a soup-and-salad meal.

Buttermilk Oat-Branana Cake

Preheat oven to 350°F (180°C)
8-inch (2 L) square baking pan, lightly greased and floured

1 cup	buttermilk	250 mL
2/3 cup	rolled oats	150 mL
1/3 cup	oat bran *or* wheat bran	75 mL
1/4 cup	butter *or* margarine	50 mL
1 cup	granulated sugar	250 mL
1	egg	1
1 tsp	vanilla	5 mL
2	ripe bananas, mashed	2
1 1/2 cups	all-purpose flour	375 mL
1 tsp	baking soda	5 mL
1 tsp	baking powder	5 mL
Glaze		
1/2 cup	granulated sugar	125 mL
1/2 cup	buttermilk	125 mL
1/4 cup	butter *or* margarine	50 mL
1/2 tsp	baking soda	2 mL

1. In a small bowl, pour buttermilk over rolled oats and oat bran. Let stand for 10 minutes.

2. In a medium bowl, cream butter and sugar. Beat in egg and vanilla. Combine bananas and buttermilk mixture with creamed ingredients. Sift together flour, baking soda and baking powder. Stir dry ingredients into banana mixture; blend well.

3. Pour batter into prepared pan. Bake in preheated oven for 45 minutes or until tester inserted in center comes out clean. Let stand for 5 minutes.

4. *Glaze:* In a small saucepan over medium heat, combine ingredients; bring just to a boil. (Watch closely; mixture will foam.)

5. Poke holes with tester (a metal skewer or a wooden toothpick) all over cake surface; pour glaze over cake while still warm. Cool cake before cutting.

PER SERVING	
Calories: 277	
Dietary Fiber: 1 g	Carbohydrate: 46 g
Fat: 9 g	Protein: 4 g

Harvest Raisin Cake

Preheat oven to 350°F (180°C)
13- by 9-inch (3.5 L) baking pan, lightly greased

1½ cups	granulated sugar	375 mL
1 cup	whole-wheat flour	250 mL
1 cup	all-purpose flour	250 mL
2 tsp	baking powder	10 mL
1 tsp	baking soda	5 mL
½ tsp	salt	2 mL
1½ tsp	ground cinnamon	7 mL
¼ tsp	ground cloves	1 mL
¼ tsp	ground nutmeg	1 mL
¼ tsp	ground ginger	1 mL
4	eggs	4
1	can (14 oz/398 mL) pumpkin purée (not pie filling)	1
½ cup	vegetable oil	125 mL
1 cup	high-fiber bran cereal	250 mL
1 cup	raisins	250 mL

1. In a large bowl, combine sugar, flours, baking powder, baking soda, salt and spices.

2. In a second bowl, beat eggs, pumpkin, oil and cereal. Add flour mixture, mixing just until combined. Stir in raisins.

3. Spread evenly in lightly greased or nonstick 13- by 9-inch (3.5 L) baking pan. Bake in preheated oven for about 40 minutes or until tester inserted in center comes out clean. Cool completely on wire rack.

PER SERVING	
Calories: 135	
Dietary Fiber: 2 g	Carbohydrate: 23 g
Fat: 4 g	Protein: 2 g

SERVES 24
....
Maryanne Cattrysse

This moist and spice-filled cake is as rich in fiber as flavor.

TIPS

You can also bake this cake in a tube pan or muffin tin. Tube pan: Bake in 350°F (180°C) oven for about 50 minutes. Muffins: Bake in 350°F (180°C) for about 20 minutes.

Makes 24 to 30 pieces in 13- by 9-inch (3.5 L) pan, 20 slices in 10-inch (25 cm) tube pan, or about 3 dozen muffins.

DIETITIAN'S MESSAGE

This cake provides both soluble and insoluble fiber. For a high-fiber meal, serve with White Bean Soup (see recipe, page 118), a green salad and fruit for dessert.

Awesome Pineapple Cake

Preheat oven to 350°F (180°C)
13- by 9-inch (3.5 L) baking pan, greased

Cake

2 cups	all-purpose flour	500 mL
1½ cups	granulated sugar	375 mL
1 cup	finely chopped pecans	250 mL
1 tsp	baking soda	5 mL
1	can (19 oz/540 mL) crushed pineapple, with juice	1
2	eggs, beaten	2
1 tsp	vanilla	5 mL

Icing

2 tbsp	butter, softened	25 mL
4 oz	light cream cheese, softened	125 g
1¼ cups	icing (confectioner's) sugar	300 mL
1 tsp	vanilla	5 mL

1. *Cake:* In a large bowl, combine flour, sugar, pecans and baking soda. In another bowl, blend together pineapple, eggs and vanilla. Make a well in the center of dry ingredients and pour in pineapple mixture; stir gently until just combined.

2. Pour batter into greased 13- by 9-inch (3.5 L) baking pan and bake in preheated oven for 40 to 45 minutes or until cake tester inserted in center comes out clean. Set aside to cool.

3. *Icing:* In a bowl, blend together butter and cream cheese until smooth. Beat in icing sugar and vanilla until smooth. Spread icing over cooled cake.

PER SERVING	
Calories: 364	
Dietary Fiber: 2 g	Carbohydrate: 62 g
Fat: 12 g	Protein: 5 g

Date Oatmeal Cake with Mocha Frosting

SERVES 16 P

Joan Triandafillou,
Dietitian

Preheat oven to 350°F (180°C)
9-inch (2.5 L) square baking pan, greased

Cake

1 cup	rolled oats	250 mL
1½ cups	boiling water	375 mL
1 cup	all-purpose flour	250 mL
1 tsp	baking soda	5 mL
¼ tsp	salt	1 mL
½ cup	margarine	125 mL
1 cup	packed brown sugar	250 mL
1 tsp	vanilla	5 mL
1 cup	chopped dates	250 mL
½ cup	chopped walnuts	125 mL

Mocha Frosting

2 tbsp	margarine	25 mL
1½ cups	sifted icing (confectioner's) sugar	300 mL
2 tsp	cocoa powder	10 mL
1 tbsp	strong coffee, cooled	15 mL
1 tsp	vanilla	5 mL

1. *Cake:* In a small bowl, combine oats and boiling water; let stand until cool.

2. In a separate bowl, combine flour, baking soda and salt. Set aside.

3. In a large bowl, cream together margarine and brown sugar until fluffy. Beat in vanilla, rolled oats mixture and flour mixture. Stir in dates and walnuts. Pour mixture into greased 9-inch (2.5 L) square baking pan and bake in preheated oven for 30 to 35 minutes or until cake tester inserted in center comes out clean. Set aside to cool.

4. *Mocha Frosting:* In a bowl, blend together margarine, sugar, cocoa, coffee and vanilla until fluffy. If necessary, thin icing with extra coffee to reach desired consistency. Spread over cooled cake.

Here's a delicious old-fashioned cake that combines dates, walnuts and oats with a yummy mocha frosting.

TIPS
Most of the dates sold in North America are dried and high in concentrated sugar. As a result, they are a great source of energy. Take some along on hikes or whenever you think you may need a power snack.

If desired, use butter instead of margarine in this recipe.

DIETITIAN'S MESSAGE
The calories and fat in this dessert are a little higher than average, so choose a smaller serving size or balance it with a lighter main course.

PER SERVING	
Calories: 252	
Dietary Fiber: 2 g	Carbohydrate: 40 g
Fat: 10 g	Protein: 2 g

For an occasional treat, pack pieces of this moist and delicious cake in lunch bags and wait for the raves at the end of the day.

TIP

It's easy to turn this recipe into pumpkin or banana cake. Just substitute 1 cup (250 mL) pumpkin purée or mashed ripe bananas (about 2 medium) for the ¾ cup (175 mL) applesauce.

DIETITIAN'S MESSAGE

Don't limit this treat to the brown baggers — it's delicious anytime!

Lunch Box Applesauce Cake with Buttercream Frosting

Preheat oven to 350°F (180°C)
8-inch (2 L) square baking pan, greased

Cake

1½ cups	all-purpose flour	375 mL
1 tsp	baking powder	5 mL
1 tsp	ground cinnamon	5 mL
½ tsp	salt	2 mL
½ tsp	baking soda	2 mL
¼ tsp	each ground nutmeg and cloves	1 mL
2	eggs	2
¼ cup	vegetable oil	50 mL
⅓ cup	granulated sugar	75 mL
⅓ cup	packed brown sugar	75 mL
¾ cup	applesauce	175 mL

Frosting

2 tbsp	butter, softened	25 mL
1 cup	sifted icing (confectioner's) sugar	250 mL
1 tbsp	milk *or* cream	15 mL
½ tsp	vanilla	2 mL

1. *Cake:* In a bowl, sift together flour, baking powder, cinnamon, salt, baking soda, nutmeg and cloves. Set aside.

2. In a large bowl with an electric mixer, blend eggs, oil, granulated sugar and brown sugar at high speed for 1 minute or until mixture is light and fluffy. Stir in applesauce; blend at medium speed for 30 seconds. Add dry ingredients; blend at medium speed for 30 seconds or until well combined. Pour into prepared pan and bake in preheated oven for 35 to 40 minutes or until tester inserted in center comes out clean. Cool in pan.

3. *Frosting:* In a medium bowl with an electric mixer, blend butter, icing sugar, milk and vanilla at high speed for 2 minutes or until light and creamy. Add additional milk as required to reach desired spreading consistency. Spread frosting on top of cake. Sprinkle with cinnamon.

PER SERVING	
Calories: 288	
Dietary Fiber: 1 g	Carbohydrate: 47 g
Fat: 10 g	Protein: 4 g

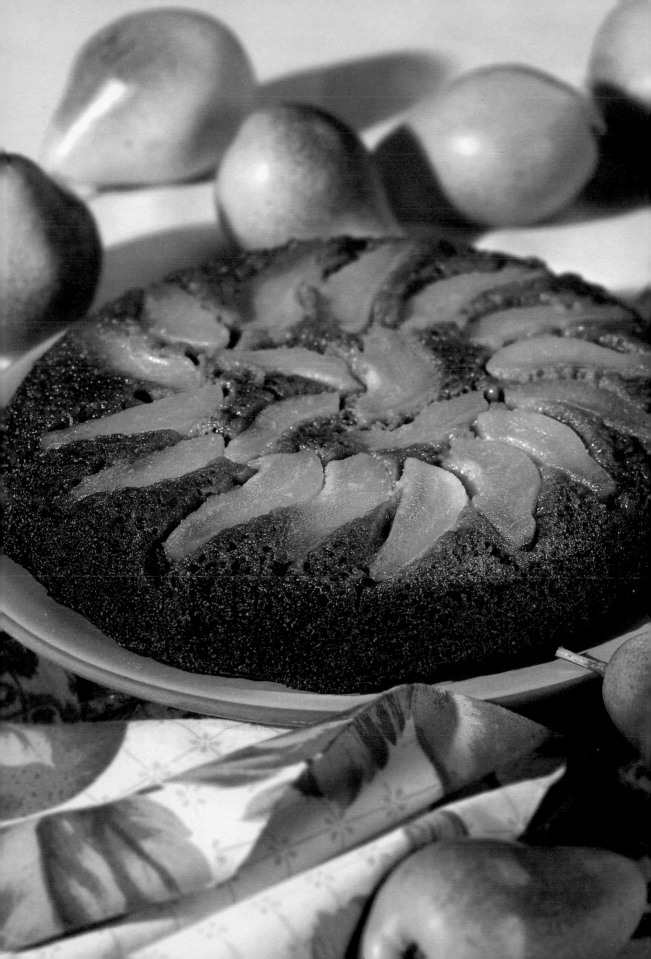

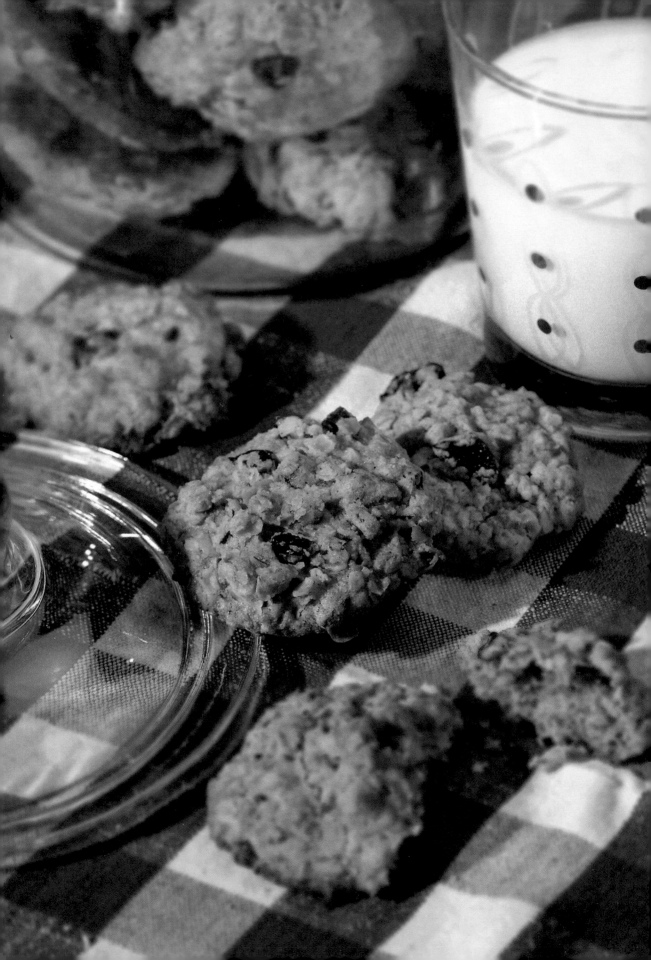

Blueberry Flan

Preheat oven to 425°F (220°C)
9-inch (23 cm) flan pan with removable bottom

1½ cups	all-purpose flour	375 mL
¼ cup	granulated sugar	50 mL
1½ tsp	baking powder	7 mL
¼ cup	soft margarine	50 mL
2	egg whites	2
¼ tsp	almond extract	1 mL
Filling		
3 cups	fresh blueberries	750 mL
⅓ cup	granulated sugar	75 mL
1 tbsp	all-purpose flour	15 mL
1 tbsp	lemon juice	15 mL
2 tsp	ground cinnamon	10 mL

1. In a bowl, combine flour, sugar and baking powder; stir in margarine, egg whites and almond extract to form dough. Press into 9-inch (23 cm) flan pan with removable bottom. Freeze for 15 minutes.

2. *Filling:* In a bowl, mix together blueberries, sugar, flour, lemon juice and cinnamon; pour over crust. Bake in preheated oven for 15 minutes. Reduce temperature to 350°F (180°C); bake for 20 to 25 minutes longer. Cool on rack. Refrigerate for at least 1 hour before serving.

PER SERVING	
Calories: 233	
Dietary Fiber: 2 g	Carbohydrate: 42 g
Fat: 6 g	Protein: 4 g

SERVES 8
....
Pamela Good, Chef
Carrie Roach, Dietitian

The flavors of blueberries, almond, lemon and cinnamon marry in this easy-to-prepare flan. Allow enough time to refrigerate the flan for at least 1 hour before serving.

TIP

Try this recipe using wild or low-bush blueberries when they are in season. They have a delicious and more intense flavor than the cultivated variety.

DIETITIAN'S MESSAGE

Blueberries are gaining in popularity because of their antioxidant properties. This delicious flan contains a minimal amount of fat.

A fluffy filling with a crunchy crust makes this pie a light, refreshing ending to a special meal. This recipe is best when served the same day it is made.

TIP

This recipe can also be made with unsweetened raspberries, which would increase the fiber content to 4 g per serving. Substitute raspberry gelatin for the strawberry, for a change of taste.

DIETITIAN'S MESSAGE

Here's another dessert that demonstrates that great-tasting food can also be light and healthful. Succulent strawberries are chilled in gelatin, and yogurt provides the creamy finish, keeping fat to a minimum. The cereal-based crust contributes fiber, as do the strawberries.

Strawberry Yogurt Pie

9-inch (23 cm) pie plate

Crust

3 tbsp	butter *or* margarine	45 mL
3 tbsp	corn syrup	45 mL
3 tbsp	firmly packed brown sugar	45 mL
2½ cups	bran flakes cereal	625 mL

Filling

1	pkg (3 oz/85 g) strawberry gelatin	1
1 cup	boiling water	250 mL
1 cup	whole strawberries, slightly thawed if frozen	1
1 cup	lower-fat plain yogurt	250 mL

1. *Crust:* In a saucepan over medium-high heat, melt butter, corn syrup and brown sugar; bring mixture to a full boil, stirring constantly. Remove from heat; stir in cereal, mixing until cereal is completely coated. Press firmly around sides and bottom of lightly greased 9-inch (23 cm) pie plate. Place in freezer while preparing filling.

2. *Filling:* Dissolve gelatin in boiling water. Cut strawberries into small pieces; stir into jelly mixture. Chill until mixture reaches the consistency of egg whites. Whisk in yogurt. Chill briefly until mixture is thick but not set. Pour into chilled pie crust. Refrigerate for about 2 hours before serving.

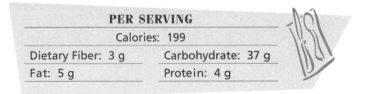

PER SERVING	
Calories: 199	
Dietary Fiber: 3 g	Carbohydrate: 37 g
Fat: 5 g	Protein: 4 g

White Chocolate Raspberry Pie

Preheat oven to 350°F (180°C)
9-inch (23 cm) pie plate

1½ cups	chocolate wafer crumbs	375 mL
¼ cup	margarine, melted	50 mL
2 tbsp	brown sugar	25 mL
Filling		
1 tsp	unflavored gelatin	5 mL
2 tbsp	cold water	25 mL
1 cup	white chocolate chips, melted	250 mL
8 oz	light cream cheese, softened	250 g
½ cup	light sour cream *or* lower-fat plain yogurt	125 mL
1 tsp	vanilla	5 mL
Raspberry Topping		
1 cup	fresh or frozen unsweetened raspberries, thawed if frozen	250 mL
⅓ cup	granulated sugar	75 mL
2 tbsp	cornstarch	25 mL
	Shaved chocolate (optional)	

1. In a bowl, combine chocolate crumbs, margarine and brown sugar; press into 9-inch (23 cm) pie plate. Bake in preheated oven for 10 to 12 minutes. Cool.

2. *Filling:* In a small saucepan or glass bowl, sprinkle gelatin over water; heat over low heat until dissolved, or microwave at High for 25 seconds. In a bowl, beat cream cheese until smooth; beat in melted chocolate, sour cream, vanilla and gelatin until smooth. Pour into pie shell. Refrigerate until set, about 3 hours.

3. *Raspberry Topping:* Drain raspberries, reserving juice. In a small saucepan, combine sugar and cornstarch; stir in juice. Cook, stirring, over medium heat until boiling; reduce heat and simmer for 1 minute. Remove from heat; stir in raspberries. Chill. Just before serving, spoon over pie. Garnish with shaved chocolate, if desired.

PER SERVING	
Calories: 423	
Dietary Fiber: 2 g	Carbohydrate: 45 g
Fat: 25 g	Protein: 7 g

SERVES 8

Janice Mitchell, Chef
Jane Henderson, Dietitian

White chocolate chips, light cream cheese and light sour cream are combined for this decadently good filling, complemented by a chocolate wafer crust and raspberry topping. For a variation, use fresh seasonal berries such as strawberries or blueberries.

TIP

White chocolate is not really chocolate — it's a product made by adding milk and flavorings to cocoa butter or vegetable shortening. The higher the percentage of cocoa butter, the better the product. It should have a creamy texture and a deep yellowish color. It shouldn't be white and waxy.

DIETITIAN'S MESSAGE

A rich dessert to end a lighter meal but worth the effort. The fruit topping provides vibrant color, and adds vitamin C and fiber to your diet.

Fresh Strawberry Pie

4 cups	hulled strawberries	1 L
⅓ cup	cold water	75 mL
¼ cup	granulated sugar	50 mL
4 tsp	cornstarch, mixed with 2 tbsp (25 mL) water	20 mL
1	prepared 9-inch (23 cm) graham cracker crumb crust	1
1 cup	whipped cream *or* Whipped Cream and Yogurt (optional) Topping (see recipe, page 427)	250 mL

1. Purée or mash 1 cup (250 mL) of the strawberries. You should have about ¾ cup (175 mL) puréed berries.

2. In a small saucepan, combine puréed strawberries, water and sugar; blend well. Bring to a boil over medium heat; whisk in cornstarch mixture. Cook, stirring constantly, for 1 minute or until slightly thickened. Remove from heat and let cool slightly.

3. Place remaining berries, stem end down, over graham cracker crust. Spoon purée mixture evenly over berries. Chill until glaze is set, about 3 hours.

4. Serve alone or, if desired, with whipped cream or Whipped Cream and Yogurt Topping.

PER SERVING	
Calories: 196	
Dietary Fiber: 2 g	Carbohydrate: 34 g
Fat: 7 g	Protein: 2 g

Carrot Pie

Preheat oven to 425°F (220°C)
Pastry for single-crust 9-inch (23 cm) pie

2 cups	thinly sliced carrots	500 mL
2	eggs, lightly beaten	2
1 cup	2% milk	250 mL
½ cup	granulated sugar	125 mL
1 tsp	ground cinnamon	5 mL
1 tsp	ground nutmeg	5 mL
½ tsp	ground ginger	2 mL
¼ tsp	salt	1 mL

1. Line pie plate with pastry; chill while preparing filling.
2. Cook carrots until tender; drain well and purée. Beat together eggs, carrot, milk, sugar and spices. Pour into prepared pie shell.
3. Bake in preheated oven for 10 minutes. Reduce heat to 350°F (180°C) and bake for about 35 minutes longer or until tester inserted in center comes out clean. Serve warm or at room temperature.

PER SERVING
Calories: 278

Dietary Fiber: 2 g	Carbohydrate: 36 g
Fat: 13 g	Protein: 6 g

SERVES 6

Laure Riendeau

Pumpkin pie lovers will also enjoy this Quebec specialty. Carrots provide a pleasing texture and appearance. The filling seems thin but it sets nicely during baking.

TIP
Chilling the pastry before baking will help to set the edges and ensure that the crust is flaky.

DIETITIAN'S MESSAGE
Here's an unusual way to increase your vitamin A intake. Serve this dessert as a finish to a lighter meal of Country Vegetable Chowder (see recipe, page 105) and bread.

Light Tiramisu

9-inch (23 cm) glass bowl

2 tsp	unflavored gelatin	10 mL
2 tbsp	frozen orange juice concentrate, thawed	25 mL
½ cup	granulated sugar	125 mL
⅓ cup	water	75 mL
6	egg whites	6
8 oz	light cream cheese	250 g
1 cup	yogurt cheese (see Tip, at left)	250 mL
½ tsp	grated orange zest	2 mL
½ tsp	vanilla	2 mL
16	soft ladyfinger cookies	16
1 cup	cold strong coffee	250 mL
2 tbsp	cocoa powder	25 mL

1. In a small saucepan, sprinkle gelatin over orange juice concentrate; cook, stirring, over low heat until dissolved. Cool.

2. In a small saucepan, combine sugar and water; cook over medium heat until syrup reaches 234° to 240°F (112° to 116°C) or soft ball stage (syrup dropped in cold water forms soft ball).

3. In a bowl, beat egg whites until soft peaks form; gradually pour in syrup, beating constantly until cool and very stiff. Beat in dissolved gelatin, beating for 30 seconds.

4. In a large bowl, beat together cream cheese, yogurt cheese, orange zest and vanilla until smooth and creamy. Fold in meringue, one-third at a time.

5. Separate ladyfingers; drizzle each with coffee and arrange half in bottom of deep 9-inch (23 cm) glass bowl. Cover with half of the meringue mixture. Sprinkle with 1 tbsp (15 mL) cocoa. Repeat layers. Cover and refrigerate for at least 4 hours until set.

PER SERVING	
Calories: 124	
Dietary Fiber: Trace	Carbohydrate: 16 g
Fat: 4 g	Protein: 6 g

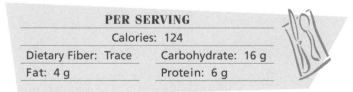

Orange Crème Caramel

Preheat oven to 350°F (180°C)
8-inch (2 L) round baking pan

½ cup	granulated sugar	125 mL
¼ cup	water	50 mL
5	eggs	5
½ cup	granulated sugar	125 mL
2½ cups	hot milk	625 mL
1 tbsp	grated orange zest	15 mL
1 tsp	vanilla	5 mL

1. In a small heavy saucepan, combine ½ cup (125 mL) sugar and water. Cook over medium heat, stirring constantly, until sugar is dissolved. (Be careful not to let the mixture boil at this stage.) Increase heat to medium-high and boil, without stirring, for 6 to 8 minutes or until mixture caramelizes and is golden in color. Pour immediately into 8-inch (2 L) round baking pan, tilting pan to cover bottom.

2. In a medium bowl, stir together eggs and ½ cup (125 mL) sugar until blended. Stir in hot milk, orange zest and vanilla; avoid overmixing. Pour into pan over caramel mixture. Place baking pan in a larger pan of boiling water. Bake in preheated oven for 40 to 45 minutes or until mixture is set. Remove from hot water. Cool on a rack. Refrigerate until ready to serve.

3. To remove from pan, run a spatula carefully around custard. Invert a rimmed serving plate over custard and turn over. Serve in wedges with caramel sauce from the pan.

PER SERVING	
Calories: 183	
Dietary Fiber: Trace	Carbohydrate: 29 g
Fat: 5 g	Protein: 6 g

SERVES 8

Canadian Egg Marketing Agency

Here's the perfect finish for a special meal with family or friends.

MAKE AHEAD
Prepare up to 2 days ahead. Cover with foil or plastic wrap and refrigerate.

DIETITIAN'S MESSAGE

This recipe is a lighter, but even tastier, variation of traditional crème caramel. It makes a nice balance to a heavier main course.

SERVES 8

Margie Armstrong

Originally developed as a recipe for using up day-old bread, bread pudding has become a cherished comfort food. This version uses apricot jam to embellish the creamy custard.

TIPS

Any day-old bread works well in this recipe.

Feel free to replace the apricot jam with your favorite fruit preserves.

DIETITIAN'S MESSAGE

All the food groups are represented in this nutritious dessert.

Apricot Bread Pudding

Preheat oven to 350°F (180°C)
10-cup (2.5 L) shallow baking dish, greased

8	slices day-old white bread	8
2 tbsp	butter, softened	25 mL
½ cup	apricot jam *or* other fruit preserves	125 mL
½ cup	raisins	125 mL
2½ cups	milk	625 mL
3	eggs	3
½ cup	granulated sugar	125 mL
1 tsp	vanilla	5 mL
1 tsp	grated orange zest	5 mL
¼ tsp	salt	1 mL

1. Spread each bread slice with butter, then apricot jam. Place 1 slice on top of another to create jam "sandwiches." With a serrated knife, cut into 1-inch (2.5 cm) cubes. Place in 10-cup (2.5 L) baking dish and stir in raisins.

2. In a bowl, whisk together milk, eggs, sugar, vanilla, orange zest and salt. Pour over bread cubes. Bake in preheated oven for 50 to 60 minutes or until custard is set in center and top is golden brown.

PER SERVING	
Calories: 295	
Dietary Fiber: 1 g	Carbohydrate: 52 g
Fat: 7 g	Protein: 8 g

Lemon Pudding

Preheat oven to 350°F (180°C)
4-cup (1 L) baking dish, lightly greased

1	medium lemon	1
⅓ cup	granulated sugar	75 mL
2 tbsp	all-purpose flour	25 mL
Pinch	salt	Pinch
2	eggs, separated	2
1 cup	2% milk	250 mL

1. With a lemon zester or grater, remove zest from lemon. Squeeze juice; set juice and zest aside.

2. In a mixing bowl, combine sugar, flour and salt. Stir in lemon juice, zest, beaten egg yolks and milk. Beat egg whites until stiff but not dry; fold into lemon mixture.

3. Pour into lightly greased 4-cup (1 L) baking dish. Place in larger pan; pour in hot water to about 1-inch (2.5 cm) depth. Bake in preheated oven for about 30 minutes or until topping is set and golden brown. Serve warm.

PER SERVING	
Calories: 150	
Dietary Fiber: Trace	Carbohydrate: 24 g
Fat: 4 g	Protein: 5 g

SERVES 4
....
Valerie Caldicott

This is a less sweet version of an old-fashioned family favorite. What's old is new again!

TIP
Placing puddings in a water bath to bake helps them to stay moist and cook evenly.

DIETITIAN'S MESSAGE

This is a lighter version of an old classic. Serve with fresh berries to add vitamins and antioxidants.

Pear Gingerbread Upside-Down Cake

Preheat oven to 350°F (180°C)
9-inch (2.5 L) square baking pan, greased

Topping

¼ cup	butter, melted	50 mL
½ cup	packed brown sugar	125 mL
1	can (28 oz/796 mL) pear halves, drained	1

Cake

¼ cup	butter, softened	50 mL
½ cup	packed brown sugar	125 mL
2	eggs	2
1 cup	applesauce	250 mL
½ cup	fancy molasses	125 mL
1½ cups	all-purpose flour	375 mL
2 tsp	ground ginger	10 mL
1 tsp	each baking powder and baking soda	5 mL
1 tsp	ground cinnamon	5 mL
½ tsp	ground cloves	2 mL
¼ tsp	salt	1 mL

1. *Topping:* In a bowl, combine butter and brown sugar; spread in bottom of prepared pan. Lay pears on top cut side up, slicing to fit if necessary.

2. *Cake:* Cream butter and brown sugar. Add eggs and beat until incorporated. Blend in applesauce and molasses.

3. In a separate bowl, combine remaining ingredients. Stir into applesauce mixture.

4. Spoon batter over pears. Bake in preheated oven for 45 minutes or until tester inserted in center comes out clean.

5. Run a knife around the edges of the cake and invert onto a serving platter. Leave the pan in place for 1 to 2 minutes to allow all of the topping to drip down.

PER SERVING	
Calories: 279	
Dietary Fiber: 2 g	Carbohydrate: 49 g
Fat: 9 g	Protein: 33 g

Pumpkin Custard

Preheat oven to 325°F (160°C)
4 large or 6 small custard cups

1 cup	2% evaporated milk	250 mL
1 cup	pumpkin purée (not pie filling, if using canned)	250 mL
2 tbsp	granulated sugar	25 mL
1	egg	1
¼ tsp	ground nutmeg	1 mL
¼ tsp	ground ginger	1 mL

1. In a blender or food processor, combine milk, pumpkin, sugar, egg and spices. Process until well blended; pour into 4 large or 6 small custard cups. Bake in preheated oven for about 30 minutes or until knife inserted in center comes out clean. Serve warm or cold.

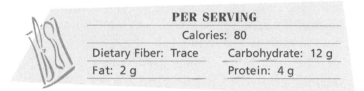

PER SERVING	
Calories: 80	
Dietary Fiber: Trace	Carbohydrate: 12 g
Fat: 2 g	Protein: 4 g

WHIPPED CREAM AND YOGURT TOPPING
This is Barbara Selley's multipurpose dessert topping: Beat ½ cup (125 mL) whipping cream until thick; add 1 tbsp (15 mL) sugar and ½ tsp (2 mL) vanilla. Whip cream until stiff. Gently fold in ½ cup (125 mL) lower-fat plain yogurt until thoroughly combined. Makes 1½ cups (375 mL).
Contains 88 calories and 7.4 g fat per ¼-cup (50 mL) serving; the same amount of regular whipped cream provides 103 calories and 11 g fat — and less calcium.

SERVES 4 TO 6

Cynthia Chace

Most baked custards have 2 or more eggs. This custard uses 2% evaporated milk and 1 egg to create a slightly softer version.

DIETITIAN'S MESSAGE

This is a superb way to use up all the pumpkin you scooped out when making the jack-o'-lantern for Halloween. The custard is rich in vitamin A and calcium and makes a good finish for a lighter meal.

**Makes 3 Dozen
Filled Cookies**

● ● ● ● ● ● ● ● ● ● ● ● ● ● ● ● ● ● ● ●

Grace Jackson

*These unsweetened
cookies taste like a
Scottish oatcake; the
sweet date filling
complements the
oatmeal. They are every
bit as warm and
comforting as when
Grandma made them.*

TIP

In this recipe, refrigerating
the cookie dough
overnight makes it easier
to slice. Remove dough
from the refrigerator
about 15 minutes
before using.

DIETITIAN'S MESSAGE

Although dates are high
in naturally-occurring
sugar, they contribute
vitamins, minerals
and fiber.

Grandma's Rolled Oat Cookies

Preheat oven to 325°F (160°C)
Cookie sheets, lightly greased

Cookie

1½ cups	all-purpose flour	375 mL
1½ cups	rolled oats	375 mL
1 tsp	baking soda	5 mL
½ cup	shortening	125 mL
½ cup	hot water	125 mL

Filling

2 cups	chopped dates	500 mL
½ cup	water	125 mL
¼ cup	granulated sugar	50 mL
1 tsp	vanilla	5 mL

1. *Cookie:* Combine flour, oats and baking soda. Cut in
   shortening until mixture resembles coarse crumbs. Add
   sufficient water to shape dough into a roll. Wrap in waxed
   paper; refrigerate overnight.

2. Cut cookie dough into thin wafers (⅛ inch/3 mm). Place
   on lightly greased or nonstick cookie sheet. Bake in
   preheated oven for about 10 minutes.

3. *Filling:* Cook dates, water and sugar on low heat for about
   30 minutes, stirring occasionally. Stir in vanilla.

4. When cookies and filling are cool, spread about 1 tbsp
   (15 mL) date filling between 2 cookies.

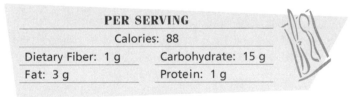

PER SERVING	
Calories: 88	
Dietary Fiber: 1 g	Carbohydrate: 15 g
Fat: 3 g	Protein: 1 g

Sunflower Cookies

Makes 5 Dozen
....
Alexa Miller

Preheat oven to 350°F (180°C)
Cookie sheets, lightly greased

½ cup	butter *or* margarine	125 mL
¾ cup	lightly packed brown sugar	175 mL
¾ cup	granulated sugar	175 mL
1	egg, beaten	1
½ tsp	vanilla	2 mL
½ tsp	baking soda	2 mL
2 tsp	hot water	10 mL
1 cup	unsalted shelled sunflower seeds	250 mL
½ cup	all-purpose flour	125 mL
½ cup	whole-wheat flour	125 mL
½ cup	large-flake rolled oats	125 mL
½ cup	chocolate chips	125 mL
½ cup	raisins	125 mL
⅓ cup	natural wheat bran	75 mL
⅓ cup	wheat germ	75 mL
1 tsp	salt	5 mL

1. In a large bowl, cream butter, brown sugar and granulated sugar until fluffy. Stir in egg, vanilla and baking soda dissolved in hot water. Add sunflower seeds, flours, oats, chocolate chips, raisins, bran, wheat germ and salt; combine thoroughly.

2. Drop batter a spoonful at a time onto lightly greased or nonstick cookie sheets. Bake in preheated oven for about 10 minutes.

The crunchiness of nuts and seeds and the sweetness of raisins and chocolate chips make this healthy cookie one that everyone will enjoy.

TIPS
Almost all cookies are ideal for freezing. They take up little space and thaw quickly. To freeze, bake cookies, cool, then wrap tightly in plastic wrap.

Since sunflower seeds are high in fat, check them for freshness before using to ensure that they haven't become rancid.

DIETITIAN'S MESSAGE
The nuts, seeds and raisins combined with chocolate chips make these cookies particularly appetizing and delicious. Serve with a cold glass of milk for a great after-school snack.

PER COOKIE

Calories: 69	
Dietary Fiber: 1 g	Carbohydrate: 9 g
Fat: 3 g	Protein: 1 g

*These classic date bars
are a perennial favorite.*

TIP
Keep a supply of these
in the freezer for
unexpected guests. They
thaw quite quickly and
are a nice treat.

DIETITIAN'S MESSAGE
These tasty bars make a
great pick-me-up. Serve
them with a glass of cold
milk or a steaming cup
of tea.

Matrimonial Cake

Preheat oven to 350°F (180°C)
13- by 9-inch (3.5 L) baking pan, lightly greased

1½ cups	all-purpose flour	375 mL
1½ cups	rolled oats	375 mL
1 cup	lightly packed brown sugar	250 mL
1 tsp	baking soda	5 mL
1 cup	butter *or* margarine	250 mL
Date Filling		
1 lb	dates, chopped (about 4 cups/1 L)	500 g
1½ cups	water	375 mL
2 tbsp	lemon juice	25 mL

1. In a large bowl, combine flour, oats, brown sugar and baking soda. Cut in butter with pastry blender or in food processor until mixture is crumbly. Press half of the crumb mixture into nonstick or lightly greased 13- by 9-inch (3.5 L) baking pan.

2. *Date Filling:* In a covered saucepan over low heat, cook dates and water for about 15 minutes or until thickened and smooth, stirring occasionally. (You may need to add extra water while cooking if mixture becomes too thick.) Stir in lemon juice. Spread over crumb layer; sprinkle with remaining crumb mixture. Bake in preheated oven for about 35 minutes or until lightly browned. Cut into bars.

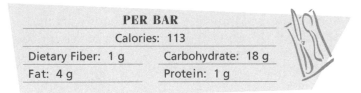

PER BAR	
Calories: 113	
Dietary Fiber: 1 g	Carbohydrate: 18 g
Fat: 4 g	Protein: 1 g

Fruit Squares

Preheat oven to 350°F (180°C)
13- by 9-inch (3.5 L) baking pan, lightly greased

2 cups	finely diced unpeeled apples	500 mL
½ cup	raisins	125 mL
½ cup	chopped dates	125 mL
2	eggs, beaten	2
¾ cup	lightly packed brown sugar	175 mL
½ cup	vegetable oil	125 mL
1 tsp	vanilla	5 mL
1 cup	all-purpose flour	250 mL
1 tsp	baking soda	5 mL
1 tsp	ground cinnamon	5 mL

1. In a medium bowl, combine apples, raisins and dates. In a large bowl, combine eggs, sugar, oil and vanilla. In a third bowl, combine flour, baking soda and cinnamon; add to egg mixture. Stir in fruit.

2. Spread in lightly greased or nonstick 13- by 9-inch (3.5 L) baking pan. Bake in preheated oven for about 25 minutes or until tester inserted in center comes out clean.

PER SQUARE	
Calories: 110	
Dietary Fiber: 1 g	Carbohydrate: 16 g
Fat: 5 g	Protein: 1 g

Makes 20 to 25 Squares

Joanne Hoyle

Pack these spicy fruit squares as a healthy treat for the brown bagger, or serve as a treat after school with a glass of milk.

TIP
In recipes using a whole egg, you can often substitute either 1 or 2 egg whites. If a recipe calls for 2 eggs, use 1 whole egg and 2 egg whites — for example in meat loaves, hamburgers, pancakes, quick breads, muffins and salad dressings. If a recipe calls for 2 egg yolks, use 1 whole egg instead. This substitution will decrease the fat and cholesterol content of the recipe.

DIETITIAN'S MESSAGE
The apples and dates in this recipe are a great way to add fruit to a lunch bag.

Lynn Roblin, Dietitian

These cookies are quick to make and fun to eat, and they're so easy that many children can make them on their own.

TIPS

If you're looking for a supply of freshly baked cookies, make up a batch of your favorite cookie dough and bake some of your favorite cookies for immediate enjoyment. Form remaining cookie dough into small balls, place on cookie sheets and freeze. When frozen, transfer to an airtight container and store in the freezer. Whenever you want a dozen freshly baked cookies, remove cookie balls from freezer, let thaw and bake.

Substitute ½ cup (125 mL) chocolate chips or your favorite chopped nuts for the dried cranberries. If using nuts, check for nut allergies before serving.

DIETITIAN'S MESSAGE

Baking cookies is a great way to get kids involved in food preparation. They are easy to make, and the result is a delicious treat for immediate consumption, with leftovers to pack up with lunch.

Cranberry Oatmeal Cookies

Preheat oven to 350°F (180°C)
Cookie sheets, greased

1 cup	all-purpose flour	250 mL
¼ cup	wheat bran	50 mL
½ tsp	baking powder	2 mL
½ cup	margarine	125 mL
½ cup	granulated sugar	125 mL
½ cup	packed brown sugar	125 mL
1	egg	1
1 tsp	vanilla	5 mL
1 cup	quick-cooking (not instant) oats	250 mL
½ cup	dried cranberries	125 mL

1. In a small bowl, combine flour, wheat bran and baking powder. Set aside.

2. In a medium bowl, cream together margarine, granulated sugar and brown sugar until light and fluffy. Add egg and mix well; stir in vanilla. Add flour mixture and blend thoroughly. Stir in oats and cranberries.

3. Drop heaping teaspoons (5 mL) of the cookie dough onto prepared cookie sheets, about 2 inches (5 cm) apart. Bake in preheated oven for 10 to 12 minutes or until edges are lightly browned.

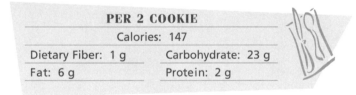

PER 2 COOKIE	
Calories: 147	
Dietary Fiber: 1 g	Carbohydrate: 23 g
Fat: 6 g	Protein: 2 g

Luscious Lemon Bars

Makes 15
....
Dairy Farmers of Canada

Preheat oven to 350°F (180°C)
8-inch (2 L) square baking pan

1⅓ cups	all-purpose flour	325 mL
1 cup	granulated sugar	250 mL
½ cup	butter, softened	125 mL
2	eggs	2
2 tbsp	all-purpose flour	25 mL
¼ tsp	baking powder	1 mL
1½ tsp	grated lemon zest	7 mL
3 tbsp	lemon juice	45 mL
	Icing (confectioner's) sugar	

1. In a medium bowl, blend together 1⅓ cups (325 mL) of the flour, ¼ cup (50 mL) of the granulated sugar and butter until mixture is crumbly. Press into bottom of 8-inch (2 L) square baking pan. Bake in preheated oven for 15 minutes or until edges are lightly browned.

2. In a small bowl, beat together remaining granulated sugar, eggs, 2 tbsp (25 mL) of the flour, baking powder, lemon zest and lemon juice. Pour filling over hot crust. Bake for 15 minutes or until filling is set. Cool in pan on wire rack. Sprinkle with icing sugar. Cut into bars.

PER SQUARE	
Calories: 161	
Dietary Fiber: Trace	Carbohydrate: 23 g
Fat: 7 g	Protein: 2 g

We all need to sit back and relax every once in a while. So take a break and enjoy one of these lemon bars with a quiet cup of tea.

TIP
The zest is the colored and flavorful portion of the lemon peel. Use a zester, which you can purchase inexpensively at kitchen stores, or a fine grater to separate the peel from the white pith underneath, which is quite bitter. Lemons and other citrus fruits are coated with wax to prevent water loss, so wash the fruit in hot water prior to zesting the lemon.

DIETITIAN'S MESSAGE
These bars are less about nutrition than pure eating pleasure. But a little indulgence practised in moderation is still an important part of healthy eating.

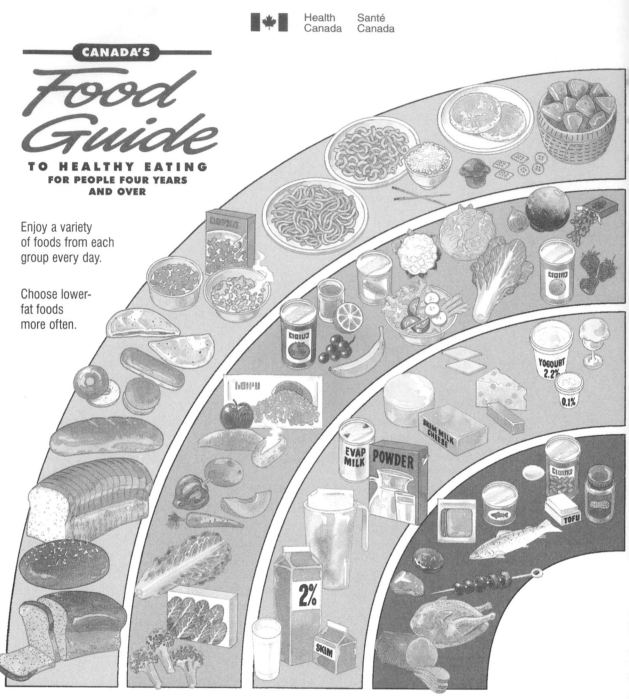

CANADA'S

Food Guide

TO HEALTHY EATING
FOR PEOPLE FOUR YEARS AND OVER

Health Canada / Santé Canada

Enjoy a variety of foods from each group every day.

Choose lower-fat foods more often.

Grain Products
Choose whole grain and enriched products more often.

Vegetables and Fruit
Choose dark green and orange vegetables and orange fruit more often.

Milk Products
Choose lower-fat milk products more often.

Meat and Alternatives
Choose leaner meats, poultry and fish, as well as dried peas, beans and lentils more often.

Canada

434

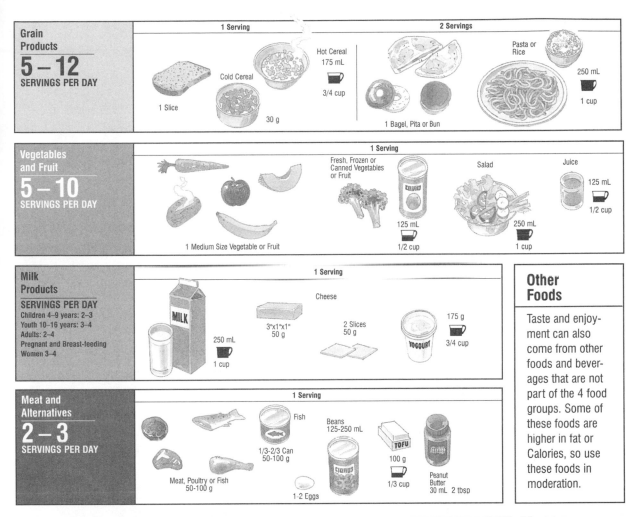

Grain Products

5 – 12
SERVINGS PER DAY

1 Serving

1 Slice

Cold Cereal
30 g

Hot Cereal
175 mL
3/4 cup

2 Servings

1 Bagel, Pita or Bun

Pasta or Rice
250 mL
1 cup

Vegetables and Fruit

5 – 10
SERVINGS PER DAY

1 Serving

1 Medium Size Vegetable or Fruit

Fresh, Frozen or Canned Vegetables or Fruit
125 mL
1/2 cup

Salad
250 mL
1 cup

Juice
125 mL
1/2 cup

Milk Products

SERVINGS PER DAY
Children 4–9 years: 2–3
Youth 10–16 years: 3–4
Adults: 2–4
Pregnant and Breast-feeding
Women 3–4

1 Serving

MILK
250 mL
1 cup

Cheese
3"x1"x1"
50 g

2 Slices
50 g

YOGOURT
175 g
3/4 cup

Meat and Alternatives

2 – 3
SERVINGS PER DAY

1 Serving

Meat, Poultry or Fish
50-100 g

Fish
1/3-2/3 Can
50-100 g

1-2 Eggs

Beans
125-250 mL

TOFU
100 g
1/3 cup

Peanut Butter
30 mL 2 tbsp

Other Foods

Taste and enjoyment can also come from other foods and beverages that are not part of the 4 food groups. Some of these foods are higher in fat or Calories, so use these foods in moderation.

Different People Need Different Amounts of Food

The amount of food you need every day from the 4 food groups and other foods depends on your age, body size, activity level, whether you are male or female and if you are pregnant or breast-feeding. That's why the Food Guide gives a lower and higher number of servings for each food group. For example, young children can choose the lower number of servings, while male teenagers can go to the higher number. Most other people can choose servings somewhere in between.

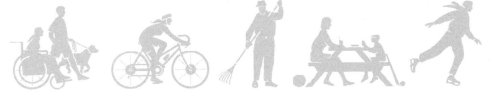

Consult *Canada's Physical Activity Guide to Healthy Active Living* to help you build physical activity into your daily life.

Enjoy eating well, being active and feeling good about yourself. That's VITALIT

© Minister of Public Works and Government Services Canada, 1997
Cat. No. H39-252/1992E   ISBN 0-662-19648-1
No changes permitted. Reprint permission not required.

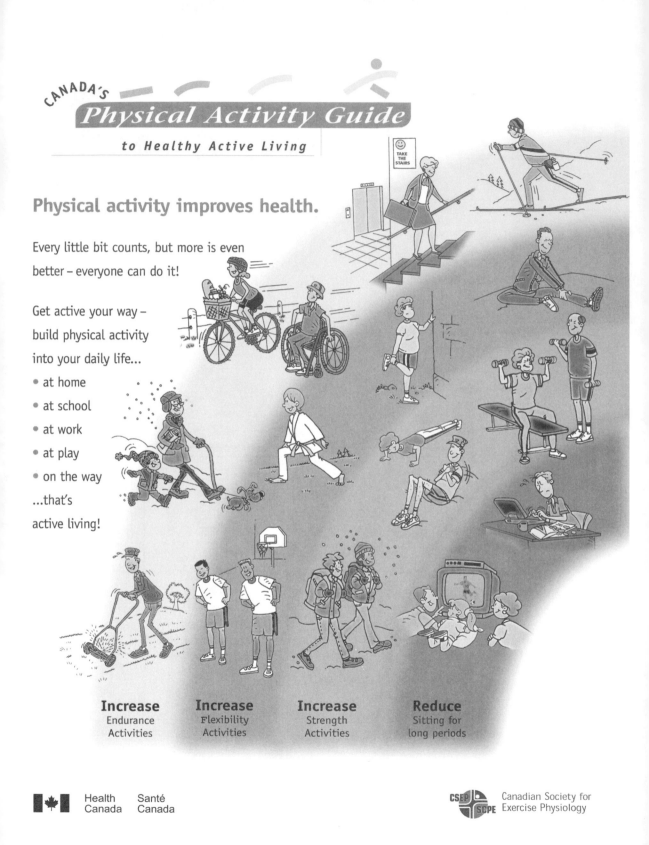

Canada's **Physical Activity Guide** to Healthy Active Living

Physical activity improves health.

Every little bit counts, but more is even better – everyone can do it!

Get active your way – build physical activity into your daily life...
- at home
- at school
- at work
- at play
- on the way
...that's active living!

TAKE THE STAIRS

Increase Endurance Activities

Increase Flexibility Activities

Increase Strength Activities

Reduce Sitting for long periods

Health Canada   Santé Canada

CSEP SCPE   Canadian Society for Exercise Physiology

Choose a variety of activities from these three groups:

Endurance

4-7 days a week
Continuous activities for your heart, lungs and circulatory system.

Flexibility

4-7 days a week
Gentle reaching, bending and stretching activities to keep your muscles relaxed and joints mobile.

Strength

2-4 days a week
Activities against resistance to strengthen muscles and bones and improve posture.

Starting slowly is very safe for most people. Not sure? Consult your health professional.

For a copy of the *Guide Handbook* and more information:
1-888-334-9769, or
www.paguide.com

Eating well is also important. Follow *Canada's Food Guide to Healthy Eating* to make wise food choices.

Get Active Your Way, Every Day—For Life!

Scientists say accumulate 60 minutes of physical activity every day to stay healthy or improve your health. As you progress to moderate activities you can cut down to 30 minutes, 4 days a week. Add-up your activities in periods of at least 10 minutes each. Start slowly... and build up.

Time needed depends on effort

Very Light Effort	Light Effort *60 minutes*	Moderate Effort *30-60 minutes*	Vigorous Effort *20-30 minutes*	Maximum Effort
• Strolling • Dusting	• Light walking • Volleyball • Easy gardening • Stretching	• Brisk walking • Biking • Raking leaves • Swimming • Dancing • Water aerobics	• Aerobics • Jogging • Hockey • Basketball • Fast swimming • Fast dancing	• Sprinting • Racing

Range needed to stay healthy

You Can Do It – Getting started is easier than you think

Physical activity doesn't have to be very hard. Build physical activities into your daily routine.

- Walk whenever you can–get off the bus early, use the stairs instead of the elevator.
- Reduce inactivity for long periods, like watching TV.
- Get up from the couch and stretch and bend for a few minutes every hour.
- Play actively with your kids.
- Choose to walk, wheel or cycle for short trips.

- Start with a 10 minute walk – gradually increase the time.
- Find out about walking and cycling paths nearby and use them.
- Observe a physical activity class to see if you want to try it.
- Try one class to start – you don't have to make a long-term commitment.
- Do the activities you are doing now, more often.

Benefits of regular activity:

- better health
- improved fitness
- better posture and balance
- better self-esteem
- weight control
- stronger muscles and bones
- feeling more energetic
- relaxation and reduced stress
- continued independent living in later life

Health risks of inactivity:

- premature death
- heart disease
- obesity
- high blood pressure
- adult-onset diabetes
- osteoporosis
- stroke
- depression
- colon cancer

ACTIVE LIVING

CANADA'S
Physical Activity Guide
to Healthy Active Living

Index